Robert A. Geffner, PhD, ABPN
Robyn Spurling Igelman, MA
Jennifer Zellner, MS
Editors

The Effects
of Intimate Partner Violence
on Children

The Effects of Intimate Partner Violence on Children has been co-published simultaneously as *Journal of Emotional Abuse*, Volume 3, Numbers (1/2) (3/4) 2003.

Pre-publication
REVIEWS,
COMMENTARIES,
EVALUATIONS . . .

"**I**MPRESSIVE. . . . Should appeal to practitioners, researchers and policy makers. For researchers it is A VALUABLE RESOURCE that presents both a review of existing research and studies that encourage new thinking and extensions of work in this area. For practitioners and program operators it PROVIDES DIRECTION FOR BEST PRACTICES AND MATERIAL INVALUABLE TO GRANT APPLICATIONS. For policy advocates the editors have included material that does a good job of capturing major themes that must be resolved in order to achieve a policy framework that truly supports the development of children exposed to partner violence."

Melissa Jonson-Reid, PhD, MSW
Associate Professor
George Warren Brown School of Social Work
Washington University

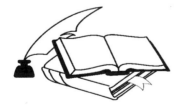

The Effects
of Intimate Partner Violence
on Children

The Effects of Intimate Partner Violence on Children has been co-published simultaneously as *Journal of Emotional Abuse,* Volume 3, Numbers (1/2) (3/4) 2003.

The *Journal of Emotional Abuse* Monographic "Separates"

Below is a list of "separates," which in serials librarianship means a special issue simultaneously published as a special journal issue or double-issue *and* as a "separate" hardbound monograph. (This is a format which we also call a "DocuSerial.")

"Separates" are published because specialized libraries or professionals may wish to purchase a specific thematic issue by itself in a format which can be separately cataloged and shelved, as opposed to purchasing the journal on an on-going basis. Faculty members may also more easily consider a "separate" for classroom adoption.

"Separates" are carefully classified separately with the major book jobbers so that the journal tie-in can be noted on new book order slips to avoid duplicate purchasing.

You may wish to visit Haworth's Website at . . .

http://www.HaworthPress.com

. . . to search our online catalog for complete tables of contents of these separates and related publications.

You may also call 1-800-HAWORTH (outside US/Canada: 607-722-5857), or Fax 1-800-895-0582 (outside US/Canada: 607-771-0012), or e-mail at:

docdelivery@haworthpress.com

The Effects of Intimate Partner Violence on Children, edited by Robert A. Geffner, PhD, ABPN, Robyn Spurling Igelman, MA, and Jennifer Zellner, MS (Vol. 3, Nos. 1/2 and 3/4, 2003). *Examines short- and long-term developments/problems facing children exposed to domestic violence.*

Bullying Behavior: Current Issues, Research, and Interventions, edited by Robert A. Geffner, PhD, ABPN, Marti Loring, PhD, LCSW, and Corinna Young, MS (Vol. 2, No. 2/3, 2001). *Shows how to stop schoolyard terror before it escalates to tragedy with timely intervention strategies and up-to-date reports on the dynamics of bullying.*

The Effects
of Intimate Partner Violence
on Children

Robert A. Geffner, PhD, ABPN
Robyn Spurling Igelman, MA
Jennifer Zellner, MS
Editors

The Effects of Intimate Partner Violence on Children has been co-published simultaneously as *Journal of Emotional Abuse*, Volume 3, Numbers (1/2) (3/4) 2003.

HMTP

The Haworth Maltreatment & Trauma Press
An Imprint of
The Haworth Press, Inc.
New York • London • Oxford

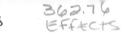

362.76
Effects

Published by

The Haworth Maltreatment & Trauma Press, 10 Alice Street, Binghamton, NY 13904-1580 USA

The Haworth Maltreatment & Trauma Press is an imprint of The Haworth Press, Inc., 10 Alice Street, Binghamton, NY 13904-1580 USA.

The Effects of Intimate Partner Violence on Children has been co-published simultaneously as *Journal of Emotional Abuse*, Volume 3, Numbers (1/2) (3/4) 2003.

Cover design by Marylouise E. Doyle.

Library of Congress Cataloging-in-Publication Data

The Effects of intimate partner violence on children / Robert A. Geffner, Robyn Spurling Igelman, and Jennifer Zellner editors.
    p. cm.
    "The effects of intimate partner violence on children has been co-published simultaneously as Journal of emotional abuse, vol. 3, nos. (1/2) (3/4) 2003."
    Includes bibliographical references and index.
    ISBN 0-7890-2160-9 (hard : alk. paper) ISBN 0-7890-2161-7 (soft : alk. paper)
    1. Children and violence. 2. Family violence–Psychological aspects. 3. Children of abused wives–Psychology. I. Geffner, Robert. II. Ingleman, Robyn Spurling III. Zellner, Jennifer. IV. Journal of emotional abuse.
Hq784.V55E34 2003
362.76–dc21
                                         200306689

Indexing, Abstracting & Website/Internet Coverage

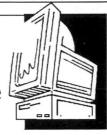

This section provides you with a list of major indexing & abstracting services. That is to say, each service began covering this periodical during the year noted in the right column. Most Websites which are listed below have indicated that they will either post, disseminate, compile, archive, cite or alert their own Website users with research-based content from this work. (This list is as current as the copyright date of this publication.)

(continued)

*Special Bibliographic Notes related to special journal issues
(separates) and indexing/abstracting:*

- indexing/abstracting services in this list will also cover material in any "separate" that is co-published simultaneously with Haworth's special thematic journal issue or DocuSerial. Indexing/abstracting usually covers material at the article/chapter level.
- monographic co-editions are intended for either non-subscribers or libraries which intend to purchase a second copy for their circulating collections.
- monographic co-editions are reported to all jobbers/wholesalers/approval plans. The source journal is listed as the "series" to assist the prevention of duplicate purchasing in the same manner utilized for books-in-series.
- to facilitate user/access services all indexing/abstracting services are encouraged to utilize the co-indexing entry note indicated at the bottom of the first page of each article/chapter/contribution.
- this is intended to assist a library user of any reference tool (whether print, electronic, online, or CD-ROM) to locate the monographic version if the library has purchased this version but not a subscription to the source journal.
- individual articles/chapters in any Haworth publication are also available through the Haworth Document Delivery Service (HDDS).

Dedicated to B. B. Robbie Rossman, PhD

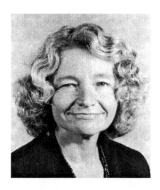

In Remembrance of B. B. Robbie Rossman, PhD, a pioneer, valued colleague, and great friend who died suddenly May 5, 2002 from cerebral aneursyms.

Robbie was a founding co-editor of the *Journal of Emotional Abuse*, and was an associate editor of the journal at the time of her death. Dr. Rossman's research interestes were in the area of children's stress and coping, specifically in children who experienced the trauma of growing up exposed to parental violence and/or personal maltreatment. She authored numerous journal articles and book chapters, and has presented papers on these subjects. This special volume is therefore dedicated to her work and efforts in promoting the importance of studying and intervening with children exposed to family violence.

Robbie was born in Esteville, Iowa. She moved to Denver in 1963 and obtained undergraduate and graduate degrees in Psychology at the University of Denver. Robbie was involved in teaching and research at The University of Denver from 1970 until her death. Her research interests focused on family violence and the impact of intimate partner violence on children. Robbie's career exemplified a passionate integration of research, clinical practice, teaching, and community service both at home and nationally. She trained numerous students and colleagues throughout the country, and always had a positive attitude.

She was Senior Clinical Professor on the Child Clinical Faculty in the Psychology Department at the University of Denver, where she taught, conducted research, and provided clinical supervision. She was a member of various professional societies, and served as a reviewer and editorial board member for several professional publications, including the *Journal of Child Sexual Abuse* and the *Family Violence and Sexual Assault Bulle-*

tin. She was senior editor of the book *Multiple Victimization of Children,* among others.

Robbie's impact goes far above her professional work noted above. Her influence professionally and personally to many of us over the years has been an inspiration attesting to the importance of working together to end abuse. Robbie always had kind words and encouragement for everyone, no matter what their views or positions were on issues. She maintained a strong commitment to the pursuit of cooperation and peace at all levels of human interaction. We share the sorrow of her loss. We dedicate and renew our efforts to her goals.

To remind us of her work and efforts, we have initiated the B. B. Robbie Rossman Annual Memorial Keynote Panel on Children Exposed to Family Violence at our annual International Conference on Family Violence each September. We have also created the B. B. Rossman Annual Memorial Student Research Award to be given during the Poster Session of this conference each year.

Robert A. Geffner, PhD
Editor

The Effects of Intimate Partner Violence on Children

CONTENTS

LEGAL ISSUES AND POLICY IMPLICATIONS

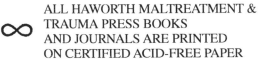

ABOUT THE EDITORS

Robert A. Geffner, PhD, ABPN, is Founder and President of the Family Violence & Sexual Assault Institute in San Diego, California. Dr. Geffner is a former Professor of Psychology at the University of Texas at Tyler, and currently is Clinical Research Professor of Psychology at the California School of Professional Psychology, Alliant International University in San Diego. A licensed psychologist and licensed marriage and family therapist, he was the Clinical Director of a large, private practice mental health clinic for over 15 years. He has a diplomate in clinical neuropsychology.

Robyn Spurling Igelman, MA, is Assistant Editor for the *Journal of Emotional Abuse* and the *Journal of Child Sexual Abuse* and is on staff at the Family Violence and Sexual Assault Institute in San Diego, California. She is currently completing her doctorate in clinical psychology at the California School of Professional Psychology, Alliant International University, San Diego and also works as a research assistant for the Chadwick Center at Children's Hospital in San Diego. Her primary research interest is in the area of treatment for child sexual abuse victims and outcomes research.

Jennifer Zellner, MS, is Assistant Editor for the *Journal of Emotional Abuse*, the *Journal of Child Sexual Abuse*, and the *Journal of Aggression, Maltreatment, & Trauma*, and is on staff at the Family Violence and Sexual Assault Institute, San Diego, California. She is currently completing her doctorate in clinical and health psychology at the California School of Professional Psychology, Alliant International University in San Diego. Ms. Zellner is also a pre-doctoral fellow at the Center for Behavioral Epidemiology and Community Health, San Diego State University. Her research interests include women's health, reproductive health, and health promotions.

ABOUT THE CONTRIBUTORS

Nicole E. Allen, PhD, is Assistant Professor of community psychology at the University of Illinois Urbana Champaign. Her research interests include intimate partner violence against women and community collaborations to stimulate social change. She is currently investigating those factors that facilitate the creation of a coordinated community response to intimate partner violence, the role of coordinating councils and other collaborative bodies in creating this response and the effect of this response on survivors and their children.

Nicholas Bala, BA, LLB, LLM, is Professor at the Faculty of Law at Queen's University in Kingston, Canada and has been Visiting Professor at Duke University. His primary area of teaching and research is Family and Children's law, with publications on issues such as child abuse, child witnesses, domestic violence, juvenile justice, divorce and the definition of the family.

Deborah I. Bybee, PhD, is Associate Professor of research in ecological/community psychology at Michigan State University. She has a primary interest in quantitative methods and how they can be used to understand complex, real-world phenomena, especially those that change over time. Substantively, she has applied her methodological interests to a variety of areas, including advocacy for women with abusive partners, intervention with children who have witnessed domestic violence, housing assistance for individuals who are homeless and mentally ill, supported education for individuals with mental illness, and mothering by women coping with a serious mental illness.

Laurel Carter, MS, LMFT, is a licensed Marriage and Family Therapist in private practice. She is also Clinical Director of the Domestic Violence Treatment Program at Family Institute in Logan, Utah. She was Project Director for the state of Utah for the Child Witness of Domestic Violence Treatment Pilot Program.

Ellen R. DeVoe, PhD, ACSW, is Assistant Professor at Columbia University School of Social Work. Her research and clinical interests are in the area of the impact of partner violence on young children, parenting among battered women, and trauma in young children.

Zvi Eisikovits, PhD, is Professor of Social Work, Dean of the Faculty of Social Welfare & Health Studies, University of Haifa, and Director of the Minerva Center for Youth Studies, University of Haifa, Israel.

Mona El-Sheikh, PhD, is a faculty member at the Human Development and Family Studies Department of Auburn University. Her research includes developmental psychopathology with a focus on associations among marital conflict, parental alcoholism, and parent-child conflict.

Jacqueline L. George, LCSW, is a licensed clinical social worker. At the time of this writing she was the Children's Treatment Program Coordinator at Weber Human Services in Ogden, Utah. Currently she is providing clinical services to children at Family & Children's Service in Harrisburg, PA.

Gabrielle Gruber is a doctoral student in social work and psychology at the University of Michigan. Her work focuses on identifying factors that reduce risk and promote resiliency among children and families. Of particular significance to her research are the impact of domestic violence on women and their children, poverty, and child abuse and neglect; and the development and evaluation of successful clinical practice and preventive interventions.

Lisa L. Harpur, PhD, MSc, BSc, is Assistant Professor in Applied Psychology at the University of Calgary where she teaches graduate level courses. She is a chartered psychologist in Alberta who maintains a clinical practice, and plays an active role in professional affairs in the College of Alberta Psychologists. Dr. Harpur has also authored or co-authored several journal articles and presentations, and has been awarded several grants for research, training and intervention programs. Her areas of interest are in Assessment, Health Psychology, Stress and Coping, FASD, Cross-cultural Psychology, and Children Exposed to Marital Violence.

Janet R. Johnston, PhD, a clinical social worker and sociologist, is Professor in the Administration of Justice Department, San Jose State University and executive director of the Judith Wallerstein Center for the Family in Transition, California. Recently, Dr. Johnston was the recipient of two prestigious honors: the John Haynes Distinguished Mediator Award from the Academy of Family Mediators, and the Stanley Cohen Distinguished Research Award from Association of Family & Conciliation Courts.

Ariel Kalil, PhD, is Assistant Professor at the Harris School of Public Policy Studies at the University of Chicago. Trained as a developmental psychologist, she is primarily interested in the effects of poverty on child development and family functioning.

Steven J. Kay, PsyD, is a psychologist living in Salt Lake City, Utah. At the time of this writing he was the Domestic Violence Treatment Program Clinical Director and is currently Adult Clinical Services Director for Cornerstone Counseling Center.

Patricia K. Kerig, PhD, is Clinical Associate Professor in the psychology department at the University of North Carolina at Chapel Hill and the Chief Psychologist in the Outpatient Clinic at the Children's Psychiatric Institute. She completed her doctoral degree at U.C. Berkeley, an internship at Stanford Children's Hospital, and a postdoctoral fellowship at the University of Colorado Medical Center. Her research focuses on developmental psychopathology and family processes, and she has carried out a number of studies of risk and resilience in children exposed to interparental conflict, divorce, and family violence.

Pamela King, MS, LMFT, is a licensed Marriage and Family Therapist. At the time of this writing she was the Domestic Violence Children's Treatment Program Coordinator. She is currently Program Coordinator of the Child Witness Treatment Program at The Family Institute of Northern Utah.

Karen M. MacMillan, BA, DipEd, MSc Counselling Psychology (University of Calgary), is Provisional Chartered Psychologist and a PhD Student in the Division of Applied Psychology at the University of Calgary.

Judee E. Onyskiw, RN, PhD, is a Postdoctoral Research Fellow in the Perinatal Research Centre, University of Alberta funded by the Canadian Institutes of Health Research, the Alberta Heritage Foundation for Medical Research, and the Perinatal Research Centre, University of Alberta.

Daniel Rosen, PhD, is Assistant Professor of Social Work at the University of Pittsburgh. He received his PhD in Sociology and Social Work from the University of Michigan.

Martha Shaffer, AB, LLB, LLM, is Associate Professor at the Faculty of Law, University of Toronto. She teaches and writes in the areas of criminal law and family law. Her research focuses on violence against women.

Erica L. Smith, MSW, CSW, is a social worker with the Children's Mental Health Alliance in New York City. Her interests include trauma in children, domestic violence and children's mental health.

Cris M. Sullivan, PhD, is Associate Professor in ecological/community psychology at Michigan State University and director of evaluation for the Michigan Coalition Against Domestic and Sexual Violence. Her research has primarily involved examining the long-term effects of community-based interventions for battered women and their children, and evaluating domestic violence and sexual assault victim service programs.

Richard Tolman, PhD, is Associate Professor of Social Work, University of Michigan. and is currently Co-Director of the Project for Research on Work, Welfare, and Domestic Violence.

Stephanie M. Whitson is a Doctoral Candidate in the Department of Psychology at Auburn University. Her research interests include child clinical psychology with a focus on associations among family conflict, children's physiological regulation, and children's adjustment and health.

Zeev Winstok, PhD, is Lecturer in the Faculty of Social Welfare & Health Studies, University of Haifa, and a Research Fellow at the Minerva Center for Youth Studies, University of Haifa, Israel.

Angela M. Wolf, PhD, is Senior Research Associate at the National Council on Crime and Delinquency. Her research interests include violence against women and children as well as interventions for high risk youth. She is currently involved with an evaluation of a national child abuse prevention project and is also part of a resource center investigating the needs of and resources available to children of incarcerated parents.

Introduction–
Children Exposed to Interparental Violence:
A Need for Additional Research
and Validated Treatment Programs

Robert A. Geffner
Robyn Spurling Igelman
Jennifer Zellner

All too often children are exposed to violence within their own homes. This violence is not limited to what children see while playing video games, watching movies or the news, or in their own neighborhood or school. Rather, a great number of children are exposed to violence between their parents. There is now wide recognition among professionals who work with abused children and maltreating families that family violence, specifically interparental or intimate partner violence, is a problem of great magnitude that can significantly impact the short- and long-term development of children who are exposed to such violence in their homes.

\ The estimates of the number of children who are exposed to or witness violence between intimate partners vary. Some estimates several years ago were as low as 3.3 million (Carlson, 1984), while others estimate the prevalence to be upwards of 10 million children each year who are exposed to intimate partner violence (Straus, 1991). Recent research

[Haworth co-indexing entry note]: "Introduction–Children Exposed to Interparental Violence: A Need for Additional Research and Validated Treatment Programs." Geffner, Robert A, Robyn Spurling Igelman, and Jennifer Zellner. Co-published simultaneously in *Journal of Emotional Abuse* (The Haworth Maltreatment & Trauma Press, an imprint of The Haworth Press, Inc.) Vol. 3, No. 1/2, 2003, pp. 1-10; and: *The Effects of Intimate Partner Violence on Children* (ed: Robert A. Geffner, Robyn Spurling Igelman, and Jennifer Zellner) The Haworth Maltreatment & Trauma Press, an imprint of The Haworth Press, Inc., 2003, pp. 1-10. Single or multiple copies of this article are available for a fee from The Haworth Document Delivery Service [1-800-HAWORTH, 9:00 a.m. - 5:00 p.m. (EST). E-mail address: docdelivery@haworthpress.com].

concerning violence against intimates, funded by the National Institute of Justice and the Centers for Disease Control and Prevention (Tjaden & Thoennes, 2000), have also concluded that children exposed to violence between intimates is a significant problem. The exact numbers are not clear, however, due to the way the questions are phrased, the methodology, utilized in different studies, and the specific measures incorporated into the research (for an excellent review of the methodological issues, see Fantuzzo & Mohr, 1999).

EFFECTS OF FAMILY VIOLENCE ON CHILDREN

As a result of better awareness among researchers and practitioners, there has been an exponential increase over the past 10 years in the amount of empirical attention that has been paid to the symptoms, outcomes, and social functioning of children exposed to family violence (e.g., see recent reviews by Geffner, Jaffe, & Sudermann, 2000; Graham-Bermann & Edleson, 2001; Holden, Geffner, & Jouriles, 1998; Rossman, Hughes, & Rosenberg, 2000). In addition, recent studies are becoming more methodologically sound, and therefore are increasing our understanding and ability to derive more definitive conclusions as to the traumatic effect that exposure to interparental violence has on children (see Graham-Bermann & Levendosky, 1998; Kerig, Fedorowicz, Brown, & Warren, 2000; Osofsky, 1999; Rossman & Ho, 2000; Rudo, Powell, & Dunlap, 1998). In this volume, Onyskiw provides an excellent updated review of the effects of domestic violence on children's adjustment.

The children who are exposed to violence between parents are believed to be at increased risk for a multitude of psychological, behavioral, social, and educational problems. In addition, children who live in a home where physical violence between parents is occurring are also more likely to be at increased risk for physical abuse themselves (O'Keefe, 1994); at times, they also exhibit aggression toward others (Holden & Ritchie, 1991). There has also been substantial research looking at the long term adverse effects of childhood maltreatment on adult functioning (for a review, see Franey, Geffner, & Falconer, 2001). The most significant and largest scale research project has been the series of studies conducted by Felitti and colleagues (1998), who reviewed records of over 9,000 patients at Kaiser Hospital in California during a six-month period. This research has been referred to as the Adverse Childhood Experiences (ACE) studies. They found numerous long-term negative effects, including a higher fatality rate, that were experienced by adults who were abused as children or grew up in abusive homes. ⁄

THEORETICAL PERSPECTIVES

Several theories have been proposed to explain why children exposed to interparental violence are at increased risk of developing social, emotional and behavioral difficulties. For example, social learning theory suggests that children who are exposed to violence learn maladaptive ways of dealing with conflict and may see aggressive behavior reinforced in the parental relationship between their parents. They then model this behavior in their interactions with peers, and possibly later in their intimate relationships. Family systems theory posits that family dysfunction and maladaptive parent-child relationships may mediate the outcomes of children living in violent families. Further, theories on the intergenerational transmission of violence propose that children who are exposed to violence between parents are at greater risk for becoming the perpetrators of violence against others or the victims of such maltreatment. Developmental psychopathology perspectives have attempted to show the detrimental effects of family violence and the variety of symptom presentation at various stages of development throughout adolescence and into adulthood. For example, infants and toddlers may have problems in attachment, sleeping, and sensory processing, and they may have difficult temperaments from being exposed to chronic trauma. Pre-school age children may have somatic complaints, enuresis, and school phobias. Latency-age children are likely to experience academic difficulties and problems of social relatedness, including trouble in the formation and maintenance of peer relationships. Indeed, the more we learn about child maltreatment and its relation to the neuropsychological functioning of those children exposed to chronic trauma, such as from family violence, the more we realize the interaction of biopsychosocial factors in the development of children (e.g., Geffner, 2002; Perry, 2001).

The interaction of exposure to family violence, trauma, and the effects on the brain can be exacerbated by other factors as well. Kalil, Tolman, Rosen, and Gruber in this volume discuss the effects of domestic violence on children's behaviors in low-income families. The combination of poverty and violence makes for a dangerous situation in the potential functioning of children in such situations. Adolescents are also adversely affected when exposed to family violence. Adolescents might suffer further in their academics, be involved in violent romantic relationships, and skip or drop out from school. They are also at risk for substance abuse. An excellent study investigating the perceptions of adolescents in Israel who have been exposed to such family violence is presented in this volume (see Winstok & Eisikovits). Their article provides a unique perspective that has not been considered very often.

RESEARCH AND METHODOLOGICAL ISSUES

Studies that have looked at the effects of interparental violence on children have not led to definitive conclusions as to the ways in which exposure to this type of violence might affect specific emotional and behavioral outcomes in children. Rudo and colleagues (1998), in a review of the literature on child victims of physical abuse and exposure to family violence, found that the symptom presentation of these children varied across studies. Methodological issues may help explain the dissimilarity between the findings. For example, such differences may depend upon the definitions of abuse and types or degrees of exposure to intimate partner violence, the method of documentation of the violence, and the degree of detail provided by the victims (Rudo et al., 1998). In addition, children who are exposed to domestic violence might also be experiencing other types of abuse as part of multiple victimizations that can lead to differing outcomes.

What is evident is that research in the field must continue in order to describe, explain, and understand the effects that exposure to interparental violence has on the development of children's social, behavioral, and emotional functioning. In this volume, Whitson and El-Sheikh discuss various moderators that affect children's adjustment and health. It is important that further information in this area is disseminated so that we can look more carefully at the dynamics of family violence such that the effects on children can be better understood.

RESILIENCY

Not all children are as negatively affected or traumatized by their exposure to family violence. Resiliency factors play a role in helping to mediate the detrimental effects of children exposed. The American Psychological Association (APA) Presidential Task Force on Violence in the Family (1996) presented a summary of the research on the various factors that seem to be involved in promoting such resiliency. These are sometimes referred to as protective factors. Some of the key factors seem to be the children's interpretation of the experience, their ability to cope with stress, the availability of a protective nonoffending parent or other support people to act as surrogate parents, psychological "hardiness" so that they can resist negative factors in the home, development of positive self-esteem and strong social skills, a sense of hope for the future, respect and empathy for others, and development of some sense of control over one's life. Heller, Larrieu, D'Imperio, and Boris (1999) also describe protective factors that are associated with resilience in their review of the literature. The protective factors they described include: dispositional/temperamental attributes of the child; global behavioral ratings and intellectual ability; sense of self-worth; internal locus of control; external attribution of blame; spirituality; ego-control and ego-resilience. Understanding and promoting protective factors are major components of the development of prevention. Therefore, these issues are also presented in this volume (see Kerig's article).

As discussed above with resiliency, it is important not to assume that all children will react or be affected the same way when exposed to family violence. Sometimes there is a tendency to minimize the trauma or significance of exposure to family violence if specific symptoms do not occur. In addition, children often attempt to cope with such trauma in different ways. Allen, Wolf, Bybee, and Sullivan (in this volume) discuss the diversity of children's coping experiences, which is an important aspect of developing interventions to ameliorate the symptoms and trauma.

ASSESSMENT AND INTERVENTION FOR CHILDREN EXPOSED TO FAMILY VIOLENCE

However, before treatment is initiated, it is important to make sure an adequate assessment is conducted since all children are not the same. It is rare, unfortunately, that programs and shelters actually conduct a comprehensive assessment. Such an assessment should focus on the children's levels of self-esteem, depression, anger, anxiety, trauma, attitudes about power and control, communication and assertiveness skills, and social skills, to name a few. In order to conduct treatment, the actual issues in need of attention must be known so that the treatment can be tailored to meet the child's varying needs. Further, assessment of the child's strengths and sources of support should also be evaluated in order for areas of resiliency to be identified and built upon in treatment. If we assume "one size fits all," then our interventions are less likely to be successful or efficient for the particular children we are attempting to help. Too often, though, this is indeed what occurs.

Unfortunately, there have not been sufficient programs to treat children or adolescents who have been exposed to family violence that have been validated by outcome research. Treatment for children exposed to domestic violence has focused on a variety of issues. One approach for treating these children is presented in this volume (Carter, Kay, George, & King). There should be different types of treatment for children exposed to family violence, depending upon their issues and the assessment. They may need psycho-educational approaches to help them break the family secret of domestic violence, to learn to express feelings, develop safety plans, improve self-esteem, and to gain support. They may need trauma treatment for Posttraumatic Stress Disorder (PTSD) to help them: understand their symptoms; cope with the trauma experiences; deal with disclosure issues; learn cognitive restructuring to deal with their feelings of helplessness, vulnerability, self-blame and guilt; and manage stress better. Some children may also need more long-term psychotherapy for the chronic conflict they have experienced, and to help them rebuild their trust, deal with their feelings, develop empathy, and improve their social skills.

When a recent National Research Council committee reviewed the research during the past decade to determine the best approaches to facilitate and promote youth development, they found several common components (Eccles & Gootman, 2002). It is interesting that many of their recommendations focus on the same issues that were found by the results of the resiliency studies mentioned above. These include a focus on psychological, social, intellectual, physical, and emotional development, and many of the specific areas parallel what appears to be needed for children exposed to family violence. The recommendations included: knowledge of essential life skills; critical thinking and reasoning skills; developing positive self-regard; development of self-regulation skills; improving nonviolent conflict resolution skills; an ability for planning for the future; development of trust with parents, peers, and some other adults; attachment to prosocial/conventional institutions; and a commitment to civic engagement. It is interesting to note that many studies in diverse fields and disciplines are formulating similar conclusions and recommendations.

The number of advocacy, prevention, and intervention programs to treat children exposed to family violence has increased in recent years. Peled (1997) emphasized that society must respond to the needs of this unique group of children. However, there have not been many studies that have investigated the outcome with well-designed research. Two such studies are reported in this volume (see Johnston as well as MacMillan & Harpur).

Further outcome research is necessary in order to determine which treatments are most effective in reducing the variety of symptoms presented, and reducing the risk that children from violent homes will perpetuate the abuse or be victimized in their own relationships as adults. It is important to fund and reinforce more of this work so that we can do a better job of developing efficient interventions. Studies on the overall family functioning of these children are necessary as well so that potential mediating factors can be identified and addressed in treatment. Similarly, an increase in research in the area of resiliency is indicated so that the associated positive factors that may potentially mediate abusive families can be identified and used to inform our treatment, practice, and understanding of the mechanisms by which exposure to domestic violence leads to either adaptive or maladaptive outcomes. We hope that this volume addresses some of the more relevant topics related to the issue of children exposed to interparental violence and becomes a valuable resource to those working with children and families in the field of family violence.

FORENSIC ISSUES, INCLUDING CHILD CUSTODY

In dealing with children exposed to family violence, it is important to also include forensic and legal issues, and the policies that are derived in dealing with aspects of these cases. DeVoe and Smith in this volume discuss the various barriers to services that are encountered by battered women and their children. It is important to review these policies so that some of these problems may be avoided in the future.

A particular forensic issue involves child custody and visitation when there has been interparental violence. Shaffer and Bala discuss these issues in this volume. Too often in many countries, there are cases in which domestic violence has been ignored in family courts by judges, attorneys, and child custody evaluators, and the children are permitted to visit unsupervised with the person who has committed the abuse. At times these offenders are even awarded custody of the children. Most often the reason (some would say the excuse) that is given in these forensic cases is that the victim of domestic violence has alienated the children from the person who has committed the abuse. There was even a term coined over a decade ago, without peer-reviewed research to validate it, to supposedly explain such a situation. It was called "parental alienation syndrome (PAS)," and it was self-published by its author (Gardner, 1992).

"PAS" has been used in many countries to remove children from battered women with no other evidence of inappropriate or unfit parenting. This circular argument often becomes a self-fulfilling prophecy in many of these court cases. It was even noted in the APA Task Force report (1996) that such pseudo-syndromes have been used to pathologize battered women in forensic cases, and that no evidence for such a syndrome exists. In fact, this Task Force even went so far as to state that one parent abusing the other is a type of child maltreatment in itself, and that the abusing parent should not have joint or sole custody of the children. The Task Force went on to indicate that such offenders should not have unsupervised visitation with their children until they have completed a specific treatment program that deals with the abusive behaviors and attitudes. Shaffer and Bala (in this volume) agree with such a view, and discuss the issues that have been involved in these cases in Canada. This does not mean that parents do not ever attempt or actually alienate their children against the other parent. However, the use of this supposed "diagnosis" or "condition" is a dangerous misuse of "junk science" to make crucial decisions in the family violence field. The decisions and recommendations are made without comprehensively reviewing or analyzing the evidence in these cases, nor taking into account the context of family violence. For recommendations concerning appropriate approaches in setting up visitation in these situations and awarding custody of the children, see Jaffe and Geffner (1998) and Lemon (2000).

CONCLUSION

It appears that the conclusions of a panel of the National Institute of Justice, Office of Juvenile Delinquency Prevention (2000) concerning children exposed to family violence is an appropriate route to focus on in beginning to eliminate family violence. This report made specific recommendations to accomplish this, including: professionals, advocates, and practitioners working together to end abuse; begin identification and interventions earlier in the lifespan of the children; begin to think developmentally and intervene accordingly; make mothers safe to keep children safe when dealing with family violence; enforce the laws that currently exist to hold the offenders accountable; make adequate resources available; work from a sound knowledge and theoretical base; and create a culture of nonviolence in each community. These are worthwhile goals in helping end the situations that cause children to be exposed to family violence. We hope this volume moves us in this direction.

REFERENCES

American Psychological Association Presidential Task Force on Violence and the Family. (1996). *Violence and the family: Report of the APA Presidential Task Force*. Washington, DC: American Psychological Association.

Carlson, E.B. (1984). Children's observations of interparental violence. In A.R. Roberts (Ed.), *Battered women and their families* (pp. 147-167). New York: Springer.

Eccles, J., & Gootman, J.A. (Eds.). (2002). *Community programs to promote youth development*. Washington, DC: National Research Council and Institute of Medicine, National Academy Press.

Fantuzzo, J.W., & Mohr, W.K. (1999). Prevalence and effects of children exposure to domestic violence. *The Future of Children: Domestic Violence and Children, 9*, 21-32.

Fellitti, V.J., Anda, R.F., Nordenberg, D., Williamson, D.F., Spitz, A.M., Edwards, V., Koss, M.P., & Marks, J.S. (1998). Relationship of childhood abuse and household dysfunction to many of the leading causes of death in adults: The Adverse Childhood Experiences (ACE) study. (1998). *American Journal of Preventive Medicine, 14 (4)*, 245-258.

Franey, K., Geffner, R., & Falconer, R. (2001). *The cost of child maltreatment: Who pays? We all do*. San Diego, CA: Family Violence & Sexual Assault Institute.

Gardner, R. (1992). *The parental alienation syndrome: A guide for mental health and legal professionals*. Creskill, NJ: Creative therapeutics.

Geffner, R., Jaffe, P.G., & Sudermann, M. (Eds.). (2000). *Children exposed to domestic violence: Current research, interventions, prevention, & policy development*. New York: The Haworth Press, Inc.

Graham-Bermann, S.A., & Edleson, J.L. (Eds.). (2001). *Domestic violence in the lives of children: The future of research, intervention, and social policy*. Washington, DC: American Psychological Association.

Graham-Bermann, S.A., & Levendosky, A.A. (1998). Traumatic stress symptoms in children of battered women. *Journal of Interpersonal Violence, 13*, 111-128.

Heller, S.S., Larrieu, J.A., D'Imperio, R., & Boris, N.W. (1999). Research on resilience to child maltreatment: Empirical considerations. *Child Abuse & Neglect, 23*, 321-338.

Holden, G., Geffner, R., & Jouriles, E. (Eds.). (1998). *Children exposed to marital violence: Theory, research, and applied issues*. Washington, DC: American Psychological Association.

Holden, G.W., & Ritchie, K.L. (1991). Linking extreme marital discord, child rearing, and child behavior problems: Evidence from battered women. *Child Development*, *62*, 311-327.

Jaffe, P.G., & Geffner, R. (1998). Child custody disputes and domestic violence: Critical issues for mental health, social service, and legal professionals. In G. Holden, R. Geffner, & E. Jouriles (Eds.), *Children exposed to marital violence: Theory, research, and applied issues* (pp. 371-408). Washington, DC: American Psychological Association.

Kerig, P.K., Fedorowicz, A.E., Brown, C.A., & Warren, M. (2000). Assessment and intervention for ptsd in children exposed to violence. *Journal of Aggression, Maltreatment & Trauma, 3(1)*, 161-184.

Lemon, N.K.D. (2000). Custody and visitation trends in the United States. *Journal of Emotional Abuse, 3 (1)*, 329-343.

National Institute of Justice (NIJ), Office of Juvenile Delinquency Prevention (OCJP). (2000). *Blueprint for action*. Washington, DC: Author.

O'Keefe, M. (1994). Racial/ethnic differences among battered women and their children. *Journal of Child and Family Studies, 3*, 283-305.

Osofsky, J.D. (1999). The impact of violence on children. *The Future of Children: Domestic Violence and Children, 9*, 33-49.

Peled, E. (1997). The battered women's movement response to children of battered women: A critical analysis. *Violence against Women, 3*, 424-446.

Perry, B.D. (2001). The neuroarcheology of childhood maltreatment: The neurodevelopmental costs of adverse childhood events. In K. Franey, R. Geffner, & R. Falconer (eds.), *The cost of child maltreatment: Who pays? We all do.* (pp. 15-37). San Diego, CA: Family Violence & Sexual Assault Institute.

Rossman, B.B.R., & Ho, J. (2000). Posttraumatic response and children exposed to parental violence. *Journal of Aggression, Maltreatment & Trauma, 3(1)*, 85-106.

Rossman, B.B.R., Hughes, H.M., & Rosenberg, M.S. (2000). *Children and the interparental violence: The impact of exposure*. New York: Taylor & Francis.

Rudo, Z.H., Powell, D.S., & Dunlap, G. (1998). The effects of violence in the home on children's emotional, behavioral, and social functioning: A review of the literature. *Journal of Emotional and Behavioral Disorders, 6*(2), 94-108.

Straus, M.A. (1991). Children as witnesses to marital violence: A risk factor for lifelong problems among a nationally representative sample of American men and women. *Children and violence: Report of the Twenty-third Ross Roundtable on Critical Approaches to Common Pediatric Problems*. Columbus, OH: Ross Laboratories.

Tjaden, P., & Thoennes, N. (2000). *Full report of the prevalence, incidence, and consequences of violence against women: Findings from the National Violence Against Women Survey*. Washington, DC: National Institute of Justice.

ADJUSTMENT IN CHILDREN EXPOSED TO INTIMATE PARTNER VIOLENCE: CLINICAL RESEARCH

Domestic Violence and Children's Adjustment: A Review of Research

Judee E. Onyskiw

SUMMARY. This article presents a review of the empirical literature on the effects of witnessing domestic violence on children's adjustment. The review includes 47 studies published in the last two decades. Although there are some inconsistent findings in early research, there is less inconsistency in more recent studies which employ standardized measures, comparison groups of children, and more sophisticated data

Address correspondence to: Judee E. Onyskiw, RN, PhD, Perinatal Research Centre, #4510 Children's Centre, Royal Alexandra Hospital, 10240 Kingsway Avenue, Edmonton, Alberta T5H 3V9 (E-mail: jonyskiw@ualberta.ca).

The author would like to thank Dr. Les Hayduk, Professor, Department of Sociology, University of Alberta, as well as the anonymous referees for their thoughtful reviews and suggestions on an earlier version of this manuscript.

[Haworth co-indexing entry note]: "Domestic Violence and Children's Adjustment: A Review of Research." Onyskiw, Judee E. Co-published simultaneously in *Journal of Emotional Abuse* (The Haworth Maltreatment & Trauma Press, an imprint of The Haworth Press, Inc.) Vol. 3, No. 1/2, 2003, pp. 11-45; and: *The Effects of Intimate Partner Violence on Children* (ed: Robert A.Geffner, Robyn Spurling Igelman, and Jennifer Zellner) The Haworth Maltreatment & Trauma Press, an imprint of The Haworth Press, Inc., 2003, pp. 11-45. Single or multiple copies of this article are available for a fee from The Haworth Document Delivery Service [1-800-HAWORTH, 9:00 a.m. - 5:00 p.m. (EST). E-mail address: docdelivery@haworthpress.com].

10.1300J135v03n01_02

analytic techniques. Results show that children exposed to domestic violence generally have more emotional and behavioral problems, less social and cognitive competence, and exhibit more health problems than children not exposed to domestic violence. Important methodological and theoretical challenges in this area of research are discussed. Suggested priority areas for future research include: studying nonshelter samples of children exposed to domestic violence, studying the effects of children's exposure to interparental verbal and other forms of aggression, conducting longitudinal research to examine the effects of domestic violence on children's long-term adjustment and to elucidate what factors, if any, ameliorate or exacerbate children's adjustment difficulties. *[Article copies available for a fee from The Haworth Document Delivery Service: 1-800-HAWORTH. E-mail address: <docdelivery@haworthpress.com> Website: <http://www.HaworthPress.com> © 2003 by The Haworth Press, Inc. All rights reserved.]*

KEYWORDS. Child witnesses, child adjustment, child behavior, domestic violence, spousal violence

Domestic violence has been characterized as a health and social issue of epidemic proportions. The actual number of children exposed to domestic violence is unclear because there has never been a national prevalence study (Edleson, 1999). Instead, estimates of the number of children exposed to this trauma have been extrapolated from surveys of violence between adult family members; adjustments are then made for the number of households with children and for the average number of children in each household. Using this strategy, Carlson (1984) estimated that at least 3.3 million children between 3 and 17 years of age were at risk of exposure to domestic violence every year, a figure based on inferences made from the first national survey of violence in American families (Straus, Gelles, & Steinmetz, 1980). Based on the second national survey, Straus (1992) maintained that as many as 10 million children may be exposed yearly. Using a similar method to project the number of children exposed to domestic violence in Canada, Johnson (1996) estimated that at least 2 million children were exposed annually, an inference based on a national survey of violence against women. Recently, a national survey of child development in Canada asked parents how often their child (aged 2 to 11 years) saw adults or teenagers in their home physically fighting, hitting, or otherwise trying to hurt others. In 1996, 8.6% of Canadian children (representing approximately 330,000 children) were reported by a parent to have witnessed some violence at home (Statistics Canada, 1997).

While estimates of the prevalence of children exposed to violence in their families are still uncertain, some facts are certain. First, there is a strong tendency to underreport domestic violence; thus, the number of children exposed to this trauma is probably underestimated (Finkelhor, 1993). Second, witnessing this trauma is stressful to children. Children rated witnessing conflict between parents as the third most distressing life stressor (Lewis, Siegel, & Lewis, 1984). Finally, there is concern among the lay public, professionals, and policy-makers about children's exposure to domestic violence (see Shaffer & Bala, 2003, for a discussion of legal issues and policy implications for children exposed to domestic violence).

The impact of witnessing domestic violence on children's adjustment has been the focus of numerous investigations over the last two decades. The purpose of this article is to review research on the effects of witnessing domestic violence on children's adjustment, behavior, functioning, and development. The objectives of the review are to: (1) summarize empirical evidence; (2) highlight important methodological and theoretical challenges with research in this area of inquiry; and (3) provide suggestions for future research.

METHOD

The studies included in this review were located through a comprehensive search of the literature. Computer searches of online databases were conducted on PsycINFO, Sociofile, Medline, and CINAHL. In conducting this search, the terms *spousal, domestic* or *family violence* (and all equivalents) were paired with a variety of keywords such as *children's adjustment, behavior, functioning,* or *development,* and limited to children. Recent issues of journals in which the impact of violence on children's adjustment tend to be reported were searched manually to locate studies not yet incorporated into the online databases. Finally, reference lists of articles were reviewed for citations to studies not yet identified through the other sources.

The conceptualization of the two phenomena of interest, domestic violence and children's adjustment, set the boundaries for the review. Studies assessing marital discord, conflict, or hostility without a clear physical component to the conflict were not included. Only studies assessing some specific aspect of children's adjustment including cognitive, social, emotional, or behavioral functioning were included. Non-English publications, dual publications of the same study, studies whose primary focus was infants, adolescents, or young adults, and expository articles that did not present data were excluded. The search resulted in 47 studies examining the relationship between domestic violence and some aspect of children's adjustment. Table 1 presents an overview of the studies reviewed highlighting the following study features: sample size, age range and child gender, setting, use of a comparison group, measures of domestic violence and children's adjustment, method of data collection, and major study findings.

RESULTS

General Overview of Studies

Most research was conducted to examine the impact on children's adjustment in two major dimensions of psychopathology: adjustment problems expressed as either internalizing or externalizing behaviors. Internalizing involves behavior that is over-controlled, anxious, and inhibited (e.g., sadness, withdrawal, and anxiety). Externalizing involves behavior that is under-controlled, aggressive, and antisocial (e.g., fighting, disobedience, and destructiveness). The distinction between these behaviors, first made by Achenbach and Edelbrock (1978), is a frequently used categorization of children's emotional and behavioral problems. Some studies also examined other important aspects of children's development such as social and cognitive competence, and physical health.

Thirty-two studies (68.1%) were conducted in the United States. Eleven studies were conducted in Canada (Copping, 1996; Jaffe, Wolfe, Wilson, & Zak, 1985, 1986a, 1986b; Kerig, 1998; Kérouac, Taggart, Lescop, & Fortin, 1986; Lehmann, 1997; Moore & Peplar, 1998; Onyskiw & Hayduk, 2001; Wolfe, Jaffe, Wilson, & Zak, 1985; Wolfe, Zak, Wilson, & Jaffe, 1986), two in Australia (Bookless-Pratz & Mertin, 1990; Mathias, Mertin, & Murray, 1995), one in Israel (Sternberg et al., 1993) and one in England (Moore, Galcius, & Pettican, 1981).

Samples

With the exception of one study based on a national survey of children, samples ranged in size from 15 to 425 children.[1] A total of 5,240

TABLE 1. Studies Examining the Link Between Domestic Violence and Children's Adjustment

Study/Year	Sample	Measures	Results
Attala & McSweeney (1997)	15 children (2-6 years) 8 boys, 7 girls Children of battered women in community were compared to shelter and comparison children from another study. (see next citation)	Mother provided ratings of spousal violence and child behavior (NSI). Developmental tests and medical exam were administered.	Children of battered women living in community had less emotional, somatic, and physical health problems and were more socially competent than shelter children. Children's developmental status was within normal range. The majority of exposed community children had normal weights, hemoglobin and lead levels but they were less likely to be up to date on their immunizations than comparison children of nonbattered women.
Attala & Summers (1999)	115 children (2-6 years) 61 boys, 54 girls Shelter children and comparison group in same social strata.	Mother provided ratings of spousal violence and child behavior (NSI). Developmental tests and medical exam were administered.	Preschool shelter children had more emotional, behavioral, and physical health problems than comparison children. They were less socially competent and had more developmental delays than comparison children.
Bookless-Pratz & Mertin (1990)	20 children (7-11 years) 11 boys, 9 girls Shelter children	Mother interviewed. Provided history of spousal violence (NSR) and child behavior. Child provided ratings of appraisal of violence (NSI) and self-concept.	55% of children fell into the high range for internalizing and externalizing behavior problems. Scores for self-concept and social competence were within normal range. No significant gender differences noted on any of the scores.
Christopoulos, Cohn, Shaw, Joyce, Sullivan-Hanson, Kraft, & Emery (1987)	80 children (5-13 years) 42 boys, 38 girls Shelter children and comparison group of similar background.	Mother interviewed. Provided ratings of spousal violence and child behavior. Child provided ratings of perceived competence. Intelligence test administered.	Shelter children had more internalizing (but not externalizing) problems than comparison children. No significant differences between groups for perceived or cognitive competence. Girls had significantly more internalizing and externalizing behaviors in the clinical range than comparison children.
Copping (1996)	75 children (3-15 years) 37 boys, 38 girls Shelter children	Mothers provided history of spousal violence (NSR). Observations by shelter staff to rate child behaviors (NSI).	Boys demonstrated more total behavior problems, more physical behaviors and more physiological complaints (i.e., headaches) than girls. Abused-child witnesses had more behavior problems than children who only witnessed abuse.
Davis & Carlson (1987)	66 children (4-11 years) 34 boys, 32 girls Shelter children	Mother provided history of spousal violence (NSR) and child behavior.	70% of children had behavior problems in the clinical range. More boys were in the clinical range during the preschool than school years, while fewer girls were in the clinical range during the preschool than school years. 53% of children were in the clinical range for depression.

15

TABLE 1 (continued)

Study/Year	Sample	Measures	Results
Fantuzzo, DePaola, Lambert, Martino, Anderson, & Sutton (1991)	107 children (3-6 years) 58 boys, 49 girls 4 groups: shelter children, home children exposed to violence, home children exposed to verbal conflict, and a comparison group matched on SES.	Mother provided ratings of spousal violence and child behavior. Child provided ratings of perceived competence.	Verbal conflict only associated with moderate level of behavior problems. Verbal plus physical conflict associated with clinical levels of conduct problems and moderate levels of emotional problems. Verbal and physical conflict plus shelter residence associated with clinical levels of conduct problems, higher level of emotional problems and lower levels of social functioning and perceived maternal acceptance.
Gleason (1995)	47 children (1-16 years) Shelter children	Mother provided ratings of spousal violence (NSR), skill development and child behavior. Shelter teacher and child care worker provided ratings of child behavior.	Shelter children had significantly lower developmental skills than standardized norms. Both mothers and teachers rated children's behavior more pathological than children in the normative database. There were no age or gender differences. Mothers rated 71% of children with problems in clinical range while teachers rated 57% with problems in the clinical range.
Graham-Berman & Levendosky (1998a)	46 children (3-5 years) 22 boys, 24 girls Shelter children and community children exposed to violence and comparison group from similar economic background.	Mother provided ratings of spousal violence, psychological abuse, maternal mental health, parenting style, and child behavior. Two observers rated child's social interactions in unstructured play.	Exposed children had significantly more internalizing and externalizing problems (including more in the clinical range) than comparison children. They also showed more negative affect, responded less appropriately to situations, were more aggressive with peers, and had more ambivalent relations with their caregivers. Emotional abuse of the mother and maternal self-esteem were the most significant predictors of child adjustment and social behavior.
Graham-Berman & Levendosky (1998b)	64 children (7-12 years) 33 boys, 31 girls Shelter children and community children exposed to spousal violence.	Mother provided ratings of spousal violence, child behavior and traumatic stress symptoms measured using diagnostic criteria for DSM-IV modified for children. Teacher provided ratings of child behavior. Child provided ratings of perceived competence.	13% of children exposed to violence qualified for a diagnosis of Posttraumatic Stress Disorder (PTSD). 52% had intrusive and unwanted remembering of traumatic events, 19% had traumatic avoidance, and 42% had traumatic arousal symptoms. No significant gender differences in symptoms. No significant differences in frequency of symptoms between abused and nonabused children. Children who experienced PTSD symptoms had higher internalizing and externalizing behavior scores than children without these symptoms.
Hershorn & Rosenbaum (1985)	45 boys (M = 9.1 years) 2 groups of children of mothers referred for marital therapy (violent and nonviolent/discordant), and comparison group.	Mother provided ratings of spousal violence, child rearing style, and child behavior.	Children from violent and nonviolent, discordant homes both had significantly more conduct problems than control children. No significant difference between children from violent and nonviolent, discordant homes. Only children exposed to violence had significantly more emotional problems than controls.

Study	Sample	Measures	Findings
Holden & Ritchie (1991)	74 children (2-8 years) 35 boys, 39 girls Shelter children and comparison group matched on age and sex.	Mother provided ratings of spousal violence, parent stress, child temperament and behavior. Teacher provided ratings of child behavior. Mother-child interactions were observed.	Shelter children had significantly more overall behavior problems and internalizing problems (not externalizing) than controls. Girls had more internalizing behaviors than boys. Younger children had fewer internalizing, externalizing, and total number of problems than older children.
Hughes (1988)	178 children (3-12 years) 86 boys, 92 girls 2 groups of shelter children (witnesses and abused-witnesses) and comparison group.	Mother provided ratings of spousal violence, anxiety, and child behavior. Child provided ratings of depression and self-esteem.	Abused-witnesses had significantly higher problem behavior scores than nonabused witnesses and controls. Both witnesses and abused-witnesses were more anxious than controls but no differences for depression. Scores for nonabused-child witnesses fell between the other groups. Preschool children had more difficulties than both middle and older children. Abused preschool children scored significantly higher than children in other two groups.
Hughes & Barad (1983)	65 children (3-13 years) 35 boys, 30 girls Shelter children	Mother provided ratings of child behavior. Child provided ratings of anxiety and self-esteem. Shelter staff and teacher provided ratings of child behavior.	Girls were more anxious than boys. School-age boys were more aggressive than girls. Preschool children had below average self-esteem when compared with normative data. Mother's ratings were more negative than staff or teacher ratings. No difference in externalizing behaviors between children and standardized norms when rated by staff.
Hughes & Luke (1998)	58 children (6-12 years) 32 boys, 26 girls Shelter children	Mother provided ratings of spousal violence, maternal mental health, externalizing child behavior, depression and anxiety. Child provided ratings of internalizing behavior, depression, anxiety and self-concept.	Results of a cluster analysis showed variability in children's adjustment. 60% of children were in the not-distressed or very mildly distressed group, while 40% of children were in clusters indicating difficulties. Children's distress was significantly associated with maternal depression, mother's verbal aggressiveness and duration of abuse. Child gender, child abuse and frequency of spousal violence did not significantly differentiate among the subgroups.
Hughes, Parkinson, & Vargo (1989)	150 children (4-12 years) Shelter children with comparison group from similar economic background.	Mother provided ratings of spousal violence and child behavior. Child provided ratings of depression and anxiety.	Abused-witnesses had significantly more internalizing and externalizing behavior problems than nonabused witnesses and comparison children. Nonabused child witnesses were significantly different from controls on total behavior problems but not anxiety, depression, or social competence.
Jaffe, Wolfe, Wilson, & Zak (1985)	100 children (4-12 years) 56 boys, 44 girls Shelter children with comparison group.	Structured interview with mothers. Mother provided ratings of spousal violence, maternal health, stress, family disadvantage, and child behavior.	Boys from violent families had significantly more behavior problems and difficulties in social competence than controls. Girls did not differ significantly on these variables. Spousal violence and maternal adjustment significantly predicted children's behavior problems.

TABLE 1 (continued)

Study/Year	Sample	Measures	Results
Jaffe, Wolfe, Wilson, & Zak (1986a)	126 children (6-11 years) 69 boys, 57 girls Shelter children with comparison group.	Mother provided ratings of spousal violence and child behavior.	Children from violent homes had more internalizing behaviors and lower levels of social competence than children from nonviolent homes; however, only boys had more externalizing behaviors than controls. Level of exposure to violence was significantly associated with greater adjustment problems in boys.
Jaffe, Wolfe, Wilson, & Zak (1986b)	65 boys (4 - 16 years) Shelter children and comparison group with similar demographic characteristics.	Mother provided ratings of spousal violence and child behavior.	Both abused and witness boys differed significantly from comparison children on measures of internalizing and externalizing problems but no difference in social competence. Abused boys had significantly more externalizing problems than boys only exposed to violence.
Johnston, González, & Campbell (1987)	56 children (4-12 years) 28 boys, 28 girls Children of families in mediation for custody disputes post-divorce.	Mother provided ratings of spousal aggression and child behavior. Child provided ratings of self-concept. Parent-child interactions were observed.	At baseline, spousal aggression did not predict child behavior problems. At follow-up (2 years later), spousal aggression significantly predicted behavior problems. Controlling for baseline level, spousal aggression at follow-up predicted additional variance. At baseline, there was no significant interaction between age and gender. At follow-up, girls in high-conflict families were more withdrawn and depressed; older children were more aggressive and had more somatic complaints.
Jouriles, Barling, & O'Leary (1987)	45 children (5-13 years) 22 boys, 23 girls Clinic referred children.	Mother provided ratings of spousal and parent-child aggression, and child behavior. Child provided ratings of depression.	Parent-child aggression significantly related to conduct problems, attention problems, anxiety-withdrawal and motor excess after controlling for age and spousal aggression. Witnessing spousal aggression was not significantly related to child behavior problems.
Jouriles, McDonald, Norwood, Ware, Spiller, & Swank (1998)	155 children (8-12 years) 84 boys, 71 girls Shelter children. 3 groups: children who observed weapons violence, children who did not observe weapons violence but weapons violence involved weapons, and those who did not observe weapons violence and violence did not involve weapons.	Mother provided ratings of interparental violence and child's externalizing behaviors. Child provided ratings of interparental violence, appraisals of conflict, and anxiety, and depression.	Children in families experiencing more severe forms of interparental violence (i.e., involving the use of knives or guns) displayed higher levels of behavior problems than children in families with less severe interparental violence, even after accounting for the frequency of interparental violence in the home. Children who observed violence using knives or guns did not differ from children who did not observe the use of knives or guns but whose mothers reported that the violence involved weapons. No gender differences in children's responses were reported.

18

Authors	Sample	Measures	Findings
Jouriles, Murphy, & O'Leary (1989)	87 children (5-12 years) 41 boys, 46 girls Children of parents in marital therapy.	Mother provided ratings of marital aggression, parent-child aggression, and child behavior.	Marital aggression significantly predicted child conduct problems, personality problems, inadequacy/immaturity and clinical levels of problematic behavior after marital discord, child age, child sex and interaction of marital discord by child sex were controlled.
Jouriles, Norwood, McDonald, Vincent, & Mahoney (1996)	*Study 1* 55 children (5-12 years) of parents in marital therapy 23 boys, 32 girls *Study 2* 199 children (5-12 years) from shelters 106 boys, 93 girls	Parents provided ratings of spousal violence and child behavior.	*Study 1* In the clinic group, both physical aggression and other forms of aggression correlated positively with children's externalizing behaviors. *Study 2* In the shelter group, both physical aggression and other forms of aggression correlated positively with internalizing and externalizing behaviors in children.
Jouriles, Spiller, Stephens, McDonald, & Swank (2000)	154 children (8-12 years) 83 boys, 71 girls Shelter children who participated in a previous study of interparental violence involving weapons (Jouriles et al., 1998).	Mother provided ratings of interparental violence, parent-child violence, and child's externalizing behaviors. Child provided rating of interparental violence, parent-child violence, appraisals of conflict, anxiety, and depression.	53% of children in clinical range for internalizing problems, 47% for externalizing problems, 23% for anxiety, and 16% for depression. Child's physical abuse was significantly associated with higher levels of externalizing problems but not internalizing problems or anxiety. Child self-blame positively correlated with maternal reports of externalizing problems. Child self-blame, threat, fear of abandonment each positively correlated with child's reports of anxiety/depression. Child age (but not gender) moderated the relationship, with appraisals more positively related to problems of older children.
Kerig (1998)	106 children (8-11 years) 58 boys, 48 girls Shelter children	Parents provided ratings of interparental violence and child's exposure to violence and child behavior. Child provided ratings of appraisal of conflict, perceived control over conflict, and anxiety.	Interparental violence significantly predicted boys' and girls' total problems and internalizing problems, and boys' externalizing problems and anxiety. Appraisals of conflict properties mediated the relationship between violence and boys' externalizing and total problems, and girls' internalizing and total problems. Some gender effects noted. Perceived threat mediated boys' anxiety while self-blame acted mediated girls' internalizing behaviors.
Kérouac, Taggart, Lescop, & Fortin (1986)	130 children (1-12 years) 76 boys, 54 girls Shelter children	Mother provided ratings of child behavior (NSR) and health.	Children described as nervous (52%), sad (48%), having problems relating to others (40%), slow learners (24%), and aggressive (13%). 51% of children were absent from school for health problems an average of 10 days in the last year compared to the national Canadian average of 10 days.

TABLE 1 (continued)

Study/Year	Sample	Measures	Results
Kolbo (1996)	60 children (8-11 years) 30 boys, 30 girls Children referred to non-shelter agencies for support.	Mother provided ratings of spousal violence and child behavior. Child provided ratings of self-worth and supportive relationships. An intelligence test was administered.	No significant gender differences in terms of supportive relationships, behavioral problems, or global self-worth. Exposure to violence positively correlated with girls' behavior or problems and negatively correlated with boys' reports of self-worth. Having supportive relationships and a higher IC was positively correlated with feelings of self-worth and negatively correlated with behavior problems.
Lehmann (1997)	84 children (9-15 years) 48 boys, 36 girls Shelter children and children referred from child protective agency.	Mother provided ratings of history of violence witnessed by child. Structured interview with child to assess posttraumatic stress symptoms. Child provided ratings of anger, depression, and anxiety.	56% of children met diagnostic criteria for Posttraumatic Stress Disorder (PTSD). There were significant differences on age, duration, and frequency of witnessing abuse between children who met PTSD criteria and those who did not. PTSD group differed significantly from the non-PTSD group on depression, assault anxiety, dissociation, anger, and negative attributions.
Levendosky & Graham-Bermann (1998)	121 children (7-12 years) 59 boys, 62 girls Shelter children and control group matched on age, ethnicity, and income.	Mother provided ratings of spousal violence, parenting stress, and child behavior.	Abuse (psychological and physical) significantly associated with higher levels of parenting stress. Parenting stress significantly predicted children's adjustment (internalizing and externalizing behaviors) after controlling for psychological and physical abuse of the mother.
Markward (1997)	134 children 72 boys, 62 girls Past shelter residents	Mother interviewed for history of spousal violence (NSR), school-related problems, and child behavior (NSR).	Mothers reported that children displayed negative behaviors. Children who were also abused behaved more negatively than children who only witnessed. The frequency with which women reported that the child was abused in spousal-abuse situations was significantly associated with the frequency of observing negative child behaviors.
Mathias, Mertin, & Murray (1995)	*Phase I* 79 6-12 year old children 47 boys, 32 girls Children were past shelter residents. *Phase II* 44 children (22 from 1st phase) and a comparison group matched on sex, age, and SES.	Mother provided ratings of spousal violence, child behavior, social skills and health. Child provided ratings of anxiety and social problem solving. Reading test was administered.	*Phase I:* 37-47% of children had behavior problems in clinical range. No gender differences noted. Only 51 to 57% of children were reading at an age-appropriate level. Children were 2.8 times more likely to have internalizing behaviors in the clinical range if they had also been abused. *Phase II:* Significant differences between child witnesses and controls for behavior problems, social competence, and tendency to choose aggressive conflict responses but no differences in anxiety. Internalizing behaviors and tendency to choose aggressive conflict responses were the variables related to spousal violence or control group membership.

Study	Sample	Measures	Findings
McCloskey, Figueredo, & Koss (1995)	365 children (6-12 years) 183 boys, 182 girls. Shelter children and community child witnesses and comparison group.	Mother given structured diagnostic interviews for maternal and child mental health. Mother provided ratings of parent-child and spousal aggression, parenting behavior, sibling support, and child behavior. Child provided ratings of parent-child aggression and parental warmth.	Significantly more children from violent homes had conduct-disorders, separation-anxiety, attention-deficits, and obsessive-compulsive disorders. Both path models using mothers' and children's reports showed direct effects of family violence on children's mental health. Although mothers showed symptoms of psychopathology, it was causally unrelated to child psychopathology. Instead, family violence accounted for most of the variance in children's mental health. Family support failed to predict child psychopathology.
Moore, Galius, & Pettican (1981)	66 children (1-18 years) 37 boys, 29 girls. Children of parents in marital therapy.	Mother provided ratings of spousal violence (NSF) and child behavior (NSR).	Children described as aggressive, anxious, withdrawn and underachieving at school.
Moore & Peplar (1998)	377 children (6-12 years) 181 boys, 196 girls. 4 groups, shelter children, exposed children living in hostels (i.e., homeless), children from one- and two-parent nonviolent homes.	Mother and child interviewed. Mother provided ratings of spousal violence and parent-child violence, stress, support, health and child behavior. Teacher and child care workers provided ratings of child behavior. Child provided ratings of locus of control. Intelligence and achievement tests were administered.	Children in the homeless group who had experienced violence were similar to shelter children in terms of the extent of emotional and behavioral problems. Gender differences noted in these groups, with more difficulties in girls. No gender differences in the other groups. A substantial portion of the shelter children had school-related difficulties. Parent-child aggression was a stronger predictor of adjustment in shelter children than witnessing domestic violence.
O'Keefe (1994)	185 children (7-13 years) 94 boys, 91 girls. Shelter children	Mothers interviewed. Provided ratings of spousal and parent-child aggression, substance abuse, family cohesion, stress, support, parenting behavior, child temperament and behavior. Child provided ratings of social competence and self-worth.	45% and 57% of children had externalizing and internalizing behaviors in the clinical range, respectively. The quality of parenting, positive child temperament, school performance, self-worth, child's age (young children more affected) and the amount of violence witnessed significantly predicted externalizing behaviors. Positive child temperament, stressful life events, sociability, and child abuse significantly predicted internalizing problems. No gender differences found.
Onyskiw & Hayduk (2001)	11,221 children (4-11 years) 5654 boys, 5567 girls who participated in a national survey of Canadian children. 8.9% of these children witnessed violence at home between parents or teens.	Mother provided ratings of intra-family aggression and child behavior.	Witnessing intra-family aggression significantly influenced children's aggression. Intra-family aggression disrupted parenting which, in turn, was associated with an increase in children's aggression, internalizing behaviors, and a decrease in prosocial behaviors. Maternal depression influenced children's internalizing behaviors. Boys used more physical aggression, less indirect aggression, and were less socially competent than girls. There was no difference in internalizing behaviors. Few age differences noted.

TABLE 1 (continued)

Study/Year	Sample	Measures	Results
Rosenbaum & O'Leary (1981)	53 boys (M = 10 years) 3 groups of children of parents in marital therapy: child witnesses living at home; children from nonviolent/discordant marriages, and comparison children.	Mother provided history of spousal violence (NSR) and child behavior.	There were no significant differences among groups for conduct disorders, personality disorders, inadequate-immature or delinquent behavior.
Rossman (1998)	425 children (4-13 years) 4 groups: child witnesses in shelters, abused child witnesses in shelters, child witnesses in community, children nonabusive, nonviolent homes.	Mother and child interviewed. Mother provided ratings of spousal violence, parent-child violence, stressful life events, and post-traumatic stress symptoms child behavior. Child provided ratings of child behavior. Vocabulary test administered.	All child witnesses had significantly higher symptomology than non-witnesses. Relative to children only exposed to violence, abused child-witnesses had greater symptomology. Generally, child witnesses exhibited more posttraumatic stress symptoms and poorer cognitive functioning. The relationship between family violence and family adversity and children's adaptive functioning was mediated by post-traumatic stress symptoms and cognitive functioning.
Rossman & Rosenberg (1992)	94 children (6-12 years) 41 boys, 53 girls 4 groups: shelter children, community children from violent homes, children from discordant homes and comparison group.	Mother provided ratings of spousal aggression, child stress and behavior. Child provided ratings of perceived competence, beliefs about control. Vocabulary test was administered.	After controlling for socioeconomic status, shelter children had more externalizing behavior problems but also more social competence than children in other groups. Shelter children reported being less accepting of their behavioral conduct than children in both nonviolent groups. No significant difference between groups on vocabulary.
Smith, Berthelsen, & O'Connor (1997)	54 children (3-6 years) 29 boys, 25 girls Children were former shelter residents.	Structured interviews with mothers. Provided ratings of spousal aggression and child behavior.	52% of children exhibited behavioral problems in the clinical range. Children divided into groups based on violence exposure and degree of behavioral problems prior to leaving abusive home. Children with behavioral problems pre-separation or who were exposed to more violence had more externalizing problems post-separation. Children who withdrew during conflict had more internalizing problems than children who responded in other ways (i.e., intervened). Mothers who reported less quality in parenting reported more behavioral problems.

22

Study	Sample	Measures	Results
Spaccarelli, Sandler, & Roosa (1994)	303 children (10-12 years) Children from inner-city schools	Mother provided history of violence (NSR), parental drinking, and child behavior. Child provided ratings of self-worth, depression, and hostility.	Using child reports, spousal violence significantly correlated with boys' and girls' self-reported depression, and with girls' conduct problems and self-esteem. Using maternal reports, spousal violence was not significantly correlated with boys' or girls' depression, anxiety, or conduct problems. Regression analyses showed that after controlling for risk factors (e.g., parental drinking), spousal violence accounted for significant unique variance in girls' self-reported conduct problems but not boys' symptomology.
Sternberg, Lamb, Greenbaum, Cicchetti, Dawud, Cortes, Krispin, & Lorey (1993)	110 children (8-12 years) 61 boys, 49 girls 4 groups of community children: abused-child, child witness, abused-witness, and a comparison group	Mothers and fathers were interviewed. Parents provided ratings of child behavior. Child provided ratings of depression and child behavior.	Using child ratings: all domestic violence (DV) groups had significantly more behavioral problems and depression than controls. Girls in the abused-child and witness-abuse groups had more externalizing behaviors than boys. Girls in the abused-witness and control group reported fewer externalizing behaviors than boys. Using maternal ratings: witness-abuse and abused-witnesses had significantly more externalizing problems than controls. Group by sex interaction: girls in all DV groups had more externalizing behaviors than boys while girls in control group had fewer problems than boys. Using paternal ratings: there were no significant differences between groups.
Westra & Martin (1981)	20 children (2-8 years) 10 boys, 10 girls Shelter children	Mother provided ratings of parental nurturance. Shelter staff provided rating of child behavior. Developmental and intelligence tests and medical exam were administered.	Children were more aggressive than standardized norms. Boys were more aggressive than girls. Children's verbal, motor, and cognitive abilities were significantly lower than standardized norms. They had more health problems including speech and hearing.
Wildin, Williamson, & Wilson (1991)	76 children (1-13 years) 39 boys, 37 girls Shelter children	Mother provided history of violence (NSR), medical and school history (NSR) and child behavior. Developmental test and medical exam were administered.	39% of children were developmentally delayed according to established norms. 46% had school-related difficulties. 87% had behavior problems, particularly, aggression, antisocial behavior and social inhibition. Six children (8%) reported suicidal attempts or ideation.
Wolfe, Jaffe, Wilson, & Zak (1985)	198 children (4-16 years) 98 boys, 100 girls Shelter children and a comparison group	Mother provided ratings of spousal and parent-child aggression, maternal health, negative life events, family crises, and child behavior.	Shelter children had significantly more internalizing and externalizing behavioral problems and were less socially competent than controls. Regression analyses revealed that both maternal stress and witnessing violence accounted for 19% of the variance in child behavior problems and 16% of the variance in social competence.

23

TABLE 1 (continued)

Study/Year	Sample	Measures	Results
Wolfe, Zak, Wilson, & Jaffe (1986)	63 children (4-13 years) 35 boys, 28 girls 3 groups: current shelter residents, former residents and a comparison group.	Mother provided ratings of spousal aggression, maternal health, negative life events, family disadvantage, and child behavior.	Current shelter residents had lower levels of social competence and school performance than former residents and control children but not significantly more internalizing or externalizing behavior problems.

Note: NSR = Non-Standardized Report; NSI = Non-Standardized Instrument; otherwise instruments were well-validated, reliable, and widely-used measures.

children comprised the subjects of this review. Children ranged in age from 2 to 18 years, although one study did include some infants in their sample. On average, children were school age ($M = 8.0$ years, $SD = 2.1$). Overall, there were slightly more boys sampled (52.7%). Mothers' average age was 31.5 years ($SD = 2.8$). The number of children per family ranged from one to eight with a mean of 2.5 ($SD = 0.5$). In terms of the ethnic composition of the samples, based on the twenty-seven studies (57.4%) that provided this information, there was some diversity, although Caucasian children were overrepresented. However, the samples included 5% to 68% of children from minority groups including African American, Hispanic, Asian, Native American, and children of mixed racial origin. In nine studies (19.1%) approximately half of the children were from minority groups. Thirty-six studies (76.6%) reported the income distribution and/or socioeconomic status of the families. Of these, 74.3% specified that children were predominantly from low income families or families classified as lower socioeconomic status, 17.1% specified that children were predominantly from low to middle income families or socioeconomic status, and 8.6% specified that children were predominantly from middle income or middle class families.

Thirty-three studies (70.2%) included children in shelters or transition houses for abused women, while four studies (8.5%) included former shelter residents (Markward, 1997; Mathias et al., 1995; Smith, Berthelsen, & O'Connor, 1997; Wolfe et al., 1986). Other studies included clinic children in therapy (Jouriles, Barling, & O'Leary, 1987; Kolbo, 1996), children of parents in marital therapy (Hershorn & Rosenbaum, 1985; Jouriles, Murphy, & O'Leary, 1989; Jouriles, Norwood, McDonald, Vincent, & Mahoney, 1996; Moore et al., 1981; Rosenbaum & O'Leary, 1981), and children of divorced parents in mediation for custody disputes (Johnston, Gonzalez, & Campbell, 1987). Eleven studies (23.4%) included children exposed to domestic violence living in the community (Attala & McSweeney, 1997; Fantuzzo, DePaola, Lambert, Martino, Anderson, & Sutton, 1991; Graham-Bermann & Levendosky, 1998a, 1998b; McCloskey, Figueredo, & Koss, 1995; Moore & Peplar, 1998; Onyskiw & Hayduk, 2001; Rossman, 1998; Rossman & Rosenberg, 1992; Spaccarelli, Sandler, & Roosa, 1994; Sternberg et al., 1993).

Measures

Violence Status. Various terms were used to connote the presence of violence in families (i.e., woman or spousal abuse; interparental, marital, domestic or family violence; interparental or marital aggression; and physical conflict). Domestic violence was assessed using a variety of methods. The majority of studies used self-report measures with pre-existing information on reliability and validity. In thirty studies (63.8%), mothers completed the Conflict Tactics Scale (CTS; Straus et al., 1980), a standardized measure to assess violence between intimate partners. The CTS has norms derived from national prevalence studies of violence in American families. In two studies (4.3%), mothers completed the O'Leary-Porter Scale (OPS; Porter & O'Leary, 1980), a scale which assesses the frequency of child exposure to interparental conflict including physical aggression. Otherwise, investigators relied on the mothers' self-reported history (23.4%) or shelter residence (8.5%) as evidence of violence status. In addition to maternal reports of violence, four studies (8.5%) also obtained assessments from the children themselves (Bookless-Pratz & Mertin, 1990; Kerig, 1998; Jouriles, McDonald, Norwood, Ware, Spiller, & Swank, 1998; Jouriles, Spiller, Stephens, McDonald, & Swank, 2000).

Child Adjustment. All studies examined the impact of domestic violence on child behavior mostly using behavior checklists. While six different behavior checklists were used to rate child behavior, the most frequently (61.7%) used instrument was the Child Behavior Checklist (CBCL; Achenbach & Edelbrock, 1978). The CBCL has good psychometric properties, normative data by age and gender, and clinical cutoffs as indices of adjustment problems. In seven studies (14.9%), investigators relied on parental reports using structured interviews designed specifically for the study without reported evidence of reliability and validity or normative data.

Mothers rated the child's behavior in forty-five studies (96.7%). Occasionally, teachers (10.6%), shelter staff (10.6%), or fathers (6.4%) rated the child's behavior usually in combination with mothers (Copping, 1996; Gleason, 1995; Graham-Bermann & Levendosky, 1998a, 1998b; Holden & Ritchie, 1991; Hughes & Barad, 1983; Moore & Peplar, 1998; O'Keefe, 1994; Westra & Martin, 1981). In seven studies (14.9%), older children also completed questionnaires on their behavior (Hughes & Luke, 1998; Jouriles et al., 1998, 2000; Moore & Peplar, 1998; O'Keefe, 1994; Rossman, 1998; Sternberg et al., 1993).

In twenty-one studies (44.7%), researchers examined the effects of domestic violence on other domains of child functioning or development (e.g., perceived competence, depression, anxiety, locus of control; self-esteem, self-concept, self-worth, and prosocial behavior) (Bookless-Pratz & Mertin, 1990; Christopoulos et al., 1987; Fantuzzo et al.,

1991; Graham-Bermann & Levendosky, 1998b; Hughes, 1988; Hughes & Barad, 1983; Hughes & Luke, 1998; Hughes, Parkinson, & Vargo, 1989; Johnston et al., 1987; Jouriles et al., 1987, 2000; Kerig, 1998; Kolbo, 1996; Lehmann, 1997; Mathias et al., 1995; Moore & Peplar, 1998; O'Keefe, 1994; Onyskiw & Hayduk, 2001; Rossman & Rosenberg, 1992; Spaccarelli et al., 1994; Sternberg et al., 1993). The scales were all well-validated, reliable, and widely-used measures developed specifically for children. Structured diagnostic interviews were conducted to assess child mental health (McCloskey et al., 1995) or traumatic stress symptoms (Graham-Berman & Levendosky, 1998b; Lehmann, 1997). In eight studies (17.0%), researchers administered standardized intelligence or developmental tests (Attala & McSweeney, 1997; Attala & Summers, 1999; Christopoulos et al., 1987; Kolbo, 1996; Mathias et al., 1995; Rossman & Rosenberg, 1992; Westra & Martin, 1981; Wildin, Williamson, & Wilson, 1991). In four studies (8.5%), medical personnel examined children to assess their physical health (Attala & McSweeney, 1997; Attala & Summers, 1999; Kérouac et al., 1986; Westra & Martin, 1981).

OVERVIEW OF STUDY FINDINGS

Although research in this area used various methodologies, instruments, and samples, the vast majority of studies reported that witnessing domestic violence was associated with a wide range of adjustment difficulties in children. Findings are summarized according to problems in major areas of child adjustment.

Externalizing Behaviors

All but one study (97.9%) examined the impact of domestic violence on children's externalizing behaviors. The vast majority reported that children exposed to domestic violence exhibited more externalizing behaviors than comparison groups of children (e.g., Graham-Bermann & Levendosky, 1998a; Hershorn & Rosenbaum, 1985; Hughes, 1988; Jaffe et al., 1985, 1986a, 1986b; Johnston et al., 1987; Jouriles et al., 1989, 1996, 1998, 2000; Levendosky & Graham-Bermann, 1998; Markward, 1997; Mathias et al., 1995; O'Keefe, 1994; Rossman & Rosenberg, 1992; Smith et al., 1997; Sternberg et al., 1993; Wolfe et al., 1985). Typically, these children were more aggressive, noncompliant, disruptive, destructive, and antisocial than comparison children from nonviolent homes. When scores for children exposed to violence were compared to normative data, a higher proportion fell into the clinical range for externalizing problems on the behavior checklists; that is, their scores fell into a range that suggests their problems were serious enough to warrant clinical intervention.

Three studies reported contradictory findings. Wolfe and his colleagues (1986) found no evidence that exposed children had more externalizing behaviors than non-exposed children. Hughes and Barad (1983) found that shelter children did not differ from standardized norms when shelter staff rated their behavior. Rosenbaum and O'Leary (1981) found that differences in conduct disorders or delinquent behavior among boys exposed to domestic violence, boys from discordant but nonviolent homes and boys from nondiscordant homes to be small in magnitude and insignificant. Other researchers reported that shelter children had significantly more internalizing behaviors than comparison children but not externalizing behaviors (Christopoulos et al., 1987; Holden & Ritchie, 1991). Finally, two researchers found links between domestic violence and externalizing behaviors in boys only (Jaffe et al., 1986a; Kerig, 1998).

Internalizing Behaviors

Forty-three studies (91.5%) examined the impact of witnessing violence on children's internalizing behaviors. There was considerable agreement among the studies that children exposed to domestic violence had more internalizing behaviors with a significant proportion of children having problems indicative of severe disturbance (Bookless-Pratz, 1990; Christopoulos et al., 1987; Davis & Carlson, 1987; Fantuzzo et al.,1991; Graham-Bermann & Levendosky, 1998a; Holden & Ritchie, 1991; Hughes, 1988; Hughes & Barad, 1983; Jaffe et al., 1986a, 1986b; Johnston et al., 1987; Jouriles et al., 1996, 2000; Mathias et al., 1995; Smith et al., 1997; Spaccarelli et al., 1994; Sternberg et al., 1993; Wildin et al., 1991; Wolfe et al., 1985). Children exposed to domestic violence were described as more anxious, sad, worried, fearful, and withdrawn than children not exposed to this disruptive environment at home. They had low self-esteem, and depressive symptoms were common. Davis and Carlson (1987) reported that 68% of preschool children and 53% of school-age children in their sample had depression scores in the clinical range, while Wildin and her colleagues (1991) reported that six school-age children in their sample of 76 had related suicidal attempts or ideation.

In contrast, Hughes (1988) found no significant difference in depression scores between exposed children and comparison children from a similar economic background; however, exposed children were more anxious than their counterparts. Likewise, Wolfe and colleagues (1986) did not find significantly more internalizing behaviors in children exposed to violence than their peers from nonviolent homes.

Social Competence

Almost half of the studies (48.9%) investigated the impact of domestic violence on children's social functioning. Children raised in violent homes had difficulty in several areas of social interaction relative to their peers from nonviolent homes (Davis & Carlson, 1987; Fantuzzo, et al., 1991; Graham-Bermann & Levendosky, 1998a; Jaffe et al., 1985, 1986a; Mathias et al., 1995; Rossman & Rosenberg, 1992; Wolfe et al., 1985, 1986). They handled their frustration poorly and had more difficulty regulating their emotions when interacting with others. They lacked effective problem-solving skills and conflict resolution strategies, often misinterpreting ambiguous interpersonal situations as potentially threatening and attributing hostile intent to the other person. Exposed children chose aggressive responses more often than their peers (Graham-Bermann & Levendosky, 1998a; Mathias et al., 1995). They also reported fewer interests and social activities, had poorer peer relations, and often suffered peer rejection (Wolfe et al., 1986).

However, some studies did not find that exposed children were less socially competent than their counterparts. Both Christopoulos and her colleagues (1987) and Jaffe and his colleagues (1986b) found no such differences between shelter children and matched controls. Interestingly, Rossman and Rosenberg (1998) found that both problem behaviors and social behaviors were higher in children exposed to domestic violence.

Cognitive Competence

Only eleven of the studies (23.4%) reviewed provided any assessment of children's cognitive functioning. The findings, though, do give some indication that children are at risk for cognitive delays. Relative to standardized norms, children exposed to domestic violence had lower developmental skills (Attala & Summers, 1999; Gleason, 1995; Rossman, 1998; Westra & Martin, 1981). Wildin et al. (1991) found that 39% of preschool children were developmentally delayed according to test criteria, and 46% of school-age children had academic problems such as failing grades, repeating grades, and/or receiving special services in school. In another study, only 51% to 57% of children were reading at an age-appropriate level (Mathias et al., 1995). Wolfe and his colleagues (1986) also reported lower school performance, as well as school-related difficulties such as distraction, inattention, frequent absences, and truancy.

In contrast, Attala and McSweeney (1997) found that the developmental status of exposed preschool children living in the community was within the normal range. Moore and Peplar (1998) found no evidence that academic performance was adversely affected by exposure to domestic violence. Finally, Christopoulos and her colleagues (1987) and Rossman and Rosenberg (1992) reported that the vocabulary scores of exposed children were not significantly different from their peers in nonviolent homes.

Physical Health

Only five studies (12.8%) described the health problems experienced by these vulnerable children. The most common problems reported were allergies and respiratory tract infections, psychosomatic complaints (e.g., headaches, stomach aches), gastro-intestinal disorders (e.g., nausea, diarrhea), and sleep disturbances (e.g., insomnia, nightmares, and sleepwalking) (Davis & Carlson, 1987; Kérouac et al., 1986; Westra & Martin, 1981; Wildin et al., 1991). Speech, hearing, and visual problems were also reported. Of the 13.8% of children who presented visual problems in one study, less than a quarter had corrective lenses (Kérouac et al., 1986). In another study, 40% of children exposed to domestic violence living in the community were not up to date on their immunizations (Attala & McSweeney, 1997). Although the majority of mothers in the Kérouac et al. (1986) study perceived their children were in good health, the children were absent from school for health problems more often in the previous year than the national average for Canadian children (10 days vs. 6.5 days).

Variables in Children's Responses to Witnessing Domestic Violence

Children's responses to witnessing domestic violence have been shown to vary according to several factors. The factors given the most attention in research to date are the child's age, gender, and whether the child is also being victimized by parents.

Child Age. Empirical evidence of developmental differences in children's responses are somewhat inconsistent. Some studies report more distress in younger children (Copping, 1996; Holden & Ritchie, 1991; Hughes, 1988; Hughes & Barad, 1983; O'Keefe, 1994) while other studies report more distress in older children (Davis & Carlson, 1987; Hughes et al., 1989). Still others report few or no age differences (Gleason, 1995; Onyskiw & Hayduk, 2001).

Child Gender. Gender differences in children's adjustment are frequently noted (Christopoulos et al., 1987; Davis & Carlson, 1987; Hughes & Barad, 1983; Jaffe et al., 1985, 1986a; Kolbo, 1996; Onyskiw & Hayduk, 2001; Spaccarelli et al., 1994) but do not appear consistently for the same type of adjustment difficulty. While most researchers found more disturbances in boys, others found more disturbances in girls (Christopoulos et al., 1987; Davis & Carlson, 1987; Kolbo, 1996; Moore & Peplar, 1998; Spaccarelli et al., 1994; Sternberg et al., 1993). Several researchers found differences in the kinds of problems experienced by each gender, with boys showing more externalizing problems and girls showing more internalizing problems (Holden & Ritchie, 1991; Kolbo, 1996; Spaccarelli et al., 1994; Sternberg et al., 1993). Other researchers report no gender differences in the kinds of problems (Bookless-Pratz & Mertin, 1990; Gleason, 1995; Graham-Bermann & Levendosky, 1998; Kerig, 1998; Mathias et al., 1995; O'Keefe, 1994).

Abuse Status. Spousal abuse and child abuse are clearly linked within families (Appel & Holden, 1998; McKay, 1994; Ross, 1996). The percentage of overlap ranges from 20% to 100% with a median rate of 40% reported in clinical samples of abused women or children (Appel & Holden, 1998). Several researchers found significantly more distress in abused children exposed to spousal violence (i.e., abused child witnesses) than in controls, with scores for nonabused children who had witnessed violence (i.e., nonabused child witnesses) falling between the two groups (Copping, 1996; Davis & Carlson, 1987; Hughes, 1988; Hughes et al., 1989; Mathias et al., 1995; McCloskey et al., 1995; Rossman, 1998). Other researchers found few differences between children who were abused and those who only witnessed abuse (Sternberg et al., 1993).

Jouriles and his associates (1987) found that the relationship between witnessing spousal violence and behavioral problems was not significant after controlling for parent-child aggression. Other researchers, however, have shown that exposure to violence still influences children's adjustment when child abuse is controlled through sampling efforts or statistical analyses (Fantuzzo et al., 1991; O'Keefe, 1994).

CRITIQUE OF EXISTING RESEARCH

Although knowledge in this area of inquiry is still developing, significant progress has been made. Early research was largely descriptive in order to portray the plight of children living with violence and to identify the serious adverse impact on their development. Comparison groups were not often used, making the credibility of findings suspect. However, methodological refinements were made over time. Researchers employed standardized and developmentally appropriate measures and comparison groups of children matched for age, sex, and family income. In lieu of comparison groups, some researchers used standardized scales that permitted comparison to normative samples.

Despite progress, many methodological and theoretical challenges remain in this important but difficult area of inquiry. Research on children who witness violence has been succinctly described as a special case of "counting hard-to-count incidents and measuring hard-to-measure activities that jeopardize the health and psychological well-being of children" (Fantuzzo, Borsch, Beriama, Atkins, & Marcus, 1997, p. 121). Some of the challenges are discussed below.

Sampling Issues

There has been a predominant use of convenience samples of children recruited from shelters and transition houses. There are obvious problems of bias associated with this method of selecting samples. For cxample, many abused women never seek refuge in shelters when they leave their partners (Rodgers, 1994; Trainor, 1999). Women who do seek refuge in shelters tend to differ from other abused women in terms of socioeconomic status, severity of the abuse they experience, how long they have endured the abuse, and the availability of support systems (Johnson, 1996; Jouriles et al., 1998; Trainor, 1999).

Children who accompany their mothers to shelters also experience stressors other than the violence. There is the upheaval associated with leaving home and familiar surroundings and adjusting to new, often chaotic, environments. Shelter children have been shown to have significantly higher levels of psychological distress and lower levels of social competence during a shelter stay than at a later time or than carefully matched children who witnessed the same amount and type of violence but were living in their own homes (Fantuzzo et al., 1991; Wolfe et al., 1986). Thus, findings from a shelter population may not generalize to all children exposed to domestic violence.

Most studies were based on small samples and often included children in a broad age range. While this no doubt reflects the inherent difficulties in recruiting subjects, it does constrain how data can be analyzed. Due to the small numbers of subjects, most researchers were not able to consider developmental or gender differences in children's responses or the possibility that gender differences in vulnerability change with age. In studies of children in the general population, externalizing behaviors are higher in boys than girls, while internalizing behaviors are similar for both genders until adolescence. The pattern then shifts and girls exhibit more internalizing behaviors than boys (Campbell, 1995; Offord, Boyle, Fleming, Blum, & Grant, 1989). The influence of age and gender warrants further investigation to resolve the uncertainties that remain. Some of the gender differences noted in children's emotional and behavioral problems in previous research may well reflect the gender differences normally seen in children in the general population that are due to socialization practices common in our society (Lytton & Romney, 1991).

Finally, researchers often reported that a large percentage of their sample (sometimes as many as half) were abused. In some studies, researchers conducted their analysis by abuse status (Hughes, 1988; Rossman, 1998) or controlled for parent-child aggression in their analysis (Jouriles et al., 1989). Others, however, only reported the percentage of children who were abused but did not take this factor into consideration when analyzing their data. Thus, researchers may be attributing adverse outcomes to the effects of witnessing violence when at least some of these effects are really associated with the child's victimization. Researchers need to control for child abuse either by screening children during recruitment and excluding these children, or alternately by controlling for the effects of direct victimization in the statistical phase of the study. Understanding the relative contribution of each of these risk factors is worthy of concerted effort.

Measurement Issues

The vast majority of studies used the CTS (Straus et al., 1980) or the OPS (Porter & O'Leary, 1980) to determine the presence of domestic violence. Neither of these measures is ideal for studies examining the effects of children's exposure to domestic violence. The CTS assesses the occurrence and frequency of specific behaviors (i.e., reasoning, verbal aggression, and physical aggression) engaged in during interpersonal conflict. Most studies used the physical aggression subscale which specifically inquires about the frequency of physically aggressive acts. The CTS, though, does not explicitly inquire about children's *exposure* to these aggressive acts, although some researchers did modify it for this purpose (Jouriles et al., 1987; O'Keefe, 1994; Rossman & Rosenberg, 1992). On the other hand, the OPS does specifically inquire about children's exposure (seen or overheard) to interparental conflict. However, it is also not an ideal measure because it covers a broad range of interparental conflict (e.g., disagreements over child-rearing) and not just physical conflict.

An additional factor to consider is that *exposure* is still only a crude measure of children's *awareness* of violence in their families. Children may well be aware of the violence without seeing or hearing any aggressive acts when they see their mother's injuries or the aftermath of violence or even just sense their mother's distress when the emotional climate in the home has changed (Jaffe, Wolfe, & Wilson, 1990). More sensitive measures of children's exposure are needed, ones that tap the various dimensions of exposure and include an assessment of the intensity, frequency, and the recency of violent events (Edleson, 1999).

Finally, most studies relied on mothers to provide information on both domestic violence and child behavior. The tendency to rely on one source for information on both constructs is always problematic but may be especially so in studies on domestic violence. Mothers' perceptions of their children's behavior may be distorted when they are experiencing crises (Hughes, 1988; Jaffe et al., 1986a, 1986b). In studies that obtained independent ratings, there was a tendency for mothers to rate their children more negatively than staff, teachers, or clinicians (Gleason, 1995; Hughes & Barad, 1983; Moore & Peplar, 1998; Sternberg et al., 1993). Thus, overreliance on maternal reports for information on both domestic violence and child behavior may be leading to stronger estimates of the relationship than when data are collected from other sources. Moreover, obtaining information from the children themselves may provide a different perspective of the difficulties they are experiencing. Researchers who study children's experiences of living with violence, using qualitative approaches, contend that children provide a unique perspective on how living with this adversity has affected their lives (Bennett, 1991; Berman, 1999; Erickson & Henderson, 1992; Humphreys, 1991; Monsma, 1988).

Theoretical Issues

Research on children exposed to domestic violence is complicated by the fact that children are rarely exposed to this one risk factor in isolation. Instead, children are often exposed to other risk factors that tend to occur with greater frequency in violent homes (Fantuzzo et al., 1997). These risk factors may contribute to children's adjustment difficulties or explain the association between domestic violence and children's adverse outcomes. For instance, alcoholism occurs with greater frequency in violent homes (Barnett & Fagan, 1993; Gelles, 1993) and children of alcoholics experience problems similar to those experienced by children exposed to domestic violence (Jaffe et al., 1990). Parental depression is also an important risk factor for a full range of child behavioral and emotional problems (Downey & Coyne, 1990; Goodman & Gotlib, 1999) and is the most common health response of abused women (Campbell, Kub, & Rose, 1996). Other social factors, including poverty, single parenting, low parental education, and large family size, are also associated with domestic violence (Fantuzzo et al., 1997). The risk of experiencing adjustment difficulties rises sharply when these risk factors accumulate and compound each others adverse effects (Rutter, 1997; Werner & Smith, 1992). The contribution of multiple risk factors needs to be systematically studied in order to learn about the relative contribution of each of these risk factors to children's adjustment.

Researchers have attempted to consider these related risk factors but most employed statistical techniques that only controlled for these other risk factors. Some studies used multivariate analysis of covariance with one or more risk factors entered as a covariate. This approach was often used to statistically equalize groups that differed on one or more family factors, so that results would not be confounded by the fact that groups differed on other family factors besides violence. For example, in one study violent families had significantly more children and marital separations than nonviolent families (Wolfe et al., 1986). Hence, these two variables were used as covariates in the analysis to eliminate these group differences. Sometimes, researchers used regression analysis with a hierarchical method of entry, first entering some important risk factors as control variables, then entering violence at the last step in order to determine if violence accounted for any unique variance in child adjustment over and above the variance attributable to these other risk factors. For example, researchers controlled for maternal alcohol problems and family size and found that spousal violence still accounted for significant unique variance in girls' conduct problems (Spaccarelli et al., 1994). In other words, spousal violence was shown to have an effect on child adjustment, with maternal alcohol problems and family size controlled or held constant.

While these statistical strategies provide a mechanism to achieve control of different risk factors, they have limited potential in terms of exploring the interplay among the various risk factors. Thus, these strategies have limitations in terms of their ability to aid researchers in developing theory to explain how children are affected by multiple stressors in their lives. Other multivariate techniques, which are extensions of regression analysis, offer more potential to assess the cascading effects of multiple risk factors. Techniques such as path analysis and structural equation modeling allow researchers to examine the simultaneous contribution of multiple risk factors to children's adjustment, to examine the relationship among these various risk factors, as well as to examine the possibility that some of these risk factors may have both direct and indirect effects on child outcomes by acting through variables which mediate the relationship between risk and outcome. In one study, researchers used structural equation modeling to examine how physical aggression in the family and several other maternal and family risk factors (e.g., maternal education, maternal depression, family size, family tension, etc.) contributed to children's adjustment. These other risk factors were hypothesized to contribute to children's adjustment indirectly through their effect on parenting. Thus, parenting was the mediating variable. With one exception, findings showed that these risk factors contributed to child adjustment indirectly through their effect on parenting. Maternal depression also had a direct effect on children's internalizing behaviors, in addition to the indirect effect operating through parenting (Onyskiw & Hayduk, 2001).

Finally, although research generally shows an association between domestic violence and child adjustment, and several studies show that domestic violence predicts child problems over and above other risk factors in children's lives, little is known about the mechanisms that underlie this association. Researchers have begun to shift their focus away from merely examining the association between domestic violence and child problems to trying to understand the mechanisms that account for this association–to understand *how* and *why* these children are at risk.

One mechanism thought to explain the link between domestic violence and child adjustment involves parenting in a mediational role, as mentioned above. Research on child adjustment in maritally conflicted (not violent) homes provides empirical support that parenting is disrupted in these families (for a review, see Krishnakumar & Buehler, 2000). However, there have been few direct investigations of parenting as a mechanism of influence in research on children exposed to domestic violence. In the Onyskiw and Hayduk study (2001), aggression in the family did disrupt parenting, at least for mothers of preschool and young schoolage children (though not for mothers of older schoolage children). Less responsive parenting (mothers) in turn, contributed to children's adjustment difficulties. In another study, McCloskey and her colleagues (1995) used structural equation modeling to test that family support and mothers' mental health mediated the relationship between family aggression and children's mental health. Although findings did show that family aggression had direct effects on both mothers' and children's mental health, neither family support nor mothers' mental health significantly contributed to children's mental health.

Although there have been few direct investigations of parenting in a mediational role, studies have provided evidence that domestic violence is linked to parent-child aggression (Hughes & Luke, 1998; Jouriles et al., 1987; Moore & Peplar, 1998; O'Keefe, 1994), as well as unresponsive and uninvolved parenting in fathers (Holden & Ritchie, 1991). Other researchers have shown that domestic violence is linked to maternal stress (Holden & Ritchie, 1991; Jaffe et al., 1985; Levendosky & Graham-Bermann, 1998; Wolfe et al., 1985) and maternal mental health problems (Hughes & Luke, 1998; Mathias et al., 1995; Moore & Peplar, 1998).

Another explanation for the link between interparental conflict and child adjustment involves children's appraisals. Scholars suggest that children's appraisals or evaluation of the event plays a vital role in determining the impact of interparental conflict (Davies & Cummings, 1994; Grych & Fincham, 1992). This hypothesis, also proposed to explain children's responses to witnessing interparental conflict, has been examined in the context of interparental violence (Jouriles et al., 2000; Kerig, 1998). In a recent investigation, Jouriles and his colleagues (2000) showed that children who tended to blame themselves for their parents' conflict had higher levels of externalizing problems, while children who blamed themselves but also felt threatened and feared abandonment had higher levels of anxiety and depression. These relationships were the same for both boys and girls, but were moderated by children's age, with appraisals being more positively related to older children's behavior. In contrast, Kerig (1998) found that interparental violence was related to appraisals in gender specific ways, with perceived threat acting as a mediator of anxiety for boys, and self-blame acting as a mediator of internalizing behaviors for girls.

While efforts to examine the processes underlying children's responses to witnessing violence are fairly recent, the shift in focus towards understanding these processes is an important one (see Kerig,

2003). An understanding of why adverse outcomes occur in children may help highlight ways that intervention and amelioration may take place (Cummings & Cummings, 1988). These perspectives need to be examined to add to theoretical knowledge in this area of inquiry as well as to inform policy, prevention, and treatment efforts.

SUGGESTIONS FOR FUTURE RESEARCH

In general, empirical findings suggest that children exposed to domestic violence are at risk for a wide range of adjustment difficulties. However, there is still some uncertainty, particularly in terms of age and gender differences in children's responses. In addition to more efforts to examine these moderating variables, as well as research to address the methodological weaknesses of past studies, there are some other suggestions for research that warrant further investigation.

Studies on domestic violence have predominantly focused on children's exposure to physical violence. In comparison, there has been relatively little attention focused on the impact of children's exposure to interparental verbal and other forms of aggression. Abused women often relate that the humiliation, intimidation, and degradation often associated with physical violence is more damaging and harder to cope with than physical acts of aggression (Johnson, 1996; Walker, 1979). Researchers have shown that other forms of aggression (e.g., insulting or swearing at a partner, throwing or destroying belongings) were associated with children's behavioral problems even after controlling for the frequency of physical aggression (Jouriles et al., 1996). In one study of preschool children, researchers found that maternal emotional abuse was one of the most important predictors of children's behavioral adjustment and social competence (Graham-Bermann & Levendosky, 1998a). In another study of preschool children, researchers investigated the additive effects of these stressors on child adjustment (Fantuzzo et al., 1991). They found that children's exposure to verbal conflict only was associated with moderate levels of behavior problems, while exposure to verbal plus physical conflict was associated with clinical levels of conduct problems and moderate levels of emotional problems. Thus, understanding the effects of exposure to these other forms of aggression is an important topic for further investigation.

Most of what is known about children is based on studies that measured children at one point in time. Most often, children were assessed at the time of shelter residence when they are also experiencing crisis and at a time when an escalation of problem behavior is likely. Information is needed to determine if children's problems persist, or subside, after they leave the shelter. Further, the cross-sectional nature of these studies impedes our ability to confidently assert that the relationship between domestic violence and children's adjustment is a causal one. Research is needed that takes into account the temporal nature of events in order to provide stronger evidence of causality. Longitudinal research is also needed to determine the effects on children's long term psychological adjustment, to understand how developmental factors interact with environmental factors to influence children's adjustment, and to elucidate any factors that may ameliorate or exacerbate children's adjustment difficulties. Many children appear to be functioning well despite this adversity in their lives. Longitudinal research is needed to understand factors that prevent adjustment problems from developing in these children.

More of the reviewed studies examined children's emotional and behavioral problems than any other domain of functioning. Additional investigative efforts are needed to more fully understand the impact on children's social and cognitive competence, academic performance, and health (see Whitson & El-Sheikh, 2003) and developmental outcomes. Further, there are fewer studies still that have examined the impact of exposure to violence on the development of adaptive or prosocial behaviors in children. Exposure to this stressor may hinder the development of these behaviors, which can have serious and long-term implications for children's development and well-being. It is critical to examine the impact of domestic violence on the development of positive, adaptive child behaviors.

Finally, much of the research has focused on the correlates of problems or pathology, little is known about the factors that promote resiliency in children. Many children exposed to violence have adapted to their difficult circumstances and are not showing signs of distress (Jaffe et al., 1990; Jouriles et al., 1989). Clearly, there are some factors which protect these children. While past research has tended to focus on maladaptive outcomes in children, there is much to be gained from understanding the factors which protect children from adverse consequences. This information is needed for scientific as well as clinical purposes since it may help clarify strategies that could be promoted to enhance children's successful adaptation to coping with domestic violence.

NOTE

These figures exclude Onyskiw and Hayduk's (2001) study, which was based on data from 11,221 children, so that the figures more accurately reflect the majority of studies reviewed. However, including the study makes no difference in terms of children's age ($M = 8.0$, $SD = 2.1$), a small difference in the gender distribution (boys = 51.1%), and improves the income distribution.

REFERENCES

Achenbach, T. M., & Edelbrock, C. S. (1978). The classification of child psychopathology: A review and analysis of empirical efforts. *Psychological Bulletin, 85,* 1275-1301.

Appel, A. E., & Holden, G. W. (1998). The co-occurrence of spouse and physical child abuse: A review and appraisal. *Journal of Family Psychology, 12*(4), 578-599.

Attala, J., & McSweeney, M. (1997). Preschool children of battered women identified in a community setting. *Issues in Comprehensive Pediatric Nursing, 20,* 217-225.

Attala, J., & Summers, S. M. (1999). A comparative study of health, developmental, and behavioral factors in preschool children of battered and nonbattered women. *Children's Health Care, 28*(2), 189-200.

Barnett, O., & Fagan, R. (1993). Alcohol use in male spouse abusers and their female partners. *Journal of Family Violence, 8,* 1-25.

Bennett, L. (1991). Adolescent girls' experience of witnessing marital violence: A phenomenological study. *Journal of Advanced Nursing, 16,* 431-438.

Berman, H. (1999). Stories of growing up amid violence by refugee children of war and children of battered women living in Canada. *Image: Journal of Nursing Scholarship, 31*(1), 57-64.

Bookless-Pratz, C., & Mertin, P. (1990). The behaviourial and social functioning of children exposed to domestic violence. *Children Australia, 15*(3), 4-7.

Campbell, J., Kub, J., & Rose, L. (1996). Depression in battered women. *Journal of the American Medical Women's Association, 51*(3), 106-110.

Campbell, S. (1995). Behavior problems in preschool children: A review of recent research. *Journal of Child Psychiatry, 36,* 113-149.

Carlson, B. E. (1984). Children's observations of interpersonal violence. In A. Roberts (Ed.), *Battered women and their families* (pp. 147-167). New York: Springer.

Christopoulos, C., Cohn, D. A., Shaw, D. S., Joyce, S., Sullivan-Hanson, J., Kraft, S. P., & Emery, R. E. (1987). Children of abused women: I. Adjustment at time of shelter residence. *Journal of Marriage and the Family, 49,* 611-619.

Copping, V. E. (1996). Beyond over- and under-control: Behavioral observations of shelter children. *Journal of Family Violence, 11*(1), 41-57.

Cummings, E. M., & Cummings, J. S. (1988). A process-oriented approach to children's coping with adults' angry behavior. *Developmental Review, 8,* 296-321.

Davies, P. T., & Cummings, E. M. (1994). Marital conflict and child adjustment: An emotional security hypothesis. *Psychological Bulletin, 116*(3), 387-411.

Davis, L. V., & Carlson, B. E. (1987). Observations of spouse abuse: What happens to the children. *Journal of Interpersonal Violence, 2*(3), 278-291.

Downey, G., & Coyne, J. C. (1990). Children of depressed parents: An integrative review. *Psychological Bulletin, 108*(1), 50-76.

Edleson, J. L. (1999). Children's witnessing of adult domestic violence. *Journal of Interpersonal Violence, 14*(8), 839-870.

Erickson, J. R., & Henderson, A. D. (1992). Witnessing family violence: The children's experience. *Journal of Advanced Nursing, 17*, 1200-1209.

Fantuzzo, J., Boruch, R., Beriama, A., Atkins, M., & Marcus, S. (1997). Domestic violence and children: Prevalence and risk in five major cities. *Journal of the American Academy of Child and Adolescent Psychiatry, 36*(1), 116-122.

Fantuzzo, J. W., DePaola, L. M., Lambert, L., Martino, T., Anderson, G., & Sutton, S. (1991). Effects of interparental violence on the psychological adjustment and competencies of young children. *Journal of Consulting and Clinical Psychology, 59*(2), 258-265.

Finkelhor, D. (1993). The main problem is still underreporting, not overreporting. In R. Gelles & D. R. Loseke (Eds.), *Current controversies on family violence* (pp. 273-287). London: Sage Publications.

Gelles, R. J. (1993). Alcohol and other drugs are associated with violence–they are not its cause. In R. Gelles & D. R. Loseke (Eds.), *Current controversies on family violence* (pp. 182-196). London: Sage Publications.

Gleason, W. J. (1995). Children of battered women: Developmental delays and behavioral dysfunction. *Violence and Victims, 10*(2), 153-160.

Goodman, S. H., & Gotlib, I. H. (1999). Risk for psychopathology in children of depressed mothers: A developmental model for understanding the mechanisms of transmission. *Psychological Review, 106*(3), 458-490.

Graham-Bermann, S. A., & Levendosky, A. A. (1998a). The social functioning of pre-school-age children whose mothers are emotionally and physically abused. *Journal of Emotional Abuse, 1*(1), 59-84.

Graham-Bermann, S. A., & Levendosky, A. A. (1998b). Traumatic stress symptoms in children of battered women. *Journal of Interpersonal Violence, 13*(1), 111-128.

Grych, J. H., & Fincham, F. D. (1990). Marital conflict and children's adjustment: A cognitive-contextual framework. *Psychological Bulletin, 108*(2), 267-290.

Hershorn, M., & Rosenbaum, A. (1985). Children of marital violence: A closer look at the unintended victims. *American Journal of Orthopsychiatry, 55*(2), 260-266.

Holden, G. W., & Ritchie, K. L. (1991). Linking extreme marital discord, child rearing, and child behavior problems: Evidence from battered women. *Child Development, 62*, 311-327.

Hughes, H. M. (1988). Psychological and behavioral correlates of family violence in child witnesses and victims. *American Journal of Orthopsychiatry, 58*(1), 77-90.

Hughes, H. M., & Barad, S. J. (1983). Psychological functioning of children in a battered women's shelter: A preliminary investigation. *American Journal of Orthopsychiatry, 53*, 525-531.

Hughes, H. M., & Luke, D. A. (1998). Heterogeneity in adjustment among children of battered women. In G. W. Holden, R. Geffner, & E. N. Jouriles (Eds.), *Children exposed to marital violence: Theory, research, and applied issues* (pp. 185-221). Washington, DC: American Psychological Association.

Hughes, H. M., Parkinson, D., & Vargo, M. (1989). Witnessing spouse abuse and experiencing physical abuse: A "double whammy"? *Journal of Family Violence, 4*(2), 197-209.

Humphreys, J. (1991). Children of battered women: Worries about their mothers. *Pediatric Nursing, 17*(4), 342-345.

Jaffe, P. G., Wolfe, D. A., & Wilson, S. K. (1990). *Children of battered women.* Sage: London.

Jaffe, P. G., Wolfe, D. A., Wilson, S. K., & Zak, L. (1985). A multivariate investigation of children's adjustment. In G. T. Hotelling, D. Finkelhor, J. T. Kirkpatrick, & M. A. Straus (Eds.), *Family abuse and its consequences: New directions in research* (pp. 229-241). Newbury Park, CA: Sage Publications.

Jaffe, P. G., Wolfe, D. A., Wilson, S. K., & Zak, L. (1986a). Family violence and child adjustment: A comparative analysis of girls' and boys' behavioral symptoms. *American Journal of Psychiatry, 143*(1), 74-77.

Jaffe, P. G., Wolfe, D. A., Wilson, S. K., & Zak, L. (1986b). Similarities in behavioral and social maladjustment among child victims and witnesses to family violence. *American Journal of Orthopsychiatry, 56*(1), 142-146.

Johnson, H. (1996). *Dangerous domains: Violence against women in Canada.* Toronto: Nelson Canada.

Johnston, J. R., Gonzàlez, R., & Campbell, L. E. G. (1987). Ongoing postdivorce conflict and child disturbance. *Journal of Abnormal Child Psychology, 15*(4), 493-509.

Jouriles, E. N., Barling, J., & O'Leary, K. D. (1987). Predicting child behavior problems in maritally violent families. *Journal of Abnormal Child Psychology, 15*(2), 165-173.

Jouriles, E. N., McDonald, R., Norwood, W. D., Ware, S. H., Spiller, L. C., & Swank, P. R. (1998). Knives, guns, and interparent violence: Relations with child behavior problems. *Journal of Family Psychology, 12*(2), 178-194.

Jouriles, E. N., Murphy, C. M., & O'Leary, D. (1989). Interspousal aggression, marital discord, and child problems. *Journal of Consulting and Clinical Psychology, 57*(3), 453-455.

Jouriles, E. N., Norwood, W. D., McDonald, R., Vincent, J. P., & Mahoney, A. (1996). Physical violence and other forms of marital aggression: Links with children's behavior problems. *Journal of Family Psychology, 10*(2), 223-234.

Jouriles, E. N., Spiller, L. C., Stephens, N., McDonald, R., & Swank, P. R. (2000). Variability in adjustment of children of battered women: The role of child appraisals of interparent conflict. *Cognitive Therapy and Research, 24*(2), 233-249.

Kerig, P. K. (1998). Gender and appraisals as mediators of adjustment in children exposed to interparental violence. *Developmental Psychology, 29*(6), 931-939.

Kerig, P. K. (2003). In search of protective processes for children exposed to interparental violence. *Journal of Emotional Abuse, 3*(3/4), 149-181.

Kérouac, S., Taggart, M., Lescop, J., & Fortin, M. (1986). Dimensions of health in violent families. *Health Care for Women International, 7,* 423-426.

Kolbo, J. R. (1996). Risk and resilience among children exposed to family violence. *Violence and Victims, 11*(2), 113-128.

Krishnakumar, A., & Buehler, C. (2000). Interparental conflict and parenting behaviors: A meta-analytic review. *Family Relations, 49*(1), 25-44.

Lehmann, P. (1997). The development of posttraumatic stress disorder (PTSD) in a sample of child witnesses to mother assault. *Journal of Family Violence, 12*(3), 241-257.

Levendosky, A. A., & Graham-Bermann, S. A. (1998). The moderating effects of parenting stress on children's adjustment in woman-abusing families. *Journal of Interpersonal Violence, 13*(3), 283-297.

Lewis, C. E., Siegel, J. M., & Lewis, M. A. (1984). Feeling bad: Exploring sources of distress among pre-adolescent children. *American Journal of Public Health, 74*, 117-122.

Lytton, H., & Romney, D. M. (1991). Parents' differential socialization of boys and girls: A meta-analysis. *Psychological Bulletin, 109*, 267-296.

Markward, M. J. (1997). The impact of domestic violence on children. *Families in Society: The Journal of Contemporary Human Services, 78*, 66-70.

Mathias, J. L., Mertin, P., & Murray, A. (1995). The psychological functioning of children from backgrounds of domestic violence. *Australian Psychologist, 30*(1), 47-56.

McCloskey, L. A., Figueredo, A. J., & Koss, M. P. (1995). The effects of systematic family violence on children's mental health. *Child Development, 66*, 1239-1261.

McKay, M. M. (1994). The link between domestic violence and child abuse: Assessment and treatment considerations. *Child Welfare, 73*(1), 29-39.

Monsma, J. (1988). Children of battered women: Perceptions, actions, and nursing care implications. In M. M. Leininger (Ed.). *Care: Discovery and uses in clinical and community nursing* (pp. 87-105). Detroit: Wayne State University Press.

Moore, J. G., Galcius, A., & Pettican, K. (1981). Emotional risk to children caught in violent marital conflict–The Basildon treatment project. *Child Abuse and Neglect, 5*, 147-152.

Moore, T. E., & Peplar, D. J. (1998). Correlates of adjustment in children at risk. In G. W. Holden, R. Geffner, & E. N. Jouriles (Eds.), *Children exposed to marital violence: Theory, research, and applied issues* (pp. 157-184). Washington, DC: American Psychological Association.

Offord, D. R., Boyle, M. H., Fleming, J. E., Blum, H. M., & Grant, N. I. (1989). Ontario Child Health Study: Summary of selected results. *Canadian Journal of Psychiatry, 34*(6), 483-491.

O'Keefe, M. (1994). Adjustment of children from maritally violent homes. *Families in Society: The Journal of Contemporary Human Services, 75*(7), 403-415.

Onyskiw, J. E., & Hayduk, L. A. (2001). Processes underlying children's adjustment in families characterized by physical aggression. *Family Relations, 50*(4), 376-385.

Porter, B., & O'Leary, D. (1980). Marital discord and childhood behavior problems. *Journal of Abnormal Child Psychology, 8*(3), 287-295.

Rodgers, K. (1994). Wife assault in Canada. *Canadian Social Trends, Statistics Canada-Catalogue 11-008E*, 3-8.

Rosenbaum, A., & O'Leary, K. D. (1981). Children: The unintended victims of marital violence. *American Journal of Orthopsychiatry, 51*(4), 692-699.

Ross, S. M. (1996). Risk of physical abuse to children of spouse abusing parents. *Child Abuse & Neglect, 20*, 589-598.

Rossman, B. B. R. (1998). Descartes's error and posttraumatic stress disorder: Cognition and emotion in children who are exposed to parental violence. In G. W. Holden, R. Geffner, & E. N. Jouriles (Eds.), *Children exposed to marital violence: Theory, research, and applied issues* (pp. 223-256). Washington, DC: American Psychological Association.

Rossman, B. B. R., & Rosenberg, M. S. (1992). Family stress and functioning in children: The moderating effects of children's beliefs about their control over parental conflict. *Journal of Child Psychology & Psychiatry, 33*(4), 699-715.

Rutter, M. (1997). Developmental psychopathology as an organizing research construct. In D. Magnusson (Ed.), *The lifespan development of individuals: Behavioral, neurobiological, and psychosocial perspectives: A synthesis* (pp. 394-423). New York: Cambridge University Press.

Shaffer, M., & Bala, N. (2003). Wife abuse, child custody and access in Canada. *Journal of Emotional Abuse, 3*(3/4), 253-275.

Smith, J., Berthelsen, D., & O'Connor, I. (1997). Child adjustment in high conflict families. *Child: Care, Health and Development, 23*(2), 113-133.

Spaccarelli, S., Sandler, I. N., & Roosa, M. (1994). History of spouse violence against mother: Correlated risks and unique effects in child mental health. *Journal of Family Violence, 9*(1), 79-98.

Sternberg, K. J., Lamb, M. E., Greenbaum, C., Cicchetti, D., Dawud, S., Cortes, R. M., Krispin, O., & Lorey, F. (1993). Effects of domestic violence on children's behavior problems and depression. *Developmental Psychology, 29*(1), 44-52.

Straus, M. A. (1992). Children as witnesses to marital violence: A risk factor for lifelong problems among a nationally representative sample of American men and women. In D. F. Schwarz (Ed.). *Children and violence: Report on the 23rd Ross Roundtable on critical approaches to common pediatric problems* (pp. 98-104). Columbus, OH: Ross Laboratories.

Straus, M. A., Gelles, R. J., & Steinmetz, S. K. (1980). *Behind closed doors: Violence in the American family*. New York: Anchor Books.

Statistics Canada. (1997). *National longitudinal survey of children and youth 1994-1995: Public use microdata file*. Ottawa: Author.

Trainor, C. (1999). Canada's shelters for abused women. *Juristat: Canadian Centre for Justice Statistics (Statistics Canada, Catalogue No. 85-002-XPE), 19*(6), 1-10.

Walker, L. (1979). *The battered woman*. New York: Plenum.

Werner, E. E., & Smith, R. S. (1992). *Overcoming the odds: High risk children from birth to adulthood*. London: Cornell University Press.

Westra, B., & Martin, H. P. (1981). Children of battered women. *Maternal-Child Nursing Journal, 10*, 41-54.

Whitson, S. M., & El-Sheikh, M. (2003). Moderators of family conflict and children's adjustment and health. *Journal of Emotional Abuse, 3*(1/2), 47-74.

Wildin, S. R., Williamson, W. D., & Wilson, G. S. (1991). Children of battered women: Developmental and learning profiles. *Clinical Pediatrics, 30*(5), 299-304.

Wolfe, D. A., Jaffe, P., Wilson, S. K., & Zak, L. (1985). Children of battered women. The relation of child behaviour to family violence and maternal stress. *Journal of Consulting and Clinical Psychology, 53*(5), 657-665.

Wolfe, D. A., Zak, L., Wilson, S., & Jaffe, P. (1986). Child witnesses to violence between parents: Critical issues in behavioral and social adjustment. *Journal of Abnormal Child Psychology, 14*(1), 95-104.

Moderators of Family Conflict and Children's Adjustment and Health

Stephanie M. Whitson
Mona El-Sheikh

SUMMARY. Emotion regulation and emotionality were examined as moderators in the associations between exposure to marital and parent-child conflict and children's adjustment and physical health. Children (6 to 11 years) and their mothers participated, and data were gathered on children's adjustment, health, emotionality, and emotion regulation. Physiological regulation measures were obtained during baseline and simulated argument conditions as components of emotion regulation. Emotion regulation variables buffered children against some of the negative health, externalizing, and internalizing outcomes associated with exposure to both marital conflict and parent-child conflict. On the other hand, higher levels of emotionality were vulnerability factors in the associations between family conflict and children's internalizing and externalizing behaviors, with more support for the latter. *[Article copies available for a fee from The Haworth Document Delivery Service: 1-800-HAWORTH. E-mail address: <docdelivery@haworthpress.com> Website: <http://www.HaworthPress.com> © 2003 by The Haworth Press, Inc. All rights reserved.]*

Address correspondence to: Mona El-Sheikh, PhD, Human Development and Family Studies, 203 Spidle Hall, Auburn University, Auburn, AL 36849 (E-mail: elshemm @auburn.edu).

The authors wish to thank all the families who participated in the study.

[Haworth co-indexing entry note]: "Moderators of Family Conflict and Children's Adjustment and Health." Whitson, Stephanie M., and Mona El-Sheikh. Co-published simultaneously in *Journal of Emotional Abuse* (The Haworth Maltreatment & Trauma Press, an imprint of The Haworth Press, Inc.) Vol. 3, No. 1/2, 2003, pp. 47-73; and: *The Effects of Intimate Partner Violence on Children* (ed: Robert A. Geffner, Robyn Spurling Igelman, and Jennifer Zellner) The Haworth Maltreatment & Trauma Press, an imprint of The Haworth Press, Inc., 2003, pp. 47-73. Single or multiple copies of this article are available for a fee from The Haworth Document Delivery Service [1-800-HAWORTH, 9:00 a.m. - 5:00 p.m. (EST). E-mail address: docdelivery@haworthpress.com].

KEYWORDS. Marital conflict, family conflict, vagal tone, emotion regulation

Children exposed to frequent and intense interparental conflict (Grych & Fincham, 2001) and parent-child aggression (see Kolko, 1992, for a review) are vulnerable to a wide array of adjustment problems and physical health difficulties (e.g., Gottman & Katz, 1989, for marital conflict; Lau, Liu, Cheung, Yu, & Wong, 1999, for child abuse). Although associations between exposure to family conflict and negative child outcomes have been established, variables and processes influencing these relationships still need to be delineated. Several conceptual formulations have been developed, including the cognitive-contextual framework (Grych & Fincham, 1990) and the emotional security hypothesis (Cummings & Davies, 1996), that incorporate emotion regulation, emotionality, and temperament as variables that may impact the association between marital discord and child functioning. This study is conceptualized from an emotion regulation framework, which proposes that the negative effects of family stressors such as marital conflict can be explained in part by disruptions in the child's emotionality and regulation associated with high levels of conflict and associated stressors (see Cummings & Davies, 1996). The present investigation builds on the literature by examining multiple measures of children's emotionality and emotion regulation as moderators of the association between family conflict (both marital and parent-child) and children's adjustment and physical health.

Children's regulation of emotion is a cornerstone within several conceptual propositions related to developmental psychopathology (e.g., Cummings & Davies, 1996; Thompson, 1994). In this context, emotional arousal is recognized for its potential adaptive value of providing the resources necessary for meeting organismic needs and environmental demands by stimulating cognitive, physiological, and behavioral processes, with the capacity to either undermine or facilitate an adaptive response in the face of stress (Cole, Michel, & Teti, 1994; Thompson & Calkins, 1996). Emotion regulation is conceptualized as a dynamic process that enables adaptive functioning by orchestrating multi-directional relationships and allocating resources among several regulatory domains (e.g., Eisenberg et al., 1997; Thompson, 1994). Emotion regulation processes are important in that they utilize emotion to facilitate an adaptive response (Cole et al., 1994; Thompson & Calkins, 1996), and emotional dysregulation may be associated with internalizing and externalizing behavior patterns such as those found among children from conflictual homes (Cicchetti, Ackerman, & Izard, 1995; Dodge & Garber, 1991). Consistent with the emotional security hypothesis (Cummings & Davies, 1996), the child's ability to adaptively regulate the experience and expression of emotion in the face of family conflict may explain some of the variability in adjustment among children exposed to family conflict.

Although emotionality and regulation are intimately intertwined and conceptually linked, variables examined in this study were grouped into these two categories to represent different facets of emotional responding (e.g., Murphy, Eisenberg, Fabes, Shepard, & Guthrie, 1999). Emotionality refers to the frequency and intensity of emotional responses (Derryberry & Rothbart, 1988; Murphy et al., 1999), and in this study, was indicated through measures of affective intensity, autonomic reactivity, anger, fear, and sadness. Emotion regulation represents monitoring and modulating the intensive and temporal features of emotional reactions (Thompson, 1994), and was examined through measures of vagal regulation, soothability, and attentional focusing and shifting. And whereas emotion regulation is posited to serve a protective function, higher levels of emotionality may be precursors to adjustment difficulties (Cummings & Davies, 1996) and may function as vulnerability factors that exacerbates negative effects associated with family conflict.

Cardiac vagal tone is conceptualized as an index of individual differences in the physiological regulation and expression of emotion (Porges, 1995, 1996) and reflects the parasympathetic nervous system's influence on the heart. The vagus nerve has sensory and motor components affecting cardiovascular, respiratory, and digestive systems and innervates several areas involved in homeostasis maintenance. When the sympathetic nervous system is aroused, the vagus nerve relays negative feedback to the peripheral autonomic system to reduce arousal and return to homeostasis (Porges, 1991). Thus, vagal tone can be conceptualized as a feedback system, orchestrating the physiological components of emotion, and indexing individual differences in regulation of arousal, temperament, and reactivity to stimulation (Borstein & Suess, 2000). Furthermore, successful emotion regulation is dependent upon appropriate vagal engagement and management of arousal (Doussard-Roosevelt & Porges, 1999).

Traditionally, two measures of vagal tone have been employed: vagal tone, calculated during baseline conditions; and vagal suppression–the difference between vagal tone during baseline and challenge conditions (Borstein & Suess, 2000; Calkins, 1997). Vagal tone indexes the individual's ability to maintain homeostasis, self-soothe, and inhibit inappropriate behavior, whereas vagal suppression indexes the individual's capacity to utilize social and attentional strategies to engage or disengage with the environment and form an organized response to stress (Huffman et al., 1998; Porges, 1984). In children, high vagal tone is associated with adaptive regulation of emotion (Porges, 1991), and better adjustment (Doussard-Roosevelt, Porges, Scanlon, Alemi, & Scanlon, 1997; Fox & Field, 1989) although discrepancies in the findings have been noted (e.g., Porges, Doussard-Roosevelt, & Maiti, 1994). Additionally, researchers have found that there are some children with high vagal tone, but poor vagal suppression who nonetheless exhibit behavioral problems (DeGangi, DiPietro, Greenspan, & Porges, 1991). Thus optimal physiological regulation involves high vagal tone and adequate suppression in response to task demands representing a rapid physiological response of limited duration, with prompt soothing (Porges et al., 1994). Furthermore, it has been proposed by several researchers that recovery or soothability of physiological response is of equal or greater importance than physiological reactivity per se (Porges et al., 1994). This study includes measures of emotion reactivity and regulation for a better elucidation of associations among family conflict and child outcomes.

The literature also suggests a relationship between vagal regulation and health. Specifically vagal disruptions have been related to respiratory (Casale, 1987) and digestive problems (Porges, 1991). High vagal tone is associated with lower incidences of physical illness (Porges, 1992), enhanced recovery from invasive medical procedures (Donchin, Constantini, Szold, Byrne, & Porges, 1992) and good health at birth (Porges, 1992, 1995). Children with high vagal tone should have a greater capacity for self-soothing and less vulnerability to the negative effects of family conflict (Katz & Gottman, 1997b; Porges, 1984). Furthermore, in the context of high levels of marital conflict and distress, vagal regulation may reduce the negative impact of this stressor on children's physical health (El-Sheikh, Harger, & Whitson, 2001; Gottman & Katz, 1989; Katz & Gottman, 1995, 1997b).

Family conflict can be considered a chronic stressor, and it is well established that exposure to such stressors has been associated with health ailments (O'Leary, 1990). In the context of family conflict, this connection can be explained at least in part by the sensitization (El-Sheikh, 1997; Hennessy, Rabideau, Cicchetti, & Cummings, 1994) and pronounced and/or chronic emotional and physiological arousal (Ballard, Cummings, & Larkin, 1993; El-Sheikh, 1994) that exposure to frequent or intense conflict elicits. Chronic arousal compromises immune and nervous system functioning and homeostasis maintenance (Henry & Stephens, 1977). Accordingly, we expected that children who are able to modulate their physiological arousal in the face of conflict may not experience sustained activation of stress systems and may be protected against health problems. On the other hand, children with higher levels of emotionality may be more at risk for the negative outcomes associated with family stressors.

In addition to physiological regulation, attentional control has been proposed as an important facet of emotion regulation due to its positive relation with adjustment (Eisenberg, Fabes, Nyman, Bernzweig, & Pinuelas, 1994; Eisenberg et al., 1996), social functioning (Eisenberg et al., 1995), and constructive anger reactions (Eisenberg et al., 1994). Attentional control can be conceptualized as the use of focusing and shifting to minimize or maximize arousal associated with impinging stimuli (Lazarus & Folkman, 1984).

Emotional intensity was also examined as a moderator in the association between exposure to family conflict and children's outcome. High emotional intensity has been associated with angry outbursts, aggression, acting out behaviors (Brody, Stoneman, & Burke, 1988; Teglasi & McMahon, 1990), and social incompetence (Eisenberg et al., 1993). Consistently, low negative emotionality has been associated with more adaptive functioning (Eisenberg et al., 1995, 1996). In the current study, children's affective intensity and autonomic reactivity, as well as dispositional anger, sadness, and fear, were explored as moderators of the family conflict-child outcomes link, and were expected to exacerbate child problems associated with family conflict. Previous studies employing the same measures found that composites including these dimensions are useful in the prediction of children's anger reactions (Eisenberg et al., 1996) and socially appropriate behavior (Eisenberg et al., 1995).

This study extends the literature in several ways. Although there is evidence that emotionality and emotion regulation are associated with children's adjustment, few studies have examined these variables as moderators of the association between family conflict and child outcomes, and even fewer studies have examined these variables across multiple responses domains. In this study, multiple measures of conflict (marital and parent-child), emotionality and regulation (based on physiological responses and self-reports), and children's adjustment and physical health are employed. Examination of children's responses across multiple domains is essential for a process-oriented understanding on children's adjustment, and is more likely to elucidate associations among variables than focusing on a single response domain (Cummings, Davies, & Campbell, 2001). Because children respond differently to verbal and physical forms of conflict with physical aggression eliciting more behavioral reactivity (Cummings, Zahn-Waxler, & Radke-Yarrow, 1981), and emotional and behavioral problems (Hershorn & Rosenbaum, 1985; Jaffe, Wolfe, Wilson, & Zak, 1986), we examined the role of emotionality and regulation in moderating the effects of both psychological and physical marital and parent-child conflict.

Based on the literature, we expected that higher levels of physiological and emotion regulation would buffer children against externalizing, internalizing, and health problems associated with exposure to both marital and parent-child aggression. On the other hand, we expected that higher levels of emotionality would be vulnerability factors and exacerbate negative outcomes associated with the conflict variables.

METHOD

Participants

Sixty-four 6-11 year-olds (31 boys and 33 girls) participated in this study. A relatively equal number of younger (ages 6-8, $n = 33$) and older (ages 9-11, $n = 31$) children were included, with a very similar representation of boys and girls in each age group. The ethnic composition of the sample was 91% Caucasian, 2% African American, 2% Native American, 2% Hispanic, and 3% other. Socioeconomic status, as determined by the four factor Hollingshead Index, ranged from Class 3 to Class 5 with a mean falling in Class 4, indicative of upper middle class social status (Hollingshead, 1975). Median yearly income fell in the category of $50,001 to $75,000. Sixty-two children (96.9%) reportedly lived in two parent households; the other two lived with their mother due to divorce and were included in the study as a result of miscommunication. Mothers' average age was 37 ($SD = 4.85$) and fathers' was 40 ($SD = 4.86$). Two children met the age and sex-normed criteria for clinically significant externalizing behavior problems (i.e., T-score ≥ 70; Achenbach, 1991) and one child met the criteria for internalizing behavior problems. Subjects were recruited from the community and were paid $10.00 for their participation. Measures and procedures used in this study were collected during a larger study on family conflict and child adjustment and only pertinent information is reported.

Procedures

In a university laboratory, parents completed questionnaires while children were taken to an adjacent room where physiological sensors were attached. Most children (91%) were accompanied to the laboratory by their mothers, and the rest were accompanied by their fathers. In order to facilitate accurate physiological recordings, a two-minute adaptation period was allowed before the three-minute baseline condition during which vagal tone was assessed. The child then listened to a one-minute audio-taped argument between a male and female concerning issues such as visiting relatives, while physiological measurements were continuously recorded in order to provide a measure of vagal suppression. The argument contained verbal conflict with no indication of physical aggression. To imply to the child that the forthcoming audio-taped interaction was real, the examiner mentioned that the child might overhear other families talking in another room. The child heard the interaction through speakers in the room. At the end of the session, a resolution to the argument was presented to ameliorate any negative effects of exposure to the conflict (e.g., El-Sheikh, Cummings, & Reiter, 1996). After the audio-taped interactions, children completed the measures subsequently mentioned via interview.

Measures

Predictor Variables

Marital Conflict. Mothers completed the Conflict and Problem Solving Scale (CPS; Kerig, 1996), which has adequate test-retest reliability at 3 months of .53 to .87, and high internal validity for the subscales ranging from .70 to .98 (Kerig, 1996). The Avoidance/Capitulation, Stalemate, Verbal Aggression, and Physical Aggression subscales were used in this study with greater scores on these scales indicating more frequent conflict and detrimental strategies. The scales were conceptually grouped according to physical and non-physical or psychological conflict tactics (i.e., Avoidance/Capitulation, Stalemate, and Verbal Aggression). Forty percent of the sample reported the use of physical aggression during marital conflict. This prevalence rate for physical aggression is greater than the lifetime rate reported by Straus and Gelles (1986) from their national sample of couples (28%), but the severity and frequency of assault in the present sample is not markedly different from the statistics reported by Kerig (1996). Two mothers reported their own, but did not report their husbands', use of various conflict tactics, and the completed portion was used as a measure of both partners' conflict.

Children reported the occurrence and frequency of various marital conflict strategies employed by their parents, using an adapted version of the Revised Conflict Tactics Scale-Couple Form (CTS2; Straus, 1995). The Verbal and Physical Aggression scales were used in this study, excluding one item ("How often has your mother/father accused your father/mother of being a bad lover?") as recommended by Straus (1995) for employing the scale with children. Although no previous published studies have used the measure with children, estimates of internal validity from previous studies for parent report on the subscales range from .79 to .95 (Straus, Hamby, Boney-McCoy, & Sugarman, 1996). The scale has acceptable construct and discriminate validity (Straus et al., 1996).

Parent-Child Conflict. To assess parent-child conflict, mothers and children completed The Parent-Child Conflict Tactics Scale (CTSPC; Straus, Hamby, Finkelhor, Moore, & Runyan, 1998). Although the authors of the scale support its use with children, we have no knowledge of work employing this measure with children. This measure was used to assess psychological and physical aggression within the context of parent-child conflict. Mothers were asked to report how often they had engaged in 18 conflict strategies toward their child in the last year. Similarly, children were asked to report the frequency of mother-child and father-child conflict. Children's reports of parent-child conflict were examined independently for each parent, as previous research has established that the sex of the perpetrator may influence the effect of parent-child conflict on child functioning (Malinsoky-Rummell & Hansen, 1993; O'Keefe, 1995). Parental report on the subscales has been found to have adequate content validity and reliability (.50 for Physical Assault and .60 for Psychological Aggression; see Straus, 1990). Mothers' responses in the present study indicated that 75% used physical aggression tactics, mainly consisting of a mild form of physical discipline (e.g., spanking) with their child in the previous year. Six mothers reported a frequency of parent-child physical aggression above the mean obtained from a national survey of 1,000 families (Straus et al., 1998). No reported aggression directed at the child was regarded as abusive.

Moderating Variables

Emotion Regulation. Children's heart rate (HR), interbeat interval (IBI; time period between successive R-spikes), and respiratory changes (expansion and compression of chest during breathing) were recorded to the nearest millisecond during the procedures to calculate vagal tone. Respiration was measured via a bellow belt around the child's chest. HR and IBI were measured by silver-silver chloride electrodes placed on the child's torso. The physiological measures were digitized using a 16 Channel A/D (James Long Co., Caroga Lake, NY). The EKG signal was amplified using a James Long Company bio amplifier (Model MME-4, James Long Co., Caroga Lake, NY). The EKG files were edited for artifact by a trained experimenter using a program that allows for visual inspection. Vagal tone was calculated and analyzed from respiratory sinus arrhythmia (RSA) data using James Long Co., IBI Analysis System Software and PHY general analysis system (James Long Co., Caroga Lake, NY). Respiratory sinus arrhythmia (RSA), the rhythmic fluctuations in heart beat that accompany phases of the respiratory cycle, is generally accepted as an accurate measurement of cardiac vagal tone when respiration variation is taken into account (Grossman, 1991). The peak-to-trough method for quantifying RSA was employed, whereby the R-R interval series (i.e., cardiac interbeat interval between successive R waves on the electrocardiogram) is used to measure heart rate differences that correspond to inspiration and expiration phases of the respiratory cycle (Grossman & Wientjes, 1986). These differences were averaged across respiratory cycles for a given measurement period (Grossman & Wientjes, 1986) in order to provide an estimate of cardiac vagal tone for the baseline and argument conditions. Vagal suppression was computed by subtracting average vagal tone during the interadult audio-taped argument from the average baseline vagal tone (Huffman et al., 1998; Katz & Gottman, 1997a). Due to technical difficulties, a small number of subjects were missing a few seconds of vagal tone and the available data in the same condition (e.g., baseline) were used to produce the average for that subject.

Mothers completed the Childhood Behavior Questionnaire (Derryberry & Rothbart, 1988; Rothbart, Ahadi, & Hershey, 1994). The scales of the CBQ have been used in similar studies related to children's emotion regulation abilities and emotionality and demonstrated adequate reliability ranging from .58 to .90 for parent and teacher reports (Eisenberg et al., 1994, 1995; Murphy et al., 1999). The CBQ items employ a 7-point Likert scale by which mothers indicated how well each item described her child. The scale is unique in that the items assessing regulation are not confounded with measures assessing the social consequences of dysregulation or emotional or behavioral disorders (Murphy et al., 1999). The Falling Reactivity/Soothability (13 items), Attentional Shifting (ability to shift attentional focus when appropriate; 5 items), and Attentional Focusing (ability to focus on task-relevant stimuli; 9 items) subscales were examined as indices of emotion regulation, and high scores on these scales indicate better regulation.

Emotionality. Emotionality was assessed using mothers' reports on (a) an adaptation of the Affective Intensity Measure (AIM; Eisenberg et al., 1997, 1996; Larsen & Diener, 1987) and (b) selected scales of the CBQ. The AIM was developed to measure adult affect intensity, but modifications of the original scale have been used in multiple studies for parental report of child behavior (Eisenberg et al., 1994, 1996). High scores indicate strong affect intensity. Eisenberg and colleagues (1994, 1995) have found the modified scale to have moderately high alpha coefficients for teachers', teachers' aides', and parents' ratings with estimates ranging from .62-.88. The CBQ's autonomic reactivity (5 items), sadness (11 items), anger/frustration (12 items), and fear (11 items) subscales were used to examine the child's negative affect with high scores representing higher levels of dispositional negative emotionality.

Outcome Variables

Child Psychological Adjustment. Mothers completed the Childhood Behavior Checklist (CBCL; Achenbach & Edlebrock, 1983) that examines child functioning using two global scales: Internalizing and Externalizing behavior problems. The CBCL has established psychometric properties including discriminate validity, high test-retest reliability (.95-.99) over a one week interval, and interparental reliability ranging from .74-.76 for the composite scales (Achenbach, 1991; Achenbach & Edlebrock, 1983).

Child Health. Mothers completed an abbreviated version of the Rand Corporation Health Insurance Survey (RHS; Eisen, Donald, & Ware, 1980) as a measure of child health. Similar adaptations have been used in previous studies (e.g., Katz & Gottman, 1997a), and the scale has been found to have adequate reliability (.57–.76) and construct validity (.34-.37; Eisen, Ware, Donald, & Brook, 1979). The survey contains four scales measuring overall health, chronic illness, acute illness, and resistance to illness.

Plan of Analysis

Regression analyses were used to test for moderation effects. Baron and Kenny (1986) define a moderator as a variable that influences "... the direction and/or strength of the relation between an independent or predictor variable and dependent or criterion variable. ... A basic moderator effect can be represented as an interaction between a focal independent variable and a factor that specifies the appropriate conditions for its operation" (p. 1174). Thus, a moderator interacts with a predictor variable so that a distinct relationship is seen between the predictor and outcome variables at various levels of the moderator. Furthermore, for a variable to qualify as a buffer, this interaction must indicate that the moderator protects against poor outcome. However, a moderator functions as a vulnerability factor if it exacerbates the association between family conflict and child outcomes.

A series of hierarchical regression analyses were conducted to examine whether various forms of family conflict interacted with emotion regulation, or emotionality to predict child outcome. Only one moderator was examined at a time for each dependent variable due to small sample size. While this approach increases the probability that Type I errors will occur, it minimizes the likelihood of Type II errors. Such an approach is appropriate in exploratory research in order to avoid unnecessarily limiting future research, but significant findings should be interpreted with caution and examined in the future among larger samples (Katz & Gottman, 1997). In the current study, the specific measure of family conflict and the moderator variable were entered first to control for direct effects. Next, the interaction term (produced by multiplying the family conflict variable by the proposed moderator) was entered. Because it is possible that interaction effects might vary by age and gender, two more steps were added in initial regression analyses to examine this possibility. The third step was an interaction term produced by multiplying gender, the family conflict variable, and the moderator. The fourth or final step entered was the product of age, family conflict, and the moderator. If either the gender or age interaction added significantly to the prediction of child outcome, the data were split according to the relevant variable, and the regression was examined separately according to the groups; otherwise, the regressions were run again without the final two steps in order to examine overall effects. Significant effects were determined using the change in R^2 as a function of the interaction term (the F-ratio for change). Statistically significant interactions that demonstrated buffering effects were further explored and interpreted by generating simple regression line plots for high (Mean + 1 SD) and low (Mean − 1 SD) values of the moderator variable (Aiken & West, 1991; Fuhrman & Holmbeck, 1995). If a variable functions as a buffer in the relation between family conflict and child outcome, one would expect the slopes of the predicted lines to differ according to the level of the moderator indicating protection by the moderating variable. On the other hand, if a moderator is a vulnerability factor, the slopes would indicate worse outcomes for children with higher levels of the moderator.

RESULTS

Preliminary Analyses

Data Reduction

Children's reports of psychological and physical marital conflict were very highly correlated, and a composite measure was used in analyses. All child-reported marital conflict variables were examined in a factor analysis and one factor emerged using a principal component extraction method and varimax rotation (loadings ranged from .70 to .94; Eigenvalue = 3.02; accounting for 75.5% of the variance), supporting the use of a composite variable of child-reported marital conflict. All composite measures were formed by averaging the pertinent scale scores after standardization.

To reduce the number of dependent variables, factor analyses were conducted on mothers' reports of child health. All RHS variables loaded highly on a single dimension (loadings ranged from .65 to .80; Eigenvalue = 2.01; accounting for 50.3% of the variance) and were subsequently standardized and aggregated into a single variable of mothers' reports of child health.

Outliers and Missing Data

Before interpreting the regressions, the measures were assessed for outliers that fell +/- 3 SDs from the Mean. Cases that were beyond this range were excluded from analyses, because such data have been found to be influential (Tabachnick & Fidell, 1991). Seven cases related to externalizing behavior and four cases involving internalizing behavior were excluded from analyses. In addition, participants with missing data due to incomplete questionnaire data or equipment failure were not included in pertinent analyses.

Primary Analyses

Three measures of marital conflict (physical, psychological, and child-reported), four measures of child-reported parent-child conflict (mother and father psychological and physical conflict), and two measures of mother-reported parent-child conflict (psychological and physical) were used in analyses. Refer to Tables 1 and 2 for descriptive statistics and correlations among the primary variables.

Buffering Effects

According to Rutter's (1990) criteria for a buffer, it is necessary to demonstrate that the protective function of the buffer cannot be accounted for by reduced exposure to the risk variable. To affirm that buffering effects could not be explained as differential exposure to risk in the present study, children were divided using a median split for each moderator, and t-tests were conducted to examine differences in exposure to the risk variable (familial conflict) among children with higher and lower levels of the hypothesized moderators. No group differences were found for vagal tone, vagal suppression, soothability, autonomic reactivity, fear, or emotionality. A few group differences were found regarding anger and sadness but were not pertinent to the significant moderation effects.

Moderators of Marital Conflict

Mother-Reported Marital Conflict. The interaction between vagal suppression and psychological marital conflict was significant in predicting child health for the entire sample (see Table 3 for β, R^2 and F statistics for marital conflict findings). The interaction plots revealed that there was a positive relation between exposure to psychological marital conflict and health problems only among children with lower vagal suppression. Among older children, the interactions between physical marital conflict and both vagal tone and vagal suppression were significant in predicting children's internalizing behavior (see Table 3). Graphs revealed that, for older children with lower levels of either vagal tone or vagal suppression, exposure to physical marital conflict was positively related to internalizing behavior. However, for children with higher vagal tone or suppression, increased exposure was not associated with higher levels of internalizing behavior.

TABLE 1. Descriptive Statistics

		Mean	SD	N
Independent Variables				
Marital Conflict	Child report of marital conflict	7.59	12.62	63
	Mother report of psychological marital conflict	65.71	18.72	56
	Mother report of physical marital conflict	1.42	2.98	59
Parent-Child Conflict	Child report of psychological mother-child conflict	4.09	4.73	63
	Child report of physical mother-child conflict	5.58	6.51	63
	Child report of psychological father-child conflict	4.52	5.16	63
	Child report of physical father-child conflict	6.06	7.23	63
	Mother report of psychological mother-child conflict	7.07	4.99	60
	Mother report of physical mother-child conflict	6.12	5.71	60
Moderating Variables				
	Vagal tone	.15	8.11E-02	61
	Vagal suppression	.14	.13	55
	Autonomic reactivity	16.38	4.56	63
	Soothability	58.32	10.95	63
	Anger	53.67	13.56	63
	Fear	37.94	11.14	63
	Sadness	50.48	7.97	63
	Affective intensity	142.79	20.96	63
Dependant Variables				
	CBCL internalizing	49.32	9.27	63
	CBCL externalizing	48.13	9.60	63
	RHS health measure	21.73	8.13	55

In addition, the interactions between autonomic reactivity (CBQ) and both psychological and physical marital conflict were significant in predicting girls' internalizing behavior (Table 3). Positive associations were found between exposure to both forms of conflict and internalizing behavior only among girls with higher autonomic reactivity.

The interaction between soothability and psychological marital conflict approached conventional levels of statistical significance in predicting externalizing behavior among older children ($p = .07$) such that positive associations between conflict and externalizing were noted only among less soothable children. Soothability demonstrated similar

TABLE 2. Correlations Among Continuous Variables

	1	2	3	4	5	6	7	8	9	10	11	12	13	14	15	16	17	18	19
1. Child report of MC	***																		
2. Mother report of psych MC	.06	***																	
3. Mother report of physical MC	.36**	.42**	***																
4. Child report of psych MCC	.42**	.05	.05	***															
5. Child report of physical MCC	.36**	-.06	.05	.75**	***														
6. Mother report of psych FCC	.40**	.02	.05	.94**	.78**	***													
7. Child report of physical FCC	.39**	-.09	.03	.78**	.93**	.80**	***												
8. Mother report of psych. MCC	-.05	.46**	.29*	.16	.02	.10	.03	***											
9. Mother report of physical MCC	-.03	.28**	.36**	.16	.16	.14	.16	.54**	***										
10. Vagal tone	-.04	-.07	.13	-.13	-.10	-.08	-.16	-.04	-.05	***									
11. Vagal suppression	.09	-.14	.15	-.10	.06	-.06	.05	-.10	-.01	.27*	***								
12. Autonomic reactivity	.15	-.06	.15	.01	-.03	-.05	-.03	-.03	.02	-.10	.36**	***							
13. Soothability	.01	-.02	-.10	-.15	.01	-.13	-.05	-.30*	-.06	.14	.12	.05	***						
14. Anger	.25	-.01	.07	.18	.05	.20	.07	.40**	.12	-.08	-.09	-.02	-.50**	***					
15. Fear	.08	-.09	-.15	.11	.05	.09	.12	.06	.06	-.33**	-.05	.12	-.21	.33**	***				
16. Sadness	.09	.02	.02	-.01	-.21	-.04	-.17	.19	.04	.02	-.08	.16	-.29*	.20	.25*	***			
17. Affective Intensity	-.03	.22	.07	.04	-.19	.01	-.20	.07	.10	.05	-.06	.14	-.15	.02	.04	.36**	***		
18. Internalizing behavior problems	.00	.23	-.11	-.11	-.16	-.08	-.15	.29*	-.03	-.09	-.06	-.10	-.24	.27*	.23	.32*	.01	***	
19. Externalizing behavior problems	.25	.27**	.13	.19	-.01	.22	.07	.47*	.11	.09	-.11	.07	-.34**	.62**	.12	.20	.09	.46**	***
20. Health	.09	.31*	-.04	.10	-.06	.15	-.04	.21	.02	.02	.01	.02	-.25	.30*	.24	.27*	.17	.25	.34*

Note. MC = Marital Conflict, MCC = Mother-child conflict, FCC = Father-child conflict.

*p ≤ .05; **p < .01; ***p < .001

TABLE 3. Marital Conflict and Child Adjustment and Health: Moderators of Outcomes

Predictors		R^2	ΔR^2	ΔF
Mother reported marital conflict				
	Child Health			
Physical MC x VS		.55	.10	5.72*
Older children	Internalizing	Behavior		
Physical MC x VT		.47	.18	5.78*
Older children	Internalizing	Behavior		
Physical MC x VS		.56	.24	7.02*
Girls	Internalizing	Behavior		
Psychological MC x AR		.33	.21	6.67*
Girls	Internalizing	Behavior		
Physical MC x AR		.19	.18	4.84*
Older children	Externalizing	Behavior		
Psychological MC x Soothability		.44	.09	3.70^{I}
Boys	Child Health			
Physical MC x Soothability		.14	.13	3.81^{I}
Child reported marital conflict				
Girls	Externalizing	Behavior		
MC x AR		.41	.18	7.08**
Girls	Internalizing	Behavior		
MC x AI		.44	.17	5.94*

Note. MC = Marital Conflict; VS = Vagal Suppression; VT = Vagal Tone; AR = Autonomic Reactivity; AI = Affective Intensity.
$^{I}p \le .07$; *$p < .05$; **$p < .01$; ***$p < .001$

buffering characteristics in the relation between physical marital conflict and child health for boys ($p = .06$; see Table 3).

Child-Reported Marital Conflict. For girls, autonomic reactivity moderated the relation between marital conflict and externalizing behavior (see Table 3), and indicated a vulnerability function. Marital conflict was positively associated with externalizing only among girls with higher autonomic reactivity. Affective intensity likewise moderated the relation between martial conflict and internalizing for girls.

Parent-Child Conflict

Mother-Reported Parent-Child Conflict. Physical conflict in the mother-child relationship interacted with vagal tone to predict internalizing behavior for older children (see Table 4 for β, R^2 and F statistics related to parent-child conflict). Specifically, exposure to conflict was positively

TABLE 4. Parent-Child Conflict and Child Adjustment and Health: Moderators of Outcomes

Predictors			R^2	ΔR^2	ΔF
Mother reported conflict					
Older children	Internalizing	Behavior			
Physical mother-child conflict x VT			.49	.23	7.67**
Girls	Externalizing	Behavior			
Psychological mother-child conflict x VS			.65	.15	5.32*
		Child Health			
Psychological mother-child conflict x Soothability			.14	.07	3.97*
Child reported conflict					
Girls	Externalizing	Behavior			
Physical father-child conflict x Soothability			.41	.20	7.55*
	Externalizing	Behavior			
Psychological father-child conflict x Soothability			.20	.05	3.57[†]
Girls	Externalizing	Behavior			
Psychological mother-child conflict x AI			.45	.15	5.12*
Girls	Externalizing	Behavior			
Psychological father-child conflict x AI			.46	.11	3.98[†]
Girls	Externalizing	Behavior			
Physical father-child conflict x AI			.63	.37	17.12***
Younger children	Internalizing	Behavior			
Psychological mother child conflict x AI			.55	.23	9.42**
	Externalizing	Behavior			
Psychological mother-child conflict x Sadness			.17	.09	6.36**
	Externalizing	Behavior			
Psychological father-child conflict x Sadness			.16	.07	4.58*
	Externalizing	Behavior			
Physical father-child conflict x Sadness			.13	.08	5.27*
Younger children	Internalizing	Behavior			
Psychological mother-child conflict x Sadness			.32	.28	10.51**
	Externalizing	Behavior			
Psychological father conflict x Anger			.46	.04	4.30*
	Externalizing	Behavior			
Physical father-child conflict x Anger			.46	.05	5.05*
Girls	Externalizing	Behavior			
Psychological mother-child conflict x Fear			.21	.19	5.42*
Girls	Externalizing	Behavior			
Psychological father-child conflict x Fear			.26	.19	5.77*

Note. VT = Vagal Tone; VS = Vagal Suppression; AI = Affective Intensity.
[†] $p \leq .06$; *$p < .05$; **$p < .01$; ***$p < .001$.

associated with internalizing only among older children with lower vagal tone. In the same manner the interaction of vagal suppression and mother-child psychological conflict was significant in predicting externalizing behavior among girls.

Child-Reported Parent-Child Conflict. For girls, the interaction between soothability and father-child physical conflict predicted externalizing behavior such that exposure to conflict was positively associated with externalizing only at lower levels of soothability. Similarly, higher soothability may have protected children (the entire sample) from externalizing behaviors associated with exposure to father-child psychological conflict tactics ($p = .06$; see Table 4).

A higher level of affective intensity was a vulnerability factor for girls in relation to externalizing behavior associated with both mother-child and father-child psychological conflict, as well as father-child physical conflict (Table 4). Positive relations were evident between exposure to parent-child conflict and children's externalizing only for children with higher affective intensity. In the same manner, affective intensity moderated the relation between mother-child psychological conflict and internalizing behavior among younger children.

For the entire sample, higher levels of dispositional sadness were vulnerability factors against children's externalizing problems associated with mother-child psychological conflict and father-child psychological and physical conflict. Positive associations were found between conflict and externalizing only for children with greater sadness. Similarly, a higher level of sadness was a vulnerability factor for younger children in relation to internalizing behaviors associated with mother-child psychological conflict.

Child anger moderated relations between both father-child psychological and physical conflict and externalizing behavior for the entire sample. Positive associations were found between exposure to conflict and externalizing behavior only among children reported to be higher in anger. In the same manner, a higher level of fear functioned as a vulnerability factor in the relations between both mother-child and father-child psychological conflict and externalizing behavior for girls.

DISCUSSION

In this study we examined indices of emotion regulation and emotionality as moderators of the relation between family conflict and child outcome. Consistent with some tenets of the emotional security hypothesis (e.g., Cummings & Davies, 1996), we expected that the child's ability to adaptively regulate the experience and expression of emotion in the face of family conflict would be protective against internalizing, externalizing, and health problems associated with exposure to marital and parent-child conflict. On the other hand, a higher level of emotionality was expected to function as a vulnerability factor in these associations. Overall, results supported our expectations and indicate that the emotionality variables were vulnerability factors, and the emotion regulation variables protective factors, for some of the negative sequelae associated with family conflict.

Emotion Regulation

Vagal tone and vagal suppression were examined as physiological components of emotion regulation and were found to act as protective factors. Higher levels of vagal suppression protected children from health problems associated with exposure to high levels of psychological marital conflict. Consistently, for older children, both vagal tone and vagal suppression were protective factors against internalizing behaviors related to exposure to physical marital conflict. Furthermore, child soothability, which was examined as another index of emotion regulation, was a protective factor in the associations between physical marital conflict and both children's health and older children's externalizing behavior. These results support previous research demonstrating the protective function of vagal tone in relation to child adjustment and health problems associated with marital discord (El-Sheikh et al., 2001; Katz & Gottman, 1995, 1997a). Previous research indicates that children who are exposed to interparental and parent-child conflict become sensitized and display more reactivity to conflict (El-Sheikh, 1994; Hennessy et al., 1994). The establishment of soothability as a protective factor against the effects of exposure to marital conflict extends the literature and is consistent with the notion that emotion regulation processes and sustained arousal play significant roles in the association between exposure to conflict and child outcomes (Cummings & Davies, 1996).

In relation to parent-child conflict, results indicated that, higher (a) vagal suppression protected girls against externalizing behavior associated with psychological mother-child conflict, (b) vagal tone buffered older children from internalizing behaviors associated with mother-child physical conflict, and (c) soothability protected against the externalizing behavior associated with father-child psychological and physical conflict. These findings extend the literature by demonstrating that these indices of physiological and emotion regulation functioned as protective factors against some of the negative outcomes generally associated with parent-child conflict. Although parent-child conflict characterized by verbal and/or physical aggression is detrimental to child functioning in behavioral and physiological domains (Fantuzzo et al., 1991; Galvin et al., 1995), the present data, especially if replicated, suggest that physiological regulation may be protective against some of the negative sequelae. The results highlight the importance of examining physiological regulation in relation to family conflict especially because many of the detrimental effects of exposure may be related to the chronic physiological arousal that frequent conflict elicits (Cohen & Willis, 1985; Porges, 1996). The activation of vagal regulation could potentially lessen or ameliorate this chronic arousal and thus allow for less detrimental outcomes (Gottman & Katz, 1989).

Emotionality

Children's emotionality as denoted by affective intensity, autonomic reactivity, sadness, anger, and fear was examined as a vulnerability factor in the relations between family conflict and child outcomes. Support for this expectation was found especially in relation to parent-child conflict and externalizing behaviors. Higher levels of dispositional anger, sadness, and fear functioned as vulnerability factors for externalizing problems in several contexts of parent-child conflict, whereas sadness was a vulnerability factor only for younger children's internalizing behaviors associated with mother-child conflict. Furthermore, higher affective intensity was also a vulnerability factor, especially for girls, for (a) externalizing behavior (and in one instance internalizing behaviors) associated with parent-child conflict, and (b) internalizing associated with marital conflict. Further, higher levels of autonomic reactivity, as reported by the parent, were vulnerability factors for girls' (a) internalizing behaviors associated with both psychological and physical marital conflict, and (b) externalizing behavior associated with child-reported marital conflict. These findings extend the literature by demonstrating the vulnerability function of several measures of emotionality in the association between both marital and parent-child conflict and children's adjustment.

General Discussion and Limitations

It is interesting that although the protective effects of emotion regulation (vagal tone, vagal suppression, and soothability) were somewhat similar across the marital and parent-child conflict contexts, the vulnerability effects of emotionality were more evident in relation to parent-child conflict versus marital discord, and for externalizing more than internalizing behaviors. Although these results should be considered as preliminary, they are consistent with observations indicating that the context and characteristics of family conflict impact children's responses to family discord (Cummings, Davies, & Campbell, 2001).

Affective intensity moderated relations between child-perceived family (marital and parent-child) conflict and child outcome, in contrast to the measures of emotion regulation, which primarily moderated relations between mother-reported family conflict and child outcome. Although emotionality and regulation are closely linked, they may index different facets of the same underlying process, and may also differentially predict child outcome. This pattern highlights the importance of obtaining information from multiple sources as different reports of the family environment may be more closely tied to particular aspects of child functioning. Investigators have also come to recognize the value of children's perceptions (see Winstok & Eisikovits, 2003) as predictive of their own functioning (Mash & Terdal, 1997). Nonetheless, the results from this study should be interpreted with caution due to the lack of convergence among sources. A related limitation is the use of mothers' reports for family conflict and child outcome. Note, however, that in all significant moderation effects, at least one variable was not assessed by mothers' reports. So the moderation results of this study cannot be solely attributed to single informant bias.

It should be noted that some of the results from the study were not expected. Many of the moderating effects of the emotion regulation and emotionality variables were selectively effective according to the gender and age of the child, with more significant buffering effects obtained for girls and older children. The differential role of the protective and vulnerability factors according to the child's gender and age should be regarded as preliminary as they are difficult to interpret and may be associated with the limitations of the study or may reflect real differences in moderation effects. In this study, the sample was relatively homogeneous, because it was composed of a disproportionate number of well-adjusted Caucasian children from relatively affluent socioeconomic backgrounds. There was also limited variability of reported marital and parent-child conflict. As previously mentioned, only six women reported higher than average physical conflict tactics in their marriage and the same number reported above average physical conflict (mostly mild physical discipline) in the parent-child relationship (Kerig, 1996; Straus, 1995). Thus, the sample was composed of relatively non-violent, non-abusive families. Although these characteristics limit the applicability of these findings to more violent populations, examination of non-abusive aggression and verbal and emotional conflict in the marital and parent-child relationship is important and pertains to a large population of children. Furthermore, because physical discipline is a prevalent practice in our culture, it is worthwhile to examine its effects on children (Graziano, 1994) and a previous study has found it to be positively associated with children's subsequent conflict towards peers (Strassberg, Dodge, Pettit, & Bates, 1994). Examination of verbal and emotional conflict within the marital relationship, apart from physical aggression, is important due to its higher frequency of occurrence and subsequent higher probability of child observance. In addition, research indicates that chronic stressors may be more to an individual than more severe but relatively rare occurrences (Holahan, Holahan, & Belk, 1984). However, given that the relationship between family conflict and child outcome is complex, divergent findings may emerge within a more diverse sample of families and children. Thus the results of this study should be considered preliminary, and interpreted with caution and in their appropriate context, pending further elucidation with larger and more diverse samples.

It may have also been the case that more moderating relationships existed but were not strong enough to be detected in this sample due to the limited number of participants and subsequent power issues. Because of the small sample size, especially when the sample was examined by gender and age, and the decision to control for Type II rather than Type I error, it could be argued that the significant relations were due to chance rather than real moderation effects. However, the substantial amount of variance accounted for by most of the interactions between various forms of conflict and the moderators argues against the proposition that all these findings were spurious. Finally, the moderation effects should be interpreted within the limitations imposed by the cross-sectional design of the study, which prevents assertions regarding direction of causality among the variables. Despite the limitations and need for replication, this study extends the literature by suggesting intra-individual variables that either reduce or increase child vulnerability to the negative effects of various contexts of family conflict.

REFERENCES

Achenbach, T. M. (1991). *Manual for the Child Behavior Checklist/4-18 and 1991 profile.* Burlington, VT: University of Vermont, Department of Psychiatry.

Achenbach, T. M., & Edelbrock, C. (1983). *Manual for the Child Behavior Checklist and Revised Child Behavior Profile.* Burlington, VT: University of Vermont, Department of Psychiatry.

Aiken, L. S., & West, S. G. (1991). *Multiple regression: Testing and interpreting interactions.* Newbury Park, CA: SAGE Publications.

Ballard, M., Cummings, E. M., & Larkin, K. (1993). Emotional and cardiovascular responses to adults' angry behavior and challenging tasks in children of hypertensive and normotensive parents. *Child Development, 64,* 500-515.

Baron, R. M., & Kenny, D. A. (1986). The moderator-mediator variable distinction in social psychological research: Conceptual, strategic, and statistical considerations. *Journal of Personality and Social Psychology, 51,* 1173-1182.

Borstein, M. H., & Suess, P. E. (2000). Child and mother cardiac vagal tone: Continuity, stability, and concordance across the first 5 years. *Developmental Psychology, 36,* 54-65.

Brody, G. H., Stoneman, Z., & Burke, M. (1988). Child temperament and parental perceptions of individual child adjustment: An intrafamilial analysis. *American Journal of Orthopsychiatry, 58,* 532-542.

Calkins, S. D. (1997). Cardiac vagal tone indices of temperamental reactivity and behavioral regulation in young children. *Developmental Psychobiology, 31,* 125-135.

Casale, T. (1987). Neuromechanisms of asthma. *Annals of Allergy, 59,* 391-398.

Cicchetti, D., Ackerman, B. P., & Izard, C. E. (1995). Emotions and emotion regulation in developmental psychopathology. *Development and Psychopathology, 7,* 1-10.

Cohen, S., & Wills, T. A. (1985). Stress, social support, and the buffering hypothesis. *Psychological Bulletin, 98,* 310-357.

Cole, P. M., Michel, M. K., & Teti, O. T. (1994). The development of emotion regulation and dysregulation: A clinical perspective. In N. Fox (Ed.), The development of emotion regulation: Biological and behavioral considerations. *Monographs of the Society for Research in Child Development,* 59 (Serial No. 204), 73-100, 250-283.

Cummings, E. M., & Davies, P. T. (1996). Emotional security as a regulatory process in normal development and the development of psychopathology. *Development and Psychopathology, 8,* 123-139.

Cummings, E. M., Davies, P. T., & Campbell, S. B. (2001). *Developmental Psychopathology and Family Process: Theory, Research, and Clinical Implications.* New York: The Guilford Press.

Cummings, E. M., Zahn-Waxler, C., & Radke-Yarrow, M. (1981). Young children's responses to expressions of anger and affection by others in the family. *Child Development, 52,* 1274-1282.

DeGangi, G. A., DiPietro, J. A., Greenspan, S. I., & Porges, S. W. (1991). Psychophysiological characteristics of the regulatory disordered infant. *Infant Behavior & Development, 14,* 37-50.

Derryberry, D., & Rothbart, M. K. (1988). Arousal, affect, and attention as components of temperament. *Journal of Personality and Social Psychology, 55,* 958-966.

Dodge, K. A., & Garber, J. (1991). Domains of emotion regulation. In J. Garber & K. A. Dodge (Eds.), *The development of emotion regulation and dysregulation.* New York: Cambridge University Press.

Donchin, Y., Constantini, S., Szold, A., Byrne, E., & Porges, S. W. (1992). Cardiac vagal tone predicts outcome in neurosurgical patients. *Critical Care Medicine, 20,* 941-949.

Doussard-Roosevelt, J. A., & Porges, S. W. (1999). The role of neurobehavioral organization in stress responses: A polyvagal model. In M. Lewis & D. Ramsey (Eds.), *Soothing and Stress* (pp. 57-76) New Jersey: Lawrence Erlbaum Associates.

Doussard-Roosevelt, J. A., Porges, S. W., Scanlon, J. W., Alemi, B., & Scanlon, K. B. (1997). Vagal regulation of heart rate in the prediction of developmental outcome for very low birth weight preterm infants. *Child Development, 68,* 173-186.

Eisen, M., Donald, C., & Ware, J. (1980). *Conceptualization and measurement of health for children in the Health Insurance Study.* R-2313-HEW. Santa Monica, CA: The RAND Corporation.

Eisen, M., Ware, J. E., Donald, C. A., & Brook, R. (1979). Measuring Components of Children's Health Status. *Medical Care, 17,* 902-921.

Eisenberg, N., Fabes, R. A., Bernzweig, J., Karbon, M., Poulin, R., & Hanish, L. (1993). The relations of emotionality and regulation to preschoolers' social skills and sociometric status. *Child Development, 64,* 1418-1438.

Eisenberg, N., Fabes, R. A., Guthrie, I. K., Murphy, B. C., Maszk, P., Holmgren, R., & Suh, K. (1996). The relations of regulation and emotionality to problem behavior in elementary school children. *Development and Psychopathology, 8,* 141-162.

Eisenberg, N., Fabes, R. A., Murphy, B., Maszk, P., Smith, M., & Karbon, M. (1995). The role of emotionality and regulation in children's social functioning: A longitudinal study. *Child Development, 66,* 1360-1384.

Eisenberg, N., Fabes, R. A., Nyman, M., Bernzweig, J., & Pinuelas, A. (1994). The relations of emotionality and regulation to children's anger-related reactions. *Child Development, 65,* 109-128.

Eisenberg, N., Guthrie, I. K., Fabes, R. A., Reiser, M., Murphy, B. C., Holgren, R., Maszk, P., & Losoya, S. (1997). The relations of regulation and emotionality to resiliency and competent social functioning in elementary school children. *Child Development, 68,* 295-311.

El-Sheikh, M. (1994). Children's emotional and physiological responses to interadult angry behavior: The role of history of interparental hostility. *Journal of Abnormal Child Psychology, 22,* 661-678.

El-Sheikh, M. (1997). Children's responses to adult-adult and mother-child arguments: The role of parental marital conflict and distress. *Journal of Family Psychology, 11,* 165-175.

El-Sheikh, M., Cummings, E. M., & Reiter, S. L. (1996). Preschoolers' responses to ongoing interadult conflict: The role of prior exposure to resolved versus unresolved arguments. *Journal of Abnormal Child Psychology, 24,* 665-679.

El-Sheikh, M., Harger, J., & Whitson, S. (2001). Exposure to Interparental Conflict and Children's Adjustment and Physical Health: The Moderating Role of Vagal Tone. *Child Development, 72,* 1617-1636.

Fantuzzo, J., DePaola, L., Lambert, L., Martino, T., Anderson, G., & Sutton, S. (1991). Effects of interparental violence on the psychological adjustment and competencies of young children. *Journal of Consulting and Clinical Psychology, 59*, 258-265.

Fox, N. A., & Field, T. M. (1989). Individual differences in preschool entry behavior. *Journal of Applied Developmental Psychology, 10*, 527-540.

Fuhrman, T., & Holmbeck, G. N. (1995). A contextual-moderator analysis of emotional autonomy and adjustment in adolescence. *Child Development, 66*, 793-811.

Galvin, M., Eyck, R. T., Shekhar, A., Stilwell, B., Fineberg, N., Laite, G., & Karwisch, G. (1995). Serum dopamine beta hydroxylase and maltreatment in psychiatrically hospitalized boys. *Child Abuse and Neglect, 19*, (821-832).

Gottman, J. M., & Katz, L. F. (1989). Effects of marital discord on young children's peer interaction and health. *Developmental Psychology, 25*, 373-381.

Graziano, A. M. (1994). Why we should study subabusive violence against children. *Journal of Interpersonal Violence, 9*, 412-419.

Grossman, P. (1991). Respiratory mediation of cardiac function within a psychophysiological perspective. In J. G. Carlson & A. R. Seifert (Eds.) *International perspectives on self-regulation and health* (pp. 17-39). New York: Plenum.

Grossman, P., & Wientjes, K. (1986). Respiratory sinus arrhythmia and parasympathetic cardiac control: Some basic issues concerning quantification, application, and implications. In P. Grossman, K. Janssen, & D. Vaitl (Eds.), *Cardiorespiratory and cardiosomatic psychophysiology* (pp. 117-138). New York: Plenum Press.

Grych, J. H., & Fincham, F. D. (1990). Marital conflict and children's adjustment: A cognitive-contextual framework. *Psychological Bulletin, 108*, 267-290.

Grych, J. H., & Fincham, F. D. (2001). *Interparental Conflict and Child Development: Theory, Research, and Application.* Cambridge University Press.

Henry, J. P., & Stephens, P. M. (1977). *Stress, health and the social environment: A sociobiologic approach to medicine.* New York: Springer.

Hennessy, K. D., Rabideau, G. J., Cicchetti, D., & Cummings, E. M. (1994). Responses of physically abused and non-abused children to different forms of interadult anger. *Child Development, 65*, 815-828.

Hershorn, M., & Rosenbaum, A. (1985). Children of marital violence: A closer look at the unintended victims. *American Journal of Orthopsychiatry, 55*, 260-266.

Holahan, C. K., Holahan, D. J., & Belk, S. J. (1984). Adjustment in aging: The roles of life stress, hassles, and self-efficacy. *Health Psychology, 3*, 315-328.

Hollingshead, A. B. (1975). *Four factor index of social status.* Unpublished manuscript.

Huffman, L. C., Bryan, Y. E., del Carmen, R., Pedersen, F. A., Doussard-Roosevelt, J. A., & Porges, S. W. (1998). Infant temperament and cardiac vagal tone: Assessments at twelve weeks of age. *Child Development, 69*, 624-635.

Jaffe, P., Wolfe, D., Wilson, K., & Zak, L. (1986). Family violence and child adjustment: A comparative analysis of girls' and boys' behavioral symptoms. *American Journal of Psychiatry, 143*, 74-77.

Katz, L. F., & Gottman, J. M. (1995). Vagal tone protects children from marital conflict. *Development and Psychopathology, 7*, 83-92.

Katz, L. F., & Gottman, J. M. (1997a). Buffering children from marital conflict and dissolution. *Journal of Clinical Child Psychology, 26*, 157-171.

Katz, L. F., & Gottman, J. M. (1997b). Spillover effects of marital conflict: In search of parenting and co-parenting mechanisms. In J. McHale & P. Cowan (Eds.), *Understanding how family-level dynamics affect children's development: Studies of two-parent families. New Directions in Child Development, 74,* (pp. 57-76). San Francisco: Jossey-Bass.

Kerig, P. K. (1996). Assessing the links between interparental conflict and child adjustment: The conflicts and problem-solving scales. *Journal of Family Psychology, 10,* 454-473.

Kolko, D. J. (1992). Characteristics of child victims of physical violence: Research findings and clinical implications. *Journal of Interpersonal Violence, 7,* 244-276.

Larsen, R. J., & Diener, E. (1987). Affect intensity as an individual difference characteristic: A review. *Journal of Research in Personality, 21,* 1-39.

Lazarus, R. S., & Folkman, S. (1984). *Stress, appraisal, and coping.* New York: Springer.

Lau, J., Liu, J., Cheung, J., Yu, A., & Wong, C. (1999). Prevalence and correlates of physical abuse in Hong Kong Chinese Adolescents: A population-based approach. *Child Abuse and Neglect, 23,* 549-557.

Malinosky-Rummell, R., & Hansen, D. (1993). Long-term consequences of childhood physical abuse. *Psychological Bulletin, 114,* 68-79.

Mash, E. J., & Terdal, L. G. (1997). Assessment of child and family disturbance: A behavioral-systems approach. In E. J. Mash & L. G. Terdal (Eds.), *Assessment of Childhood Disorders* (pp. 3-68). New York, NY: The Guilford Press.

Murphy, B. C., Eisenberg, N., Fabes, R. A., Shepard, S., & Guthrie, I. K. (1999). Consistency and change in children's emotionality and regulation: A longitudinal study. *Merrill-Palmer Quarterly, 45,* 413-444.

O'Keefe, M. (1995). Predictors of child abuse in martially violent families. *Journal of Interpersonal Violence, 10,* 3-25.

O'Leary, A. (1990). Stress, emotion, and human immune function. *Psychological Bulletin, 108,* 363-382.

Porges, S. W. (1984). Heart rate oscillation: An index of neural mediation. In M. G. H. Coles, J. R. Jennings, & J. A. Stern (Eds.), *Psychophysiological perspectives* (pp. 229-241). New York: Van Nostrand Reinhold.

Porges, S. W. (1991). Vagal tone: An autonomic mediator of affect. In Garber, J. & Dodge, K. D. (Eds.), *The development of emotional regulation and dysregulation.* New York: Cambridge University Press.

Porges, S. W. (1992). Vagal tone: A physiological marker of stress vulnerability. *Pediatrics, 90,* 498-504.

Porges, S. W. (1995). Orienting in a defensive world: Mammalian modifications of our evolutionary heritage. A polyvagal theory. *Psychophysiology, 32,* 301-318.

Porges, S. W. (1996). Physiological regulation in high-risk infants: A model for assessment and potential intervention. *Development and Psychopathology, 8,* 29-42.

Porges, S. W., Doussard-Roosevelt, J. A., & Maiti, A. K. (1994). Vagal tone and the physiological regulation of emotion. In N. A. Fox (Ed.), The development of emotion regulation. *Monographs of the Society for Research in Child Development, 59* (Serial No. 240), 167-186, 250-283.

Rothbart, M. K., Ahadi, S. A., & Hershey, K. L. (1994). Temperament and social behavior in childhood. *Merrill-Palmer Quarterly, 40,* 21-39.

Rutter, M. (1990). Psychosocial resilience and protective mechanisms. In J. Rolf, A. S. Masten, D. Cicchetti, K. H. Neuchterlein, & S. Weintraub (Eds.), *Risk and protective factors in the development of psychopathology* (pp. 181-214). New York: Cambridge University Press.

Strassberg, Z., Dodge, K. A., Pettit, G. S., & Bates, J. E. (1994). Spanking in the home and children's subsequent aggression toward kindergarten peers. *Development and Psychopathology, 6,* 445-461.

Straus, M. A. (1990). Measuring intrafamily conflict and violence: The Conflict Tactics (CT) Scales. In M. A. Straus & R. J. Gelles, *Physical violence in American families: Risk factors and adaptations to violence in 8,145 families* (pp. 29-48). New Brunswick, NJ: Transaction Publications.

Straus, M. A. (1995). *Manual for the Conflict Tactics Scale.* Durham, NH: Family Research Laboratory, University of New Hampshire.

Straus, M. A., & Gelles, R. J. (1986). Societal change and change in family violence from 1975-1985 as revealed by two national surveys. *Journal of Marriage and the Family, 48,* 465-479.

Straus, M. A., Hamby, S. L., Boney-McCoy, S., & Sugarman, D. B. (1996). The Revised Conflicts Tactics Scale (CTS2): Development and preliminary psychometric data. *Journal of Family Issues, 17,* 283-316.

Straus, M. A., Hamby, S. L., Finklehor, D., Moore, D. W., & Runyan, D. (1998). Identification of child maltreatment with the Parent-Child Conflict Tactics Scales: Development and psychometric data for a national sample of American parents. *Child Abuse and Neglect, 22,* 249-270.

Tabachnick, B. G., & Fidell, L. S. (1991). Software for advanced ANOVA courses: A survey. *Behavior Research Methods, Instruments, & Computers, 23,* 208-211.

Teglasi, H., & McMahon, B. H. (1990). Temperament and common problem behaviors of children. *Journal of Applied Developmental Psychology, 11,* 331-349.

Thompson, R. A. (1994). Emotion regulation: A theme in search of definition. In N. Fox (Ed.), The development of emotion regulation: Biological and behavioral considerations. *Monographs of the Society for Research in Child Development, 59* (Serial No. 240), 25-52, 250-283.

Thompson, R. A., & Calkins, S. D. (1996). The double-edged sword: Emotional regulation for children at risk. *Development and Psychopathology, 8,* 163-182.

Winstok, Z., & Eisikovits, Z. (2003). Divorcing the parents: The impact of adolescents' exposure to father-to-mother aggression on their perceptions of affinity with their parents. *Journal of Emotional Abuse, 3*(1/2), 103-121.

Domestic Violence and Children's Behavior in Low-Income Families

Ariel Kalil
Richard Tolman
Daniel Rosen
Gabrielle Gruber

SUMMARY. This paper uses data from a representative sample ($N =$ 443) of mothers with pre-school and school-age children who were randomly selected from the welfare caseload in one urban county in Michi-

Address correspondence to: Ariel Kalil, Irving B. Harris Graduate School of Public Policy Studies, University of Chicago, 1155 East 60th Street, Chicago, IL 60637 (E-mail: a-kalil@uchicago.edu).

Special thanks are due to WES survey manager Bruce Medbury and the interviewing staff. The authors appreciate the helpful comments of Sandra Graham-Bermann, Jeff Edleson, and Alytia Levendosky on previous drafts of the manuscript.

The Women's Employment Study is an ongoing study conducted at the Poverty Research and Training Center at the University of Michigan. Support for this research was provided in part by grants from the Charles Stewart Mott and Joyce Foundations and the National Institute of Mental Health (R24-MH51363) to the Social Work Research Development Center on Poverty, Risk, and Mental Health, the Office of the Vice-President for Research at the University of Michigan to the Program on Poverty and Social Welfare Policy, and by a grant from the National Institute of Child Health and Human Development (F-32 HD08145-01) to the first author.

A previous version of this paper was presented at the Annual Research Conference of the Population Association of America, March, 1999, New York, NY.

gan in early 1997. We investigate how mothers' experiences of severe physical abuse relate to maternal reports of children's internalizing and externalizing behavior problems. Mothers experiencing domestic violence did not differ from other mothers on punitive discipline or emotional warmth towards their children, but they did experience more parenting stress and had higher rates of mental health and substance abuse disorders. Controlling for an array of demographic characteristics, results suggest that children of abused mothers display significantly higher levels of externalizing, but not internalizing, behavior problems. The association of domestic violence and externalizing behaviors is only partially mediated by maternal psychological characteristics. *[Article copies available for a fee from The Haworth Document Delivery Service: 1-800-HAWORTH. E-mail address: <docdelivery@haworthpress.com> Website: <http://www.HaworthPress.com> © 2003 by The Haworth Press, Inc. All rights reserved.]*

KEYWORDS. Domestic violence, child adjustment, woman abuse, child witness, welfare recipients

Approximately 1.8 million women (about 3.2%) are severely beaten each year in the United States, and some estimate that at least one out of three children in the U.S. has witnessed domestic violence (Straus, 1992; Straus & Gelles, 1990). In recent years, researchers have become concerned with the adjustment of children in violent homes–the so-called "indirect" victims of family violence (Kolbo, Blakely, & Engleman, 1996). Children of abused mothers are at risk for a variety of adjustment difficulties; these are most often measured in terms of acting-out behavior (e.g., aggression, overt disobedience, destructiveness) and over-controlled symptomatology (e.g., anxiety, withdrawal, depression, and somatic complaints; Edleson, 1999)

Children's behavioral adjustment problems may relate to a variety of correlates of maternal abuse. Recent reviews of the literature (see, e.g., Edleson, 1999) describe three major hypotheses. First, children's behavior may be disrupted due to the psychological trauma of "witnessing" (i.e., seeing or hearing) violence perpetrated against their mothers. Second, mothers' abusers may themselves victimize children. Third, children's adjustment may be associated with the traumatic aftereffects of maternal abuse. These aftereffects could include events such as moving to a shelter or having contact with the police. Aftereffects could also be characterized in terms of the increased psychological distress or disrupted parenting behavior of mothers that has been linked to inter-adult violence and discord. Support for each of these hypotheses is equivocal, due in part to sampling and methodological problems characterizing many studies in the field. Small sample sizes and over-reliance on shelter-based samples limit the generalizability of many existing studies.

In this paper, we draw on a new, large-scale representative sample of mothers with young children to examine the links between mothers' experiences of severe physical violence and children's behavioral adjustment. In addition to examining the direct effects of domestic violence on children's behavior, our data allow us to assess whether maternal psychological well-being and parenting behavior mediate the association between their exposure to domestic violence and their children's behavioral adjustment. This hypothesis is particularly important to test in a large-scale, random design study because of the common perception in the literature that maternal "aggression" and "emotional availability" are major explanatory factors in the behavioral adjustment of children of abused mothers. This perception holds forth despite the dearth of empirical studies on this topic and has been characterized as "mother-blaming" by some (Sullivan, Nguyen, Allen, Bybee, & Juras, 2000). If mothers' psychological characteristics and parenting behaviors are found to be important factors linking maternal abuse to children's adjustment, this has implications for service provision and social policies. On the other hand, if these factors do not seem to account for the association between maternal abuse and children's adjustment, this suggests that future research and intervention efforts may need to be focused elsewhere.

BACKGROUND

Numerous studies link maternal experiences of domestic violence to children's adjustment in multiple domains. Children who witness domestic violence are at-risk for maladaptation in behavioral, emotional, social, cognitive, and physical realms. Links between domestic violence and children's outcomes appear to be strongest in the areas of children's emotional and cognitive functioning. For example, children exposed to domestic violence exhibit lower social competence, more anxiety, lower self-esteem, more anger, greater temperament problems, more rejection from peers and less skill in understanding how others feel (Edleson, 1999; Kolbo et al., 1996; Levendosky & Graham-Bermann, 1998).

Explanatory Factors

Despite consistent findings that children of physically abused women are at an increased risk for negative physical and behavioral outcomes, actual percentages of children suffering negative outcomes varies from 25 to 70 percent across different studies (Holden, Geffner, & Jouriles, 1998). Three positions have been advanced to explain the heterogeneity in outcomes among these children. These include variations in the extent of witnessing violence, whether the child is victimized him- or herself, and variations in exposure to traumatic aftereffects including the psychological distress and disrupted parenting of the abused mothers. Evidence for each of these positions is presented below.

Witnessing violence has been variously defined as seeing or hearing violent episodes, but it can also include being threatened, coerced, or used as a pawn during a violent incident (Edleson, 1999). Any of these experiences could result in physical or psychological trauma. Children themselves may also be the direct recipients of abuse. Estimates of the co-occurrence of spouse and child physical abuse range from 6% in representative samples to between 20% and 100% in clinical samples of battered women or physically abused children (Appel & Holden, 1998). Margolin (1998) notes that children exposed to domestic violence are at increased risk for sexual abuse (especially from the mother's partner) and community violence. Among studies that have been able to distinguish between actual child abuse and witnessing abuse, children who both witnessed violence and were abused had greater problems than children who had "only" witnessed abuse (the "double whammy" effect; Hughes, Parkinson, & Vargo, 1989).

Finally, children's behavioral adjustment may be related to the mental health and parenting disruptions known to occur among mothers who have experienced abuse. Abused women are more likely to suffer from psychological disorders, including post-traumatic stress disorder, major depression, anxiety disorders, and substance problems (Bassuk et al., 1996; Plichta, 1996; Tolman & Rosen, 2001). Mothers who experience physical violence also report higher levels of parenting stress (Levendosky & Graham-Bermann, 1998; Wolfe, Jaffe, Wilson, & Zak, 1985). Others have proposed that abused mothers may be less emotionally available to their children. Living in a hostile environment is hypothesized to be emotionally draining, leaving mothers with less energy to devote to children's needs.

Mothers living with domestic violence may also modify their parenting in an effort to prevent harm. Osofsky (2000) notes the consistent finding that a strong relationship with a positive adult, often a parent, can buffer children from adversity, such as exposure to domestic violence. She also points out that children need a balance between autonomy to explore one's world and protection by caregivers to develop basic trust and security, but that parents living in an unsafe environment may limit their children's autonomy. Thus, a mother who is physically abused by an intimate partner and who discourages her children's independence may be protecting herself and her children from further abuse. In one study, one-third of the battered women in the sample reported altering their disciplinary practices based on whether or not the batterers were present (Holden & Ritchie, 1991). While these behaviors may be protective of the safety of women and their children, limited autonomy and inconsistent discipline also may involve costs to the adjustment of the children.

These mental health and parenting characteristics have important implications for child conduct problems (Patterson, DeBaryshe, & Stouthamer-Loeber, 1989) and behavioral and psychological well-being (Conger, Ge, Elder, Lorenz, & Simons, 1994). Warm and supportive parenting, positive parent-child relationships, and consistent, non-coercive discipline behaviors have been linked to positive psychosocial development and low levels of behavior problems and internal distress in children (e.g., Lamborn, Mounts, Steinberg, & Dornbusch, 1991; Maccoby & Martin, 1983; Patterson et al., 1989; Steinberg, Lamborn, Dornbusch, & Darling, 1992). Maternal psychological well-being is a key component of these effective parenting practices (McLoyd, 1990) and can also be directly associated with children's emotional adjustment (Thompson, 1998).

Subgroup Differences

Some research has found differential effects of maternal experiences of physical violence on the behavioral adjustment of boys versus girls, but results in this area remain inconclusive. Theoretical models from developmental psychopathology suggest that boys may be more vulnerable to psychosocial stress (Zaslow, 1988) and that this may have biological roots (Rutter, 1990). However, other theories argue that basic gender differences in interpersonal orientation predispose girls toward being more negatively affected by witnessing violence. For example, girls have been shown to develop greater interpersonal sensitivity to the affective cues and states of others (Zahn-Waxler, 1993) and may be more likely to engage in behaviors that diffuse or mitigate conflict.

Thus, they may be more likely than boys to respond behaviorally to domestic violence. Other theories propose that because children identify with the same-sex parent, they will develop self-concepts that mirror the self-concepts of their same-sex parent (Chodorow, 1991). Girls, then, may be particularly susceptible to the depressed mood of their abused mothers.

Empirical results from early studies indicated that boys who had been exposed to domestic violence exhibited more externalizing symptomatology while girls displayed more internalizing problems (Hughes, 1988; Porter & O'Leary, 1980; Wolfe et al., 1985). More recent studies have also reported higher scores for girls on behavior problem checklists, particularly with respect to internalizing problems (Cummings, Pepler, & Moore, 1999). However, Graham-Bermann (1996) found that boys who witnessed domestic violence evidenced more internalizing problems than girls who had also been exposed, and in a different study, Graham-Berman and Levendosky (1998) did not find significant differences in adjustment between pre-school-aged boys and girls exposed to domestic violence. Cummings et al. (1999) report that shelter-residing girls receive more verbal aggression from fathers than do boys, suggesting one explanation for gender differences. More studies are needed to further our understanding of the role of gender in moderating the effects of exposure to domestic violence, although the balance of evidence points to greater maladjustment in girls compared to boys who have witnessed violence.

Methodological Issues

A limitation of existing studies is an over-reliance on convenience sampling from battered women's shelters or clinics. There is very little evidence concerning the association between domestic violence against women and children's adjustment among families who are not currently residing in shelters or who are randomly sampled from the community. In the majority of available research, volunteer samples of mothers and children are drawn from shelters and matched with non-sheltered controls (Edleson, 1999; Kolbo et al., 1996; Morley & Brennan, 1999). Yet, mothers and children who use shelters represent only a small fraction of the domestic violence population, and reliance on this sampling method presents several selection biases. First, the effects of domestic violence may be confounded with living in a shelter. Shelter residence involves additional salient stresses such as residential instability or separation from friends and neighbors. Fantuzzo et al. (1991) found that sheltered children had significantly higher levels of internalizing problems than children of battered mothers who had previously been sheltered but were residing at home at the time of the survey. Margolin (1998) similarly asserts that sampling from identified or treatment samples (as opposed to community samples) has been associated with different outcomes, indicating the importance of this distinction. Second, mothers who are able to marshal the resources necessary to utilize shelters may differ in important ways from abused women who remain in their own homes. Thus, unmeasured characteristics of mothers may be associated with differences in children's adjustment. Studying representative community samples and non-clinical samples where family violence has occurred is among the most pressing needs for research in this area (Appel & Holden, 1998).

Our study advances knowledge in the field in several important ways. Morley and Brennan's (1999) exhaustive review of the literature revealed only one study (Sternberg et al., 1993) that sampled families who were living at home. That study was conducted in Israel. Eighteen of the 28 studies reviewed sampled from shelters for battered women and nine sampled from outpatient clinics. It is impossible to know the extent to which observed effects in these studies are due to the trauma and stress associated with leaving home, changing schools, or adjusting to shelter life. Our study is a large-scale survey of non-sheltered low-income mothers randomly sampled from one urban community. Second, our survey offers excellent data with which to test one of the three major hypotheses linking maternal experiences of abuse to children's behavior; namely, that the linkages occur via maternal psychological problems and parenting behaviors. Most studies examining these links have focused on single measures of mothers' parenting, typically a measure of parenting stress (Morley & Brennan, 1999). We assess the role of parenting stress in addition to several other dimensions of parenting behavior. Third, we assess the effects of the timing of children's potential exposure to physical violence against their mothers by distinguishing between physical abuse that occurred within the past 12 months versus that which occurred at any point in the mother's lifetime. Finally, we examine children's adjustment as a function of age. Fantuzzo and Mohr (2000) summarize past findings, noting that approximately half of the studies on children's exposure to domestic violence to date have included school-age children only. Moreover, of the studies that included school-age children as well as younger children, only three examined whether outcomes differed by age and developmental stage (see Winstok & Eisikovits, 2003, for a discussion of how adolescents may be affected by father-to-mother physical aggression). Our sample is large enough to allow us to examine interactions based on preschool relative to school-age children, and for boys as well as girls.

HYPOTHESES

In this study of maternal experiences of physical violence and children's behavioral adjustment, we hypothesize that mothers' experience of violence will be positively associated with children's internalizing and externalizing behavior problems. We define maternal abuse as severe physical abuse (e.g., having been kicked, punched, assaulted with a weapon), hypothesizing that children will be more aware of and potentially more traumatized by violence that may result in physical injury to the mother. We test the hypothesis that mothers' psychological functioning and parenting practices mediate the effects of domestic violence on children's behavior. However, because we lack data on whether the children themselves were abused, the nature and extent of their "witnessing," and other caregivers' (e.g., fathers') mental health and parenting, we expect that maternal factors will account for some, but not all, of this association.

Due to the equivocal findings regarding associations of domestic assault of their mothers with adjustment in boys versus girls, we do not make specific hypotheses in this regard. However, we predict that children of mothers who have experienced domestic violence in the past 12 months (i.e., recently) will have poorer adjustment than children whose mothers have experienced violence in their lifetime but not in the past 12 months, who will in turn display poorer adjustment than those whose mothers have never experienced violence. There have been too few studies of children of different ages to develop specific hypotheses about effects for pre-school versus school-age children. We consider these analyses exploratory.

METHOD

Participants

We use data from the Women's Employment Study (WES), a random sample of 753 mothers who were receiving cash welfare assistance in an urban Michigan county in February 1997. The purpose of the study was to measure barriers to employment among low-income women. Women's experiences of domestic violence and assessment of their mental health and family conditions were a major focus of the study. The sample was systematically selected with an equal probability from an ordered list of the universe of active single mother cases of the Michigan Family Independence Agency, the state welfare agency. Women younger than 18 or older than 55 years of age were not included in the sample. In-home, face-to-face interviews, lasting about one hour, were completed between September and December 1997 by trained interviewers. Completed interviews represent an 86% response rate. Mothers were paid $20 for their participation (see Danziger et al., 2000, for further detail).

Information about children's emotional well-being and social adjustment, as well as maternal parenting practices and mother-child relationships, was collected if the mother had at least one child between the ages of 2 and 10 (designated the "focal child"). Seventy-six percent ($N = 575$) of the mothers interviewed had a focal child. Of these, 443 were in the appropriate age range (3-10) for the child behavior measures of interest in this study.

The mean age of the mothers in this sample of 443 was approximately 30 years old and the average child's age was 5.45. Fifty-six percent of the children were preschoolers (ages 3-5). Fifty-three percent of the children were girls. Fifty-five percent of mothers are Black and 45 percent are White. The average family size was 3.9 individuals. Although all women were unmarried at the time the sampling frame was drawn, 23 percent of mothers had married or were living (or continuing to live) as unmarried partners with a male by the time the interview occurred. Seventy-two percent of the mothers had a high school degree or its equivalent and 64 percent were employed.

MEASURES

Domestic Violence

Predictor Variables. Domestic violence is measured by items drawn from the Conflict Tactics Scale, a widely used measure of family violence (Straus & Gelles, 1990). A 6-item index of severe physical violence was used that yields information about women's lifetime and recent experiences of having been threatened with a harmful object, physically assaulted, choked or beaten up, threatened or assaulted with a weapon, or forced into sexual activity by a romantic partner. Total scores were calculated by summing the number of affirmative responses to each of the six questions. The internal consistency of this scale was .97. This scale was recoded and subgroups were created to distinguish mothers who have never experienced any of these forms of violence ($n = 207$, 46%) from those who have (a) experienced at least one of these forms of physical violence at some point in their lifetime but not in the past 12 months ($n = 170$, 39%) and (b) experienced at least one of these forms of physical violence in the past 12 months ($n = 66$, 15%). In regression analyses (described below), the "never experienced violence" group is the reference category.

Control Variables. A variety of family demographic and socioeconomic characteristics were statistically controlled. Control variables include whether mothers are currently married or living as unmarried partners with a male partner, maternal education, age, race (Black, White), and employment status. The family's economic well-being was assessed with an income-to-needs ratio. Income-to-needs is a measure of household income adjusted for family size that indicates distance above or below the 1998 poverty threshold for a family of that size (values greater than 1.0 are above the poverty threshold; values less than 1.0 are below it). Separate analyses (described below) were conducted for preschool and school-age boys and girls.

Maternal Characteristics

Mental Health. Maternal psychological characteristics were assessed using diagnostic screening batteries from the University of Michigan Composite International Diagnostic Interview Short Screening Scales (UM-CIDI; Kessler & Mroczek, 1993). These diagnostic screening scales are based on the National Comorbidity Study (NCS), the first nationally representative survey to administer a structured psychiatric interview (Kessler et al., 1994). The short form of the CIDI (CIDI-SF) used in the first wave of WES measures the DSM-III-R disorders of depression (MDE), generalized anxiety disorder (GAD), and alcohol and drug dependence (ADP and DDP) in the past 12 months. The CIDI-SF scales correctly classify between 77% and 100% of CIDI cases, and between 94% and 99% of CIDI non-cases in the NCS. For the scales used in this study, overall classification accuracy ranges from 93% for depression to 99% for generalized anxiety disorder (Kessler, Andrews, Mroczek, Ustun, & Wittchen, in press). Post-traumatic stress disorder (PTSD) was also measured using a modification of the UM-CIDI long form, which determines the lifetime prevalence of PTSD based on women's responses to the most upsetting traumatic event (not limited to domestic violence experiences). It was then determined which women with lifetime PTSD have symptoms that persist into the past 12 months. To reduce the number of predictor variables, we created one variable indicating the presence of any mental health disorder in the past 12 months (i.e., MDE, GAD, or PTSD) and another variable indicating the presence of substance dependence (i.e., ADP or DDP).

Mastery. Mothers' mastery is assessed with the Pearlin Mastery scale (Pearlin, Menaghan, Lieberman, & Mullan, 1981), a seven-item summary scale ($\alpha = .74$) that measures the extent to which mothers report feeling efficacious and in control of their life. Representative items include "I can do anything I set my mind to," and "What happens in the future depends on me." Items are scored on a four-point scale where "1" indicates "strongly disagree" and "4" indicates "strongly agree" with each statement. The theoretical range of the scale is from 7 to 28 and higher scores indicate greater mastery.

Parenting Stress. The parenting stress scale is an 8-item index that measures the degree of stress or irritation the mother perceives in relation to her interactions with her child. This scale explores mothers' subjective sense of difficulty specifically with regard to the parenting role and has been related to child maltreatment. Items for this scale were taken from or adapted from Abidin's Parenting Stress Index (PSI; Abidin, 1983) and from the New Chance Study of disadvantaged young mothers (Morrison, Zaslow, & Dion, 1998). A sample item is "I find that being a mother is much more work than pleasure." Items are measured on a 5-point scale and are coded such that 1 = "never" and 5 = "almost always." The theoretical range of the scale is from 8 to 40, with higher scores indicating greater parenting stress. Cronbach's alpha for this scale was .75.

Maternal Emotional Warmth. This three-item maternal report captures the extent to which mothers (a) praise their children, (b) do something special with them, and (c) play games, hobbies, or sports together. Maternal warmth is associated with teacher ratings of fewer behavior problems as well as greater social competence in young elementary school children. It is also an important protective factor in diminishing the likelihood of later psychopathology (Morrison et al., 1998). The three items, developed for the present study, were based on items used in the New Chance study (Morrison et al., 1998) and Block's Child Rearing Practices Report (CRPR; Block, 1965). Items are measured on a five-point scale with 1 = "never" and 5 = "every day." The scale has a theoretical range of 3 to 15, with higher scores indicating warmer and

more positive parent-child interactions. Cronbach's alpha for the entire sample for this scale was .61.
Maternal Punitive Discipline. This three-item summary measure assesses the extent to which mothers report (a) yelling, (b) threatening to spank, and (c) spanking their children as a means of discipline. These types of discipline strategies predict children's social competence with peers in childhood and adolescence (Maccoby & Martin, 1983). These items were created for the present study. Items were measured on a three-point scale with 1 = "never" and 3 = "often." The scale has a theoretical range of three to nine and higher scores indicate more punitive discipline behaviors. Cronbach's alpha for this scale for the entire sample was .56. Maternal warmth and maternal punitive discipline were not highly correlated with each other ($r = -.14, p < .01$).

Criterion Variables

Children's adjustment was assessed with maternal reports of children's behavior. The survey contained a subset of items based on the Behavioral Problems Index (BPI) described in Chase-Lansdale, Mott, Brooks-Gunn, and Phillips (1991) and the Adaptive Social Behavior Index (ASBI; Hogan, Scott, & Bauer, 1992). Identical or similar items have been used in other studies of low-income children (Hogan et al., 1992). Unfortunately, due to space constraints, the survey did not include the entire 28-item BPI (itself based on the longer Child Behavior Checklist; Achenbach & Edelbrock, 1983). However, principal components factor analysis with varimax rotation revealed the presence of two underlying factors reflective of what Achenbach and Edelbrock (1983) term "internalizing" and "externalizing" behavioral syndromes.

The 10-item externalizing behaviors scale ($\alpha = .82$) is characterized by disobedience, defiance, and aggressiveness. For example, it measures the extent to which children follow family rules, cooperate, share toys or possessions, or bully or are cruel to others. Items were coded such that 1 = "never" and 3 = "often." The scale has a theoretical range of 10 to 30 and higher scores indicate more externalizing behavior. The 5-item internalizing scale ($\alpha = .76$) measures the extent to which children, for example, feel that no one loves them, are withdrawn, or are unhappy, sad, or depressed. Items were coded such that 1 = "not true of child" and 3 = "often true of child." The scale has a theoretical range of 5 to 15, with higher scores indicating greater internalizing behaviors. The two children's outcome measures are moderately correlated with each other ($r = .55; p < .01$).

RESULTS

Descriptive Statistics

Table 1 presents descriptive statistics on all study variables. With respect to the maternal characteristics, about one-third of mothers have at least one mental health disorder and six percent are dependent on drugs or alcohol. Mothers' average scores on the mastery scale are in the upper half of the scale, while average scores on the parenting stress scale are at about the theoretical midpoint. With respect to children's outcomes, on the average mothers reported relatively low levels of both internalizing and externalizing behavior problems. It should be noted that the actual range of internalizing behavior problems reported by mothers is quite limited, although the range of scores on externalizing behavior problems is greater.

Bivariate Analyses. Table 2 presents means and standard deviations of the hypothesized mediators and child outcome variables in each of the three domestic violence categories. Omnibus tests of group differences were conducted using one-way analysis of variance procedures. For all analyses in which the overall F-test was significant, we present the pairs of means that are significantly different at the .05 level, based on the LSD multiple comparison procedure (Klockars & Sax, 1986). These differences are indicated in the far right column. For clarity, the three groups of domestic violence experience are hereafter referred to as "never," "lifetime," and "recent" violence groups.

In general, significant differences reflect expectations based on previous research. Mothers in the never violence group are less likely to have a mental health disorder or be substance dependent than their counterparts with any violence experience. In addition, mothers in the recent violence group are more likely to have a mental health disorder than those in the lifetime violence group. Mothers in the never violence group have lower levels of parenting stress than other mothers. There are no differences among the groups on mastery. With respect to children's outcomes, mothers with recent violence reported more externalizing behavior problems among their children than the never-violence group.

Multiple Regression Analyses

To assess the association of maternal lifetime and recent experiences of violence with children's behavior problems and the association of maternal characteristics with those problems, we conducted

TABLE 1. Descriptive Statistics

Variables	%	M	SD	Min	Max
Maternal Age		29.98	6.57	19.00	54.00
Child Age		5.45	2.12	3.00	10.00
Child Gender (female)	53				
Household Size		3.90	1.48	2.00	11.00
Income-to-Needs Ratio		0.93	0.55	.05	4.28
Parenting Stress		22.06	5.70	8.00	39.00
Mastery		21.82	3.14	14.00	28.00
Emotional Warmth		12.19	2.04	4.00	15.00
Punitive Discipline		6.49	1.29	3.00	9.00
Behavior Problems (Internal)		5.73	1.40	5.00	15.00
Behavior Problems (External)		15.93	4.05	10.00	30.00
Mother is Black	55				
Mother is Cohabiting	23				
Less than High School	28				
Employed	64				
Severe Domestic Violence (12 month)	15				
Severe Domestic Violence (Lifetime)	39				
Mother Substance Dependent	06				
Any Mental Health Diagnosis	34				

TABLE 2. Group Differences Among Violence Groups

Mediators	Never		Lifetime		Recent		Significance
	%		%		%		
Mother Substance Dependent	3.30		6.30		12.10		b**
Any Mental Health Diagnosis	20.30		41.70		60.60		a***, b***, c**
	Mean	SD	Mean	SD	Mean	SD	
Parenting Stress	20.80	5.36	23.00	5.61	23.74	6.17	a***, b***
Mastery	22.10	3.12	21 71	3.25	21.27	2.87	
Emotional Warmth	12.33	2.13	12.11	1.96	12.00	1.97	
Punitive Discipline	6.34	1.24	6.60	1.33	6.68	1.29	
Child Behavior Outcomes							
Behavior Problems (Internal)	5.60	1.27	5.32	1.51	5.90	1.47	
Behavior Problems (External)	15.35	3.71	16.04	4.17	17.54	4.40	b***

* $p < .05$ ** $p < .01$ *** $p < .001$
Notes to table:
a = "never" significantly different from "lifetime"
b = "never" significantly different from "recent"
c = "lifetime" significantly different from "recent"

89

pre-planned hierarchical regression analyses. We include all the hypothesized control variable and mediators in the regression (see Table 3), despite the bivariate results that indicate that some (notably parenting practices and mastery) are not associated with domestic violence. These maternal variables and other control variables may account for child outcomes. In Step 1 of each model, we entered the set of demographic control variables and the two violence variables to assess their association with children's outcomes. In Step 2 we entered the maternal psychological well-being and parenting characteristics. Finally, we entered interaction terms to see if the associations of domestic violence and children's behavior differ for boys and girls, and for preschoolers relative to school-age children. We were particularly interested in the change in strength of the association between the violence variables and children's behavioral adjustment once maternal characteristics and parenting were included in the model.

Externalizing Behavior Problems. Results for this analysis are presented in Table 4. In Step 1, only the coefficient for recent violence variable was significant; as expected, mothers who had experienced domestic violence in the past 12 months reported significantly higher levels of externalizing behavior problems with their children. Adding the maternal characteristics and parenting at Step 2 further improved the model. The significant variables in this group were parenting stress, mastery and maternal warmth, and punitive discipline. Mothers who reported lower levels of parenting stress and higher levels of mastery reported that their children had significantly lower levels of externalizing behavior problems. Likewise, those with higher levels of warmth and lower levels of punitive discipline reported lower levels of externalizing behavior problems. The coefficient for recent violence remained significant in the final model. The gender by recent domestic violence interaction and age by recent domestic violence interactions were not significant. Through all the models, child's age and gender were significantly associated with externalizing behavior problems. Younger children and boys were more likely to have externalizing behavior problems. Mother's education and employment were also significantly associated with externalizing behavior problems. Children of mothers who did not complete high school, and who were not employed had higher levels of externalizing behavior problems.

Internalizing Behavior Problems. Results for this analysis are presented in Table 5. In Step 1, domestic violence variables with the set of control variables did not account for significant variance. When maternal characteristics were added in Step 2, the model was improved and

TABLE 3. Intercorrelations Among Independent Variables

Variable	1	2	3	4	5	6	7	8	9	10	11	12	13	14	15	16	17
1. Recent D.V.	—																
2. Past D.V.	**.33**	—															
3. Mother's Age	-.09	**.12**	—														
4. Child Age	-.05	.03	**.43**	—													
5. Sex of Child	.01	.00	-.00	.04	—												
6. Cohabiting	-.07	.06	-.03	-.02	.03	—											
7. African American	-.07	**-.15**	-.05	-.02	-.01	**-.30**	—										
8. Household Size	-.03	**.10**	.09	-.08	-.06	**.28**	.02	—									
9. Less than High School	-.01	.01	-.04	**-.18**	.03	**-.11**	-.02	**.11**	—								
10. Employed	.00	.02	-.01	**.10**	-.01	-.02	-.01	**-.11**	**-.31**	—							
11. Income-to-Needs	.05	-.01	.01	.05	-.07	**.33**	**-.21**	**-.12**	**-.21**	**.29**	—						
12. Parenting Stress	**.12**	**.13**	.04	.01	.03	.05	-.05	**.10**	-.04	-.07	.08	—					
13. Mastery	-.07	-.03	**-.14**	-.00	-.08	-.07	.10	-.07	**-.17**	**.15**	**.10**	**-.27**	—				
14. Substance Dependent	**.11**	.02	-.01	-.01	.02	.05	-.06	-.00	.09	-.02	.02	**.27**	**-.17**	—			
15. Mental Health Disorder	**.22**	**.14**	.09	-.01	-.04	-.02	-.06	.06	.03	**-.11**	-.05	**.33**	**-.25**	**.23**	—		
16. Emotional Warmth	-.04	-.03	**-.09**	**-.21**	.03	-.05	-.04	-.07	.06	-.06	-.02	**-.26**	**.11**	-.06	-.05	—	
17. Punitive Discipline	.06	.07	**-.17**	**-.23**	**-.13**	-.03	.09	.00	.01	.02	.04	**.31**	-.08	**.14**	**.14**	**-.14**	—

Bold indicates correlation is significant at .05 level or less.

TABLE 4. Hierarchical Regression Analysis for Domestic Violence and Maternal Characterisics Predicting Children's External Behavior Problems (N = 443)

Variable	B	SE B	β
Model 1			
Demographic Controls			
Mother Age	7.64E-03	.03	.01
Child Age	−.32	.10	−.17*
Sex of Child	−.92	.37	−.11*
Cohabiting	.70	.52	.07
African American	4.68E-02	.40	.01
Household Size	−1.8E-02	.14	−.01
Less than High School	.90	.44	.10*
Employed	−1.04	.41	−.12*
Income-to-Needs Ratio	5.36E-04	.39	.00
Violence Experience			
Recent	2.21	.56	.19***
Lifetime	.71	.41	.09

Variable	B	SE B	β
Model 2			
Mother Age	1.20E-02	.03	.02
Child Age	−.30	.09	−.16*
Sex of Child	−.77	.33	−.10*
Cohabiting	.56	.47	.06
African American	−.20	.36	−.03
Household Size	−9.20E-02	.12	−.03
Less than High School	.88	.40	.10*
Employed	−.95	.37	−.11ᐟ
Income-to-Needs Ratio	−.21	.35	−.03
Violence Experience			
Recent	1.48	.52	.13**
Lifetime	.19	.37	.02
Maternal Variables			
Parenting Stress	.13	.03	.19***
Substance Dependence	.86	.75	.05
Mastery	−.13	.06	−.10*
Mental Health Disorder	−.64	.39	−.07
Punitive Discipline	.75	.14	.24***
Emotional Warmth	−.34	.09	−.17***

Note: R^2 = .12 for Step 1, ΔR^2 = .20 for Step 2 (p < .001). In Step 3 Age by Recent Domestic Violence interaction and Gender by Recent Domestic Violence interactions were added. Neither interaction was significant, ΔR^2 = .003 (ns).
*p < .05   **p < .01   ***p < .001

TABLE 5. Hierarchical Regression Analysis for Domestic Violence and Maternal Characterisics Predicting Children's Internal Behavior Problems (N = 443)

Variable	B	SE B	β
Model 1			
Mother Age	1.82E-02	.01	.09
Child Age	3.67E-02	.04	.06
Sex of Child	−7.35E-02	.13	−.03
Cohabiting	.12	.19	.04
African American	3.13E-02	.14	.01
Household Size	1.78E-02	.05	.02
Less than High School	−.10	.16	−.03
Employed	−.42	.15	−.15**
Income-to-Needs Ratio	.11	.14	.04
Vlolence Experience			
Recent	.33	.20	.08
Lifetime	.20	.15	.07
Variable	B	SE B	β
Model 2			
Mother Age	1.64E-02	.01	.08
Child Age	5.42E-02	.03	.08
Sex of Child	−4.10E-02	.13	−.02
Cohabiting	5.00E-02	.18	.02
African American	−6.55E-03	.14	−.00
Household Size	1.05E-02	.05	.01
Less than High School	−.18	.15	−.06
Employed	−.38	.14	−.13**
Income-to-Needs Ratio	8.78E-02	.13	.03
Violence Experience			
Recent	4.88E-02	.20	.01
Lifetime	3.94E-02	.14	.01
Maternal Variables			
Parenting Stress	2.04E-02	.01	.08
Substance Dependence	.80	.28	.13**
Mastery	−6.36E-02	.02	−.14**
Mental Health Disorder	−7.10E-04	.15	.00
Punitive Discipline	.22	.05	.20***
Emotional Warmth	−4.37E-02	.03	−.06

Note: R^2 = .04 for Step 1 ($p < .001$), ΔR^2 = .13 for Step 2 ($p < .001$). In Step 3, Age by Recent Domestic Violence interaction and Gender by Recent Domestic Violence interactions were added. Neither interaction was significant, ΔR^2 = .004 (*ns*).
*$p < .05$ **$p < .01$ ***$p < .001$

indicated that mothers who reported less mastery, had a substance abuse problem, and used more punitive discipline reported significantly higher levels of internalizing behavior problems with their children. In contrast to the regression predicting externalizing problems, the only control variable that remained significant in the models was maternal employment. Employed mothers reported lower levels of internalizing behavior problems for their children. Age and gender of the child were not significantly associated with internalizing problems, nor were the interactions of gender or age by recent violence.

DISCUSSION

Mothers' recent experiences of domestic violence are associated with their children's externalizing behavior problems. Domestic violence was not associated with mothers' reports of children's internalizing behavior problems. Lifetime violence was not associated with reports of children's behavior problems. Overall, these results support previous studies that have shown that domestic violence can have a deleterious effect on children's behavior. Notably, this study finds support for the harmful effects of domestic violence in a community sample of non-service seeking women.

While boys were more likely to have externalizing problems, we did not find a significant gender by violence interaction. Previous research has been equivocal about differential effects of domestic violence on children by gender. At this point, our research does not support any interactions of gender and exposure to domestic violence.

Overall, maternal well-being and parenting did account for a substantial proportion of the variance in children's behavior problems. While our results indicate that mothers' well-being and parenting only partially mediate the effects of domestic violence on children's behavior problems, they do indicate that mothers' well-being impacts their children. Therefore, efforts to help mothers become safe from abuse and recover from its traumatic effects would be important for increasing the well-being of their children as well.

These results regarding parenting and child outcomes may shed new light on the relationship between the well-being and parenting practices of battered women and their children's adjustment. We found that parenting stress is associated with externalizing behavior problems of children but we did not find similar results for internalizing problems. It is possible that children with greater levels of problem behavior pose a greater challenge to mothers, leading to higher levels of parenting stress. Women experiencing domestic violence had higher levels of parenting stress than those who did not and parenting stress partially mediated the association of recent violence and externalizing problems of children. This finding is consistent with Graham-Bermann and Levendosky (1998) who found that domestic violence (as a continuous variable) was significantly related to parenting stress. Sullivan et al. (2000b) conducted a path analysis that revealed that although abuse did not directly increase mothers' parenting stress, the abuse towards mothers directly increased children's level of behavior problems, which in turn increased mothers' parenting stress.

Although mothers experiencing domestic violence reported greater parenting stress, they were not more likely to use harsh punitive discipline on their children. They did not differ from non-abused mothers on levels of emotional warmth towards their children. This also supports the work of Sullivan and her colleagues (2000b), who found that mothers who had a history of recent domestic violence were emotionally and physically available to their children and used non-corporal punishment more often than corporal punishment. The picture that emerges from our data is that the traumatic effects of violence may be associated with greater stress on mothers, but that this stress is not associated with harsher treatment or less warmth towards their children. Our findings also may suggest that children's exposure to violence against their mothers may have a direct adverse impact on their behavioral adjustment, which may in turn lead to greater maternal stress. Future research should develop and test models that examine the complex mechanisms by which children can be impacted by domestic violence and how these impacts can be shaped by and shape their relationships with their mothers. Longitudinal data will be particularly helpful in examining these issues. Furthermore, future studies should explore the ways in which battered women mobilize internal and external resources to care for their children, despite the trauma and stress they experience.

We did not find, as hypothesized, an association of domestic violence and children's internalizing problems. As mentioned above, the internalizing measure had limited variation in the sample and may not have been sensitive to differences. However, the literature to date has shown inconsistent findings for the effects of domestic violence on internalizing behaviors. For example, Sternberg and colleagues (1993) also found no link between domestic violence and internalizing problems. It is also possible that shelter samples may differ from community samples in terms of the level of internalizing problems children exhibit.

Our sample was drawn from women who had recently received welfare benefits. Changes in the welfare system have drawn attention to domestic violence within this population. In 1996, the Personal Responsibility and Work Opportunity Reconciliation Act (PRWORA) was passed, making several notable changes in welfare. Specifically, lifetime time-limits on welfare receipt were imposed, rapid engagement in paid labor was mandated, and the federal entitlement to welfare benefits for those in need was rescinded. The Family Violence Option, an amendment to PRWORA which has been adopted in almost every state, encourages states to screen and identify battered women on welfare caseloads and to assist battered women by providing services and exemptions from some of the requirements imposed by the new welfare law. Our results would support efforts to screen for and identify domestic violence within the welfare system as a way of potentially benefiting children living in families where domestic violence occurs. If such identification leads to effective help for abused mothers and their children rather than punitive sanctions, then children may be benefited by the effort. Further, our finding of behavioral effects of domestic violence in a non-service seeking community sample supports community prevention and early intervention efforts. Many children affected by domestic violence are not likely to be provided services through the formal help-seeking of their mothers (see DeVoe & Smith, 2003). Therefore, efforts to identify and assist children in other settings can broaden the potential for help for those impacted by domestic violence.

As mentioned previously, a limitation of this study is that information on the male partners of these mothers was not gathered; as such, it is important to note that mothers' current male partners or spouses may not be the same males who perpetrated the recent abuse. Future research should be directed at understanding the ways that these men and their behavior might be associated with children's adjustment. This issue is particularly important because focusing on maternal characteristics alone can inadvertently support a view that mothers alone are responsible for the behavior of their children. While our data support the importance of maternal well-being for understanding children's emotional and behavioral outcomes, the impact of paternal or male caregivers is critical to development of more complete models. Sullivan, Juras, Bybee, Nguyen, and Allen (2000a), for example, found that the adjustment of children of abused mothers depended on the abuser's biological relationship to the child. Abusers who were the children's biological fathers or father figures were significantly more abusive to the mothers than were non-father figures. Similarly, children whose fathers were the abusers witnessed more violence than did children whose mothers' assailants were non-father figures. Accordingly, children whose mothers' assailants were not fathers or father figures showed significantly higher levels of social competency, scholastic competency, and feelings of self-worth.

The differences in results observed for the different referent periods point out the importance of measuring multiple time periods when violence might have occurred. Given that mothers' experiences of violence do not appear to be associated with children's behavior via maternal psychological characteristics and parenting behaviors, it is not surprising that lifetime violence was not significantly associated with children's behavior problems. Rather, it is possible that violence is associated with children's behavior via concurrent events, perhaps by children's identifying with the mood of their parents, being abused themselves, or being affected by related ongoing stressors and disruptions. Given these findings on the relevance of referent period, it would be important for future studies to gather even more detail in this regard.

Given that our sample is drawn from an exclusively low-income sample, it is possible that differences between the groups experiencing domestic violence and those that do not are diminished by the presence of high rates of external stressors that families in poverty experience. In other words, the effect size for the relationship between child outcomes and domestic violence may be somewhat more constricted in this sample than in the general population.

The present study is among the few that have examined the effects of domestic violence on children drawn exclusively from the community and that used a random sample. Previous studies, focusing primarily on shelter samples, might be expected to have larger effect sizes, given that mothers who use shelters are likely to experience high levels of repeated severe violence and their children are almost certain to be made aware of the violence. At the same time, while our sample for the most part did not seek shelter in response to violence, three-quarters of the victims of recent violence had sought help of some sort in the previous year. Help-seeking actions among this group included calling the police, seeking medical help for injuries, and getting a protection order (data not reported here). We can be relatively certain, therefore, that many of the children whose mothers experienced domestic violence in the past 12 months were exposed in some way to the violence, the conflict surrounding it, or to its impact on their mothers. Nevertheless, it is clearly important for future studies to gather information regarding whether children were witnesses to the violence when it occurred.

REFERENCES

Abidin, R. R. (1983). *Parenting Stress Index–Manual*. Charlottesville, VA: Pediatric Psychology Press.

Achenbach, T., & Edelbrock, C. (1983). *Manual for the child behavior checklist and revised child behavior profile*. Burlington, VT: University of Vermont.

Appel, A. E., & Holden, G. W. (1998). The co-occurrence of spouse and physical child abuse: A review and appraisal. *Journal of Family Psychology, 12*, 578-599.

Bassuk, E., Weinreb, L., Buckner, J., Browne, A., Salomon, A., & Bassuk. S. (1996). The characteristics and needs of sheltered homeless and low-income housed mothers. *The Journal of the American Medical Association, 276*, 640-646.

Block, J. H. (1965). *The Child-Rearing Practices Report (CRPR): A set of Q items for the description of parental socialization attitudes and values*. Berkeley, CA: University of California, Institute of Human Development.

Chase-Lansdale, P. L., Mott, F. L., Brooks-Gunn, J., & Phillips, D. A. (1991). Children of the National Longitudinal Survey of Youth: A unique research opportunity. *Developmental Psychology, 27*, 918-931.

Chodorow, N. J. (1991). *Feminism and psychoanalytic theory*. London: Yale University Press.

Conger, R. D., Ge, X., Elder, G. H., Lorenz, F. O., & Simons, R. (1994). Economic stress, coercive family process, and developmental problems of adolescents. *Child Development: Special Issue: Children and poverty, 65*, 541-561.

Cummings, J. G., Pepler, D. J., & Moore, T. E. (1999). Behavior problems in children exposed to wife abuse: Gender differences. *Journal of Family Violence, 14*, 133-156.

Danziger, S., Corcoran, M., Danziger, S., Heflin, C., Kalil, A., Levine, J., Rosen, D., Seefeldt, K., Siefert, K., & Tolman, R. (2000). Barriers to the employment of welfare recipients. In R. Cherry & W. Rodgers (Eds.), *Prosperity for all? The economic boom and African Americans* (pp. 245-278). New York: Russell Sage.

DeVoe, F. R., & Smith, E. L. (2003). Don't take my kids: Barriers to service delivery for battered mothers and their young children. *Journal of Emotional Abuse, 3*(3/4), 277-294.

Edleson, J. L. (1999). Children's witnessing of adult domestic violence. *Journal of Interpersonal Violence, 14*, 839-870.

Fantuzzo, J. W., De Paola, L. M., Lambert, L., Martino, T., Anderson, G., & Sutton, S. (1991). Effects of interparental violence on the psychological adjustment and competencies of young children. *Journal of Consulting and Clinical Psychology, 59*, 258-265.

Fantuzzo, J. W., & Mohr, W. K. (2000). Prevalence and effects of child exposure to domestic violence. *The Future of Children. Domestic Violence and Children, 9*, 21-32.

Graham-Bermann, S. A. (1996). Family worries: Assessment of interpersonal anxiety in children from violent and nonviolent families. *Journal of Clinical Child Psychology, 25*, 280-287.

Graham-Bermann, S. A., & Levendosky, A. A. (1998). The social functioning of preschool-age children whose mothers are emotionally and physically abused. *Journal of Emotional Abuse, 1*, 59-84.

Hogan, A. E., Scott, K. G., & Bauer, C. R. (1992). The Adaptive Social Behavior Inventory (ASBI): A new assessment of social competence in high-risk three-year olds. *Journal of Psychoeducational Assessment, 10,* 230-239.

Holden, G. W., Geffner, R., & Jouriles, E. N. (1998). *Children exposed to marital violence. Theory, research, and applied issues.* Washington, DC: American Psychological Association.

Holden, G. W., & Ritchie, K. L. (1991). Linking extreme marital discord, child rearing, and child behavior problems: Evidence from battered women. *Child Development, 62,* 311-327.

Hughes, H. M. (1988). Psychological and behavioral correlates of family violence in child witnesses and victims. *American Journal of Orthopsychiatry, 58,* 77-90.

Hughes, H. M., Parkinson, D., & Vargo, M. (1989). Witnessing spouse abuse and experiencing physical abuse: A "double whammy"? *Journal of Family Violence, 14,* 197-209.

Kessler, R., Andrews, G., Mroczek, D., Ustun, B., & Wittchen, H. (in press). The World Health Organization Composite International Diagnostic Interview Short-Form (CIDI-SF). *International Journal of Methods in Psychiatric Research.*

Kessler, R., & Mroczek, D. (1993). *Scoring the UM-CIDI short forms.* Unpublished memorandum, University of Michigan: Ann Arbor, MI.

Kessler, R. C., McGonagle, K. A., Zhao, S., Nelson, C. B., Hughes, M., Eshleman, S., Wittchen, H. U., & Kendler, K. S. (1994). Lifetime and 12-month prevalence of DSM-III-R psychiatric disorders in the United States: Results from the National Comorbidity Study. *Archives of General Psychiatry, 51,* 8-19.

Klockars, A. I., & Sax, G. (1986). *Multiple comparisons.* Newbury Park: Sage.

Kolbo, J. R., Blakely, E. H., & Engleman, D. (1996). Children who witness domestic violence: A review of empirical literature. *Journal of Interpersonal Violence, 11,* 281-293.

Lamborn, S. D., Mounts, N. S., Steinberg, L., & Dornbusch, S. M. (1991). Patterns of competence and adjustment among adolescents from authoritative, authoritarian, indulgent, and neglectful families. *Child Development, 62,* 1049-1065.

Levendosky, A. A., & Graham-Bermann, S. A. (1998). The moderating effects of parenting stress on children's adjustment in woman-abusing families. *Journal of Interpersonal Violence, 13,* 383-397.

Maccoby, E. E., & Martin, J. A. (1983). Socialization in the context of the family: Parent-child interaction. In E. M. Hetherington (Ed.), P. H. Mussen (Series Ed.), *Handbook of Child Psychology, Vol. 4. Socialization, Personality, and Social Development.* New York: Wiley.

Margolin, G. (1998). Effects of domestic violence on children. In P. K. Trickett & C. J. Schellenbach (Eds.), *Violence against children in the family and the community* (pp. 57-101). Washington, DC: American Psychological Association.

McLoyd, V. C. (1990). The impact of economic hardship on Black families and children: Psychological distress, parenting, and socioemotional development. *Child Development: Special Issue: Minority children, 61,* 311-346.

Morley, E., & Brennan, E. (1999, March). *No safe refuge: An HBSE module on child witnesses of domestic violence.* Paper presented at the Annual Meeting of the Council on Social Work Education, San Francisco, CA.

Morrison, D., Zaslow, M., & Dion, R. (1998). Completing the portrayal of parenting behavior with interview-based measures. In M. Zaslow & C. Eldred (Eds.), *Parenting behavior in a sample of young mothers in poverty*. New York: Manpower Demonstration Research Corporation.

Osofsky, J. D. (2000). The impact of violence on children. *The Future of Children. Domestic Violence and Children, 9*, 33-49.

Patterson, G. R., DeBaryshe, B. D., & Ramsey, E. (1989). A developmental perspective on antisocial behavior. *American Psychologist: Special Issue: Children and their development: Knowledge base, research agenda, and social policy application, 44*, 329-335.

Pearlin, L. I., Menaghan, E. G., Lieberman, M. A., & Mullan, J. T. (1981). The stress process. *Journal of Health & Social Behavior, 22*, 337-356.

Plichta, S. B. (1996). Violence and abuse: Implications for women's health. In M. M. Falik & K. Scott-Collins (Eds.), *Women's Health: The Commonwealth Fund Survey* (pp. 237-270). Baltimore: Johns Hopkins University Press.

Porter, B., & O'Leary, K. D. (1980). Marital discord and childhood behavior problems. *Journal of Abnormal Child Psychology, 8*, 287-295.

Rutter, M. (1990). Psychosocial resilience and protective mechanisms. In J. E. Rolf, A. S. Masten, D. Cicchetti, K. H. Nuechterlein, & S. Weintraub (Eds.), *Risk and protective factors in the development of psychopathology* (pp. 181-214). New York: Cambridge University Press.

Steinberg, L., Lamborn, S. D., Dornbusch, S. M., & Darling, N. (1992). Impact of parenting practices on adolescent achievement: Authoritative parenting, school involvement, and encouragement to succeed. *Child Development, 63*, 1266-1281.

Sternberg, K. J., Lamb, M. E., Greenbaum, C., Cicchetti, D., Dawud, S., Cortes, R. M., Krispin, O., & Lorey, F. (1993). Effects of domestic violence on children's behavior problems and depression. *Developmental Psychology, 29*, 44-52.

Straus, M. (1992). Children as witnesses to marital violence: A risk factor for lifelong problems among a nationally representative sample of American men and women. *Report of the Twenty-third Ross Roundtable*. Columbus, OH: Ross Laboratories.

Straus, M. A., & Gelles, R. J. (1990). *Physical Violence in American Families: Risk Factors and Adaptations to Violence in 8,145 Families*. New Brunswick, NJ: Transaction Books.

Sullivan, C. M., Juras, J., Bybee, D., Nguyen, H., & Allen, N. (2000a). How children's relationship to their mother's abuser affects their adjustment. *Journal of Interpersonal Violence, 15*, 587-602.

Sullivan, C. M., Nguyen, H., Allen, N., Bybee, D., & Juras, J. (2000b). Beyond searching for deficits: Evidence that battered women are nurturing parents. *Journal of Emotional Abuse, 2*(1), 51-72.

Thompson, R. A. (1998). Early sociopersonality development. In W. Damon (Series Ed.) & N. Eisenberg (Vol. Ed.) *Handbook of child psychology: Vol. 3. Social, emotional, and personality development* (5th ed., pp. 25-104). New York: J. Wiley.

Tolman, R. M., & Rosen, D. (2001). Domestic violence in the lives of women receiving welfare: Health, mental health and well-being. *Violence Against Women, 7*(2), 126-140.

Winstok, Z., & Eisikovits, Z. (2003). Divorcing the parents: The impact of adolescents' exposure to father-to-mother aggression on their perceptions of affinity with their parents. *Journal of Emotional Abuse, 3*(1/2), 103-121.

Wolfe, D. A., Jaffe, P., Wilson, S. K., & Zak, L. (1985). Children of battered women: The relation of child behavior to family violence and maternal stress. *Journal of Consulting and Clinical Psychology, 53*, 657-665.

Zahn-Waxler, C. (1993). Warriors and worriers: Gender and psychopathology. *Development and Psychopathology: Special Issue: Toward a developmental perspective on conduct disorder, 5*, 79-89.

Zaslow, M. J. (1988). Sex differences in children's response to parental divorce. I. Research methodology and postdivorce family forms. *American Journal of Orthopsychiatry, 58*, 355-378.

Divorcing the Parents:
The Impact of Adolescents' Exposure
to Father-to-Mother Aggression
on Their Perceptions of Affinity
with Their Parents

Zeev Winstok
Zvi Eisikovits

SUMMARY. This study explores the impact of adolescents' exposure to father-to-mother aggression on their perceptions of affinity with their parents, using a probability sample of 1,014 Jewish Israeli youth between the ages of 13-18 years. It was hypothesized that adolescents' exposure to interparental violence reduces affinity, a notion that may explain one link between exposure to interparental violence and adolescent development. We theorized that when the affinity between adolescents and their parents decreases, the role of the latter as a developmental resource will be diminished. It was assumed that affinity is represented by two factors: parent-adolescent closeness and resemblance. Findings demonstrated a negative correlation between father-to-mother aggression

Address correspondence to Zeev Winstok, PhD, Minerva Center for Youth Studies, University of Haifa, Mount Carmel, Haifa 31905, Israel (E-mail: zeevwin@ research.haifa.ac.il).

[Haworth co-indexing entry note]: "Divorcing the Parents: The Impact of Adolescents' Exposure to Father-to-Mother Aggression on Their Perceptions of Affinity with Their Parents." Winstok, Zeev, and Zvi Eisikovits. Co-published simultaneously in *Journal of Emotional Abuse* (The Haworth Maltreatment & Trauma Press, an imprint of The Haworth Press, Inc.) Vol. 3, No. 1/2, 2003, pp. 103-121; and: *The Effects of Intimate Partner Violence on Children* (ed: Robert A. Geffner, Robyn Spurling Igelman, and Jennifer Zellner) The Haworth Maltreatment & Trauma Press, an imprint of The Haworth Press, Inc., 2003, pp. 103-121. Single or multiple copies of this article are available for a fee from The Haworth Document Delivery Service [1-800-HAWORTH, 9:00 a.m. - 5:00 p.m. (EST). E-mail address: docdelivery@haworthpress.com].

10.1300J135v03n01_05

and adolescents' perceptions of affinity with their family, so that as aggression increased, affinity decreased. Interparental aggression was found to have a significant and direct negative impact on closeness. Its impact on resemblance was negative and mediated by closeness. The theoretical and practical implications of these findings are discussed in terms of developmental resources and opportunities. *[Article copies available for a fee from The Haworth Document Delivery Service: 1-800-HAWORTH. E-mail address: <docdelivery@haworthpress.com> Website: <http://www.HaworthPress.com> © 2003 by The Haworth Press, Inc. All rights reserved.]*

KEYWORDS. Child and adolescent witnessing interparental violence, violence against women, parent-adolescent relationships, conflicts in intimate relationships, developmental risk factors

INTRODUCTION

Adolescents, more than any other age group, are preoccupied with identity construction in terms of who they are and where their place is in the world (Brown, Dykers, Steele, & White, 1994; Josselson, 1987; Markus & Nurius, 1986; Rosenberg, 1989; Snow & Anderson, 1987). The process of identity construction shapes and represents their experience both within and outside their family (Mahabeer, 1993; Osborne, 1996; Tomori, 1994). During childhood, the parents' contribution to image development is central and almost exclusive (Osborne, 1996). As children grow older, they are increasingly exposed to extra-familial influences. Yet, family members in general, and parents in particular, remain highly influential on their development, and serve as an important source of strength, support and belonging. This is especially so during the period of adolescence (Becker, 1992; Dacey & Kenny, 1997; Dunlop, Burns, & Bermingham, 2001; Erikson, 1965, 1968; Gecas, 1971; Hunter, 1984; Schave & Schave, 1989; Thomas, Gecas, Weigert, & Rooney, 1974; Tomori, 1994). As such, the home environment can be seen as a launching pad from which adolescents take off, and to which they return (Eisikovits, Winstok, & Enosh, 1998).

There are significant differences between the experiences of children and adolescents who live in families with physical and/or psychological aggression, and those who live in a non-aggressive family environment (Eisikovits, Winstok, & Enosh, 1998). Such experiences have a formative influence on the ways in which they perceive their relationship with their parents. Yet, the influence of interparental violence on the relationship between parents and their adolescent children has received only scant research attention (Goldblatt, 2001a, 2001b; Holden, Geffner, & Jouriles, 1998). This is especially conspicuous in view of the extensive literature on the critical effect of the parent-child relationship on adolescent development (e.g., Grotevant & Cooper, 1986; Henry, Sagar, & Plunkett, 1996; Laible, Carlo, & Raffaelli, 2000; Peterson & Leigh, 1990; Silverberg & Gondoli, 1996).

The aim of this study was to explore the impact of adolescents' exposure to father-to-mother aggression on their perceptions of affinity with their parents. It may be assumed that from the adolescents' viewpoint, parents involved in escalatory conflicts cannot provide them with the necessary developmental resources, such as supervision and support. Accordingly, in such situations the interpersonal distance between adolescents and their parents may widen beyond normatively acceptable boundaries. This dynamic may prove to be one of the missing links between interparental violence and adolescent development. It should be emphasized, however, that such distancing might be socially and culturally dependent (Triandis, McCusker, & Hui, 1990).

There is growing evidence that a large number of children are negatively affected by interparental violence, and that such exposure carries severe physical, cognitive, emotional, and behavioral consequences. These include emotional distress, such as anxiety, depression, mood swings, post-traumatic reactions, and suicidal thoughts (Anderson & Cramer-Benjamin, 1999; Cantrell, MacIntyre, Sharkey, & Thompson, 1995; Davies & Windle, 1997; Silva, Alpert, Monuz, Matzner, & Dummit, 2000); reduced social and academic competence (Davis & Carlson, 1987; Walter, Trainham, & LeDoux, 1997); aggression and other behavior problems, such as running away and alcohol abuse (Downs, Smyth, & Miller, 1996; Martin, Sigda, & Kupersmidt, 1998; O'Keefe, 1996); and a range of violent expressions toward parents (Brezina, 1999; Feindler & Becker, 1996; Micucci, 1995), including parricide (Berliner, 1993; Heide, 1993; Hillbrand, Alexandre, Young, & Spitz, 1999; Mones, 1993).

There are recent studies indicating that the development of some children who live in a violent interparental reality remains unharmed (Beeman, 2001; Goldblatt, 2001a, 2001b; Hughes, Graham-Bermann, & Gruber, 2001; Osofsky, 1999). These findings demonstrate that the implications of children's and adolescents' exposure to interparental violence are non-deterministic. Thus, it may be assumed that the familial context affects child and adolescent development and influences how they experience interparental violence.

Most studies on the impact of interparental violence on children have employed a fairly narrow theoretical framework, despite the fact that theoretical formulations using a wide yet integrative approach have been suggested in this field. For instance, Grych and Fincham (1990) proposed a conceptualization of the cognitive-contextual processing of marital conflict by children. Their model was composed of marital conflict variables, contextual variables, primary and secondary cognitive processes, coping behavior, and affect. However the model was not specifically designed for understanding children's experience of interparental violence. Similarly, Cummings (1998) suggested a conceptualization of children's adjustment to interparental conflict in terms of "emotional security" as articulated by emotion regulation, internal representation of family relations, and regulation of exposure to family affect. Graham-Berman (1998) proposed an expanded conceptual model based on factors influencing the adjustment of children exposed to domestic violence, including maternal stress and mental health, positive and negative social networks, and child adjustment. These conceptualizations broaden our understanding of the interrelationships among variables in the family ecology and conflict or violence, as well as the ways in which children's construction of meaning is affected by their cognitive and emotional reactions to the conflicts.

What is unique about interparental relationships in which conflicts escalate to violence? In these relationships, the ontological basis of the couple as a collective entity is gradually eroded. As such, the sense of "we-ness" is substituted by mutual antagonism. Through intimate violence, the partners come to define each other as enemies, living in a state of varying degrees of hostility towards each other (Gergen, 1994). Children and adolescents in such situations learn about themselves and their environment through hostility and conflict, rather than through harmony and intimacy, and must mobilize their resources accordingly in an attempt to make their lives tolerable and livable. In line with the rigid, black-and-white worldview that they may develop, they may also come to see people as divided into winners and losers, perpetrators and victims, predators and prey. Intimacy and closeness are thereby redefined as dangerous (Eisikovits & Winstok, 2001; Eisikovits et al., 1998).

Previous research dealing with the experience of such children and adolescents focused on violent events as the topic under scrutiny. We argue that throughout the process of reality construction (i.e., children's and adolescents' attempts to understand what happened, why, and what it means), their perceptions and relationships with family members are reshaped. Therefore, studying how these children and adolescents perceive their relationships with their parents seems promising, not only for the understanding of their experience but also for understanding its influence on their development.

A recent study on the subject (Winstok, Eisikovits, & Karniely-Miller, 2002) explored the differential influence of the father's level of aggression towards the mother on adolescents' perceptions of their parents and of themselves, and how these perceptions are interrelated. The findings showed that adolescents held a coherent image of family members in those families where conflicts were resolved non-aggressively. However, with the emergence of and increase in aggression, this sense of coherence deteriorated. In cases of mild aggression, adolescents tended to identify with their fathers, whereas in cases of severe aggression, the adolescents tended to identify more with the victim. These findings are supported by additional studies (Goldblatt, 2001a, 2001b; Peled, 1997).

Based on the recent studies discussed above, we theorized that interparental violence affects the affinity between adolescents and their parents such that the more severe and frequent the violence, the weaker the affinity. This affinity is articulated by closeness and resemblance which taken together, represent the adolescents' extent of physical and psychological affinity with their family of origin. Although we recognize that a weaker affinity between adolescents and their parents may have far-reaching effects on their development, this is not the focus of the present study. Here we explore the assumption that interparental violence distances the adolescent from the family. This notion may provide one link between exposure to interparental violence and development. Based on the previously mentioned literature on the relationships between adolescents and their parents we assume that affinity (closeness and resemblance) serves to channel the resources to be used by the adolescent during development. When the affinity between adolescents and their parents decreases, the role of the latter as a developmental resource is diminished. As a result the adolescent turns to alternative resources, which then increases developmental risks (Erikson, 1968). Figure 1 heuristically describes the proposed model. It emphasizes the direct negative impact of interparental violence on closeness and the indirect negative impact on resemblance.

The present study explores the following hypotheses: (1) a negative correlation will be found between the level of father-to-mother aggression and the adolescent's perception of closeness to the parents. That is, the higher the aggression level, the greater the distance of the adolescent

FIGURE 1. Proposed Model of the Impact of Interparental Violence on Closeness and Resemblance

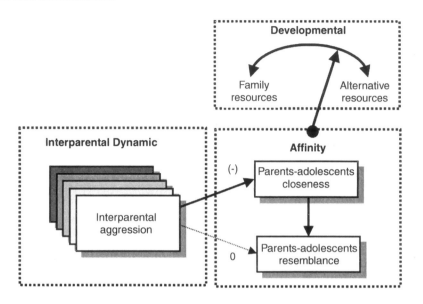

from his/her parents. (2) The relationship between the level of father-to-mother aggression and the adolescent's perception of resemblance to each parent will be positively mediated by the adolescent's perception of closeness to the parents. In other words, closeness mediates the relationship between aggression and resemblance. (3) There will be a positive correlation found between closeness and resemblance. That is, the higher the adolescent's perception of closeness, the greater the perception of resemblance to his/her parents.

METHOD

Participants

The sample was originally comprised of 68 neighborhoods (56 Jewish and 12 Arab), which were randomly selected from the list of the Central Bureau of Statistics utilizing special computer software. Each neighborhood's probability of being included in the sample depended on the number of adolescents in the age group of 13-18 years living in the neighborhood. Two ultra-orthodox Jewish neighborhoods were eliminated from the sample, due to lack of willingness of the interviewees to cooperate. Therefore, the final sample consisted of 54 Jewish and 12 Arab neighborhoods, in which a random sampling of streets and house numbers was performed for each neighborhood.

Interviews were conducted with 19 adolescents in each Jewish neighborhood and 20 adolescents in each Arab neighborhood. About 75% of the 1,700 adolescents who were asked to participate in the study cooperated. The sample consisted of 1,273 participants, including 1,038 Jewish and 231 Arab youths. The Israeli population is composed of two major groups: Jews who make up the majority (80%), and Arabs who are divided among several religious groups: Moslems (75%), Christians (16%), and others (9%) (Smooha, 1993). It is widely accepted that Jewish secular families in Israel maintain Western values (Lavee & Katz, 2002), while Arab families in general and Moslems in particular retain traditional ones (Al-Haj, 1989, 1991). Given the above, we opted for a homogeneous sample in the present study and decided to address the Jewish youths only.

The final study sample consisted of 1,014 Jewish youths, after 24 questionnaires were disqualified due to inconsistencies in participants' answers. The sample consisted of 49% males and 51% females. The average age was 16 years ($SD = 1.4$), with 36% of the sample comprised of adolescents between the ages of 13-15 years, and 64% between the ages of 16-18 years.

Measures

The instrument administered to participants was a structured self-report questionnaire, originally designed to measure a wide range of attitudes in various aspects of adolescents' lives (Sherer, Karniely-Miller, Eisikovits, & Fishman, 2001). Five items from the instrument were identified as proxy measures for the three constructs derived from the previously described conceptual framework. They were phrased in a simple and straightforward manner. Both the structural equation modeling and the clustering statistics used in this study provide support for the validity and reliability of the measures.

Aggression. Two questions were asked to measure adolescents' perceptions of the frequency of their father's physical/verbal aggression towards their mother. The first referred to verbal aggression: "During the last year, did your father yell at, curse, insult, or threaten your mother?" The second item was related to physical aggression: "During the last year, did your father hit, shove, slap, punch, or kick your mother?" The answers were scored on a 4-point scale, as follows:

(1) did not happen at all; (2) I don't know; (3) seldom; (4) often. The questions were phrased using content categories from the Conflict Tactics Scale (Straus, Hamby, Boney-McCoy, & Sugarman, 1996). The two questions were positively correlated ($r = .6$), supporting the assumption that both represent the same underlying construct of aggression, or that those who are physically aggressive are also likely to be verbally aggressive (Straus et al., 1996). The rates of aggression reported in this study were similar to those reported by the National Survey of Domestic Violence in Israel conducted during the same year (Fishman, Eisikovits, Mesch, & Gusinsky, 2001).

Closeness. Two questions were asked to measure adolescents' perceptions of their closeness to their parents. The first question was: "How close would you like to be to your parents?" The answers were scored on the following 3-point scale: (1) I would not like to be close to either of my parents; (2) I would rather be close to one of my parents (father or mother); (3) I would rather be close to both of my parents. The second question was: "How close do you think your parents would like to be to you?" The answers to this question were also scored on a 3-point scale: (1) Neither of my parents would like to be close to me; (2) One of my parents would like to be close to me; (3) Both of my parents would like to be close to me. The two questions were positively correlated ($r = .5$), supporting the assumption that both represent the same underlying construct of closeness.

Resemblance. One question was asked to measure adolescents' perceptions of their resemblance to their parents: "Who of your parents do you resemble in personality?" The answers were scored on a 3-point scale: (1) I do not resemble any of my parents in personality; (2) I resemble one of my parents in personality (my father or my mother); (3) I resemble both of my parents in personality.

Procedure

The University Research Ethics Committee authorized the protocol for the interviews and procedures to secure informed consent. The interviewers were undergraduate social work students who were trained both individually and in small groups. The training included a detailed explanation of the content and form of the instrument and sampling procedures as well as contact and process information. They were blind to the hypotheses of the study. The interviewers were instructed to obtain informed consent from the participants. Incentives such as movie tickets were distributed among the youths that participated in recognition of their time spent with the interviewers. The interviewers offered help in cases where the adolescent encountered difficulties in completing the questionnaire, such as understanding the questions, answers, and method of marking the answers. The study was conducted over a period of six months.

RESULTS

Descriptive Statistics

When examining the descriptive statistics on perceived exposure to father-to-mother aggression, we found that 27% of the adolescents did not know whether their father verbally abused their mother (could not deny or confirm verbal aggression). Only 7% of the adolescents took this position regarding their father's physical aggression. Among those who confirmed their father's physical aggression towards their mother, 87% responded similarly when asked about verbal aggression. Only 1% of those who denied verbal aggression did not deny the use of physical aggression. Regarding the existence of verbal aggression, 7% did not deny or confirm it, whereas this was so in only 3% of the cases for physical aggression. We also examined the relations between age, gender, and verbal and physical aggression, and found no significant correlations between these variables.

When examining the descriptive statistics on adolescents' perceptions of closeness, we found that 64% wanted to be close to their parents and 60% thought that their parents wanted to be close to them. Regarding adolescents' perceptions of resemblance, only 36% felt that they resembled both parents.

Structural Equation Model

Structural equation models (SEMs) represent a general approach to the statistical examination of how theoretical models fit empirical data. SEMs with latent variables, as used in this study, embody simultaneous equations with multiple exogenous and endogenous variables (path analysis), along with measurement error models (confirmatory factor analysis).

Preparation for CFA Analysis. The measurement level of the research model indicators is ordinal (3 or 4 levels). Some problems may arise when non-continuous variables are analyzed with CFA (Kline,

1998). One of the options for overcoming these problems is to use a special statistical procedure to correct the observed covariance prior to CFA analysis (e.g., Bollen, 1989). In the present study, PRELIS2 (Joreskog & Sorbom, 1996) was used to prepare a corrected covariance matrix for non-continuous variables. An SEM analysis was conducted using the AMOS program (Arbuckle, 1999), based on this corrected covariance matrix.

First, the model was tested without posing any constraint. This model yielded a significant chi-square statistic: $\chi^2(3, N = 950) = 13.90$, $p = .003$. However, the significance may have been due to the large sample size. In such cases, the fit indices may offer a more reasonable estimation of the fit of the model (Kaplan, 1990; MacCallum, 1990; MacCallum, Browne, & Sugawara, 1996; Sugawara & MacCallum, 1993). The fit indices suggested that the model fit the data very well: NFI = .98; RFI = .93; CFI = .99; RMSEA = .06.

Second, the path between aggression and resemblance was constrained to "0." This model yielded a significant chi-square statistic as well: $\chi^2(4, N = 950) = 15.88$; $p = .003$, which again was likely due to the large sample size. Here, too, the fit indices suggested that the model fit the data very well: NFI = .98; RFI = .93; CFI = .99; RMSEA = .06. As demonstrated, the constraint did not produce a significant change ($\Delta\chi^2 = 2 \Delta$, df = 1), indicating that aggression does not influence resemblance directly.

Findings indicate that the factor loadings (standardized regression weights) of father-to mother aggression, represented by verbal and physical aggression, and parent-adolescent closeness, represented by adolescent to parents and parents to adolescent closeness were adequate ($\beta > 0.6$). Father-to-mother aggression accounted for 60% of the variance in parent-adolescent closeness. Parent-adolescent closeness accounted for 19% of the variance in parent-adolescent resemblance. As previously mentioned, father-to-mother aggression had no direct influence on parent-adolescent resemblance. Figure 2 presents the model and its estimates. In sum, the model supported our assumptions that interparental aggression influences closeness directly and negatively and that its influence on resemblance is negative and fully mediated by closeness.

Clustering. In order to overcome problems that may arise when non-continuous variables are analyzed with CFA, we used a special statistical procedure to correct the observed covariance before they were analyzed. As described, the data fit the model. We used K-means cluster analysis as a way to provide additional support for the research hypoth-

FIGURE 2. Model of Relationship Between Interparental Agression, Closeness, and Resemblance

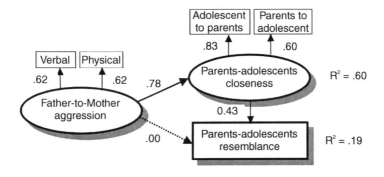

Path between aggression and resemblance was constrained to "0" and did not produce a significant change ($\Delta\chi^2 = 2$ Δdf = 1).
χ^2 (4, $N = 950$) = 15.88, $p = .003$, NFI = .98, RFI = .93, CFI = .99, RMSEA = .06
$p < 0.001$ in all estimates

eses and model. This statistical procedure forms groups with similar characteristics, as based on the "Nearest Centroid Sorting" (Andenberg, 1973). We specified three clusters for all five research variables. Figure 3 summarizes the results. Cluster "a" consists of the largest group, which is characterized by high adolescent-parent affinity and a low level of aggression. Cluster "c" is completely opposite, representing the smallest group and characterized by low adolescent-parent affinity and a high level of aggression. The characteristics of Cluster "b" fall in between clusters "a" and "c."

DISCUSSION

This study demonstrates that adolescents' perceptions of affinity with their family may decrease as father-to-mother aggression increases. Affinity was found to be represented by two factors: parent-adolescent closeness and resemblance. Aggression significantly affected closeness both directly and negatively, while its influence on resemblance was indirect and mediated by closeness. As the father's aggression against the mother became more frequent, closeness between the adolescent and the parents weakened, and resemblance decreased accordingly. There was a significant positive association between closeness and resemblance.

FIGURE 3. Results of K-Means Cluster Analysis

Variables (adolescents' perceptions)	Cluster Centers		
	#a	#b	#c
1 Father-to-mother verbal aggression	1.05	2.95	3.25
2 Father-to-mother physical aggression	1.02	1.05	3.03
3 Adolescents' closeness to their parents	2.32	2.11	1.72
4 Parents' closeness to adolescents	2.66	2.37	1.95
5 Adolescents' resemblance to their parents	2.64	2.49	1.95
Number of cases in each cluster	716	186	40

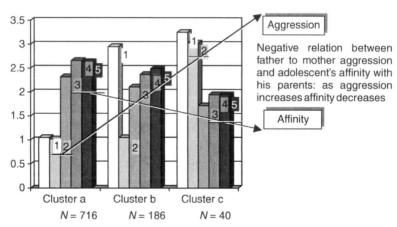

Aggression

Negative relation between father to mother aggression and adolescent's affinity with his parents: as aggression increases affinity decreases

Affinity

Cluster a   Cluster b   Cluster c
N = 716   N = 186   N = 40

It is important to reiterate that the present research design does not allow for causal inferences to be made; however, these findings do support the notion that, from the perspective of an adolescent, interparental violence may erode their sense of belonging, while possibly forcing him/her out of the family. Such distancing may have developmental implications for one of the most critical periods in life when self-identity is being formed (e.g., Brown, Dykers, Steele, & White, 1994; Erikson, 1950; Markus & Nurius, 1986; Rosenberg, 1989; Snow & Anderson, 1987). This is a difficult and complex task for any adolescent, but especially for those who are additionally challenged by interparental violence (Edleson, 1999).

As previously mentioned, interparental dynamics are a central factor that regulates the adolescent's position in the family. The more negative these dynamics are, the further away the adolescent will position himself/herself from the family. However, the distancing associated with loss of parental supervision and support does not necessarily carry an exclusively negative effect on development. Adolescents in such situations may indeed seek alternatives. In recent years, some evidence points to indicators of resilience among youths who grow up in violent families (Beeman, 2001; Goldblatt, 2001a, 2001b; Hughes, Graham-Bermann, & Gruber, 2001; Osofsky, 1999). It is certainly possible that these adolescents manage to find alternative sources of support that compensate for the reduction in parental support and guidance. Still, it is noteworthy that in most cases, an absence of family resources correlates with an absence of personal resources and with limited, and usually negative, opportunities (Jaffe, 1998).

Theoretically, this study emphasizes the central role of affinity in adolescent development. Affinity is primarily affected by interparental and parent-adolescent relationships, but it should not be considered as the sole factor mediating between interparental aggression and its developmental effects. Other factors inherent in personality and/or socio-cultural environment may have an influence on the course of child development. Practically, the present study identifies a central component in the dynamics influencing adolescent development, and as such it emphasizes the importance of developing personal resources and positive opportunities to counterbalance being pushed away from the family of origin. Our conclusions are in line with the current movement in the field which emphasizes a systemic orientation, advocates for a "coordinated community response" (Pence & Shepard, 1999), and suggests taking into account the intra and extra familial needs and resources when intervening.

Limitations

This study has a few major limitations, of which one is related to measurement. Proxy measures were used to represent the three constructs derived from the conceptual framework. This poses two problems. The first is that a limited number of variables represent each construct, and the second is that the variables were non-continuous with a small number of levels. In order to overcome these problems, a special statistical procedure was used to correct the observed covariance prior to CFA analysis. Since this study has identified the importance of affinity, subsequent studies should develop more accurate measurements of the constructs derived from the present conceptual framework.

Another limitation of this study has to do with sampling. The present study is based on a probability sample. There is a negative correlation between aggression level and the number of subjects, with the number of subjects becoming smaller as aggression grows. Although a relatively large sample was used, the number of subjects reporting a high occurrence of severe violence was relatively limited. Future studies need to be based on samples with an over-representation of the phenomenon. Such samples may enhance our ability to generalize. In addition, similar studies need to be carried out in other ethnic groups and inter-group comparisons need to be performed in order to identify the similarities and differences among them.

The methodology used in this study does not allow causal inference, though theoretical reasoning definitely supports causal relationships. While a longitudinal study is essential, although not sufficient to establish causality, it will allow for the exploration of interparental dynamics over time, their effects on perceptions of affinity, and the influence of affinity on adolescent development. It is also important to continue studying the resources and opportunities available to adolescents in order to deepen our understanding of potential resilience factors (see Kerig, 2003, for a discussion of protective processes and resiliency factors).

Finally, this study did not explore the effects of adolescents' age and gender or parents' gender on the correlation between interparental violence and the affinity of adolescents with their family of origin. These variables may prove to be of great influence on parent-adolescent relationships, especially in families where interparental conflicts escalate into violence.

CONCLUSION

This study was a preliminary attempt to explore the impact of adolescents' exposure to father-to-mother aggression on their perceptions of affinity with their parents. The concept of affinity was articulated in this study by closeness and resemblance, which, taken together, represent the adolescents' physical and psychological position in their family of origin. It was argued that interparental violence reduces affinity, and that when the affinity between adolescents and their parents decreases, the role of the latter as a developmental resource becomes limited. In such cases adolescents may turn to alternative resources, which increases developmental risks. Thus, studying affinity in these families may provide the link between exposure to interparental violence and development. Findings of this study substantiated our theoretical framework. For the children who are exposed to interparental violence, home may not serve as a launching pad from which they can take off and to which they can return. This study was limited to the examination of the impact of father-to-mother aggression on the adolescent's sense of affinity. Future studies need to address the effect of reduced affinity on adolescent development.

REFERENCES

Al-Haj, M. (1989). Social research on family lifestyles among Arabs in Israel. *Journal of Comparative Family Studies, 20*, 175-195.

Al-Haj, M. (1991). *Education and social change among the Arabs in Israel.* Tel-Aviv, Israel: The International Center for Peace in the Middle East.

Andenberg, M. R. (1973). *Cluster analysis for applications.* New York: Academic Press.

Anderson, S. A., & Cramer-Benjamin, D. B. (1999). The impact of couple violence on parenting and children: An overview and clinical implications. *The American Journal of Family Therapy, 27*, 1-19.

Arbuckle, J. L. (1999). AMOS (Version 4.0) [Computer software]. Chicago: SmallWaters Corporation.

Becker, C. S. (1992). *Living and relating.* Newbury Park, CA: Sage.

Beeman, S. K. (2001). Critical issues in research on social networks and social supports of children exposed to domestic violence. In S. A. Graham-Berman & J. L. Edleson (Eds.), *Domestic violence in the lives of children* (pp. 219-234). Washington, DC: American Psychological Association.

Berliner, L. (1993). When should children be allowed to kill abusers? *Journal of Interpersonal Violence, 8*, 269-301.

Bollen, K. A. (1989). *Structural equation modeling with latent variables.* New York: Wiley.

Brezina, T. (1999). Teenage violence toward parents as an adaptation to family strain. *Youth and Society, 30*, 416-444.

Brown, J. D., Dykers, C. R., Steele, J. R., & White, A. B. (1994). Teenage room culture: Where the media and identities intersect. *Communication Research, 21(6)*, 813-827.

Cantrell, P. J., MacIntyre, D. I., Sharkey, K. J., & Thompson, V. (1995). Violence in the marital dyad as a predictor in the peer relationships of older adolescents/young adults. *Violence and Victims, 10*, 35-41.

Cummings, E. M. (1998). Children exposed to marital conflict and violence: Conceptual and theoretical directions. In G. W. Holden, R. Geffner, & E. N. Jouriles (Eds.),

Children exposed to marital violence: Theory, research, and applied issues (pp. 55-93). Washington, DC: American Psychological Association.

Dacey J., & Kenny, M. (1997). *Adolescent development.* Madison, WI: Brown & Benchmark.

Davies, P. T., & Windle, M. (1997). Gender-specific pathways between maternal depressive symptoms, family discord, and adolescent adjustment. *Developmental Psychology, 33,* 657-668.

Davis, L. V., & Carlson, B. E. (1987). Observations of spouse abuse: What happens to the children? *Journal of Interpersonal Violence, 2,* 278-291.

Downs, W. R., Smyth, N. J., & Miller, B. A. (1996). The relationship between childhood violence and alcohol problems among men who batter: An empirical review and synthesis. *Aggression and Violent Behavior, 1,* 327-344.

Dunlop, R., Burns, A., & Bermingham, S. (2001). Parent-child relations and adolescent self-image following divorce: A 10 year study. *Journal of Youth and Adolescence, 30*(2), 117-134.

Edleson, J. L. (1999). Children's witnessing of adult domestic violence. *Journal of Interpersonal Violence, 14,* 839-870.

Eisikovits, Z., Winstok, Z., & Enosh, G. (1998). Children's experience of interparental violence: A heuristic model. *Children and Youth Services Review, 20,* 547-568.

Eisikovits, Z., & Winstok, Z. (2001). Researching children's experience of interparental violence: Towards a multidimensional conceptualization. In S. A. Graham-Bermann & J. L. Edleson (Eds.), *Domestic Violence in the Lives of Children: The Future of Research, Intervention and Social Policy.* (pp. 203-218). Washington, DC: American Psychological Association.

Erikson, E. H. (1950). *Childhood and society.* New York: W. W. Norton and Company.

Erikson, E. H. (1965). *The challenge of youth.* Garden City, NY: Doubleday.

Erikson, E. H. (1968). *Identity: Youth and crises.* New York: Norton.

Feindler, E. L., & Becker, J. V. (1996). Interventions in family violence involving children and adolescents. In L. D. Eron, J. H. Gentry, & P. Schlegel (Eds.), *Reason to hope–a psychosocial perspective on violence and youth* (pp. 405-430). Washington, DC: American Psychological Association.

Gecas, V. (1971). Parental behavior and dimensions of adolescent self-evaluation. *Sociometry, 34(4),* 466-482.

Gergen, K. J. (1994). *Realities and relationships.* Cambridge, MA: Harvard University Press.

Goldblatt, H. (2001a). *The meaning of interparental violence for adolescents.* Unpublished doctoral dissertation, University of Haifa, Israel (in Hebrew).

Goldblatt, H. (2001b). *Strategies of coping among adolescents experiencing interparental violence.* Manuscript submitted for publication.

Grotevant, H. D., & Cooper, C. R. (1986). Individuation in family relationships. *Human Development, 29,* 82-100.

Grych, J. H., & Finchman, F. D. (1990). Marital conflict and children's adjustment: A cognitive-contextual framework. *Psychological Bulletin, 108,* 267-290.

Heide, K. M. (1993). Parents who get killed and the children who kill them. *Journal of Interpersonal Violence, 8,* 531-544.

Henry, C. S., Sager, D. W., & Plunkett, S. W. (1996). Adolescents'perceptions of family system characteristics, parent-adolescent dyadic behaviors, adolescent qualities and adolescent empathy. *Family Relations, 45,* 283-292.

Hillbrand, M., Alexandre, J. W., Young, J. L., & Spitz, R. T. (1999). Parricides: Characteristics of offenders and victims, legal factors, and treatment issues. *Aggression and Violent Behavior, 4,* 179-190.

Holden, G. W., Geffner, R., & Jouriles, E. N. (Eds.). (1998). *Children exposed to marital violence: Theory, research, and applied issues.* Washington, DC: American Psychological Association.

Hughes, H. M., Graham-Bermann, S. A., & Gruber, G. (2001). Resilience in children exposed to domestic violence. In S. A. Graham-Berman & J. L. Edleson (Eds.), *Domestic violence in the lives of children* (pp. 67-90). Washington, DC: American Psychological Association.

Hunter, F. T. (1984). Socializing procedures in parent-child and friendship relations during adolescence. *Developmental Psychology, 20*(6), 1092-1099.

Jaffe, M. L. (1998). *Adolescence.* New York: J. Wiley & Sons.

Joreskog, K. G., & Sorbom, D. (1996). *PRELIS2: User's reference guide.* Chicago. Scientific Software International.

Josselson, R. (1987). *Finding herself.* San Francisco: Jossey-Bass Publications.

Kaplan, D. (1990). Evaluating and modifying covariance structure models: A review and recommendation. *Multivariate Behavioral Research, 25,* 137-155.

Kerig, P. K. (2003). In search of protective processes for children exposed to interparental violence. *Journal of Emotional Abuse, 3*(3/4), 149-181.

Laible, D. J., Carlo, G., & Raffaelli, M. (2000). The differential relations of parent and peer attachment to adolescent adjustment. *Journal of Youth and Adolescence, 29,* 45-59.

Lavee, Y., & Katz, R. (2002). Division of labor, Perceived fairness and marital quality: The effect of gender ideology. *Journal of Marriage and Family, (February),* 27-39.

MacCallum, R. C. (1990). The need for alternative measures of fit in covariance structure modeling. *Multivariate Behavioral Research, 25,* 157-162.

MacCallum, R. C., Browne, M. W., & Sugawara, H. M. (1996). Power analysis and determination of sample size for covariance structure modeling. *Psychological Methods, 1,* 130-149.

Mahabeer, M. (1993). Correlations between mothers' and children's self-esteem and perceived familial relationships among intact, widowed, and divorced families. *Psychological Reports, 73,* 483-489.

Markus, H., & Nurius, P. (1986). Possible selves. *American Psychologist, 41,* 954-969.

Martin, S. L., Sigda, K. B., & Kupersmidt, J. B. (1998). Family and neighborhood violence: Predictors of depressive symptomatology among incarcerated youth. *The Prison Journal, 78,* 423-438.

Micucci, J. A. (1995). Adolescents who assault their parents: A family systems approach to treatment. *Psychotherapy, 32,* 154-161.

Mones, P. (1993). When the innocent strikes back–abused children who kill their parents. *Journal of Interpersonal Violence, 8,* 297-299.

O'Keefe, M. (1996). The differential effects of family violence on adolescent adjustment. *Child and Adolescent Social Work Journal, 13*, 51-68.

Osborne, R. E. (1996). *Self: An eclectic approach.* Boston: Allyn and Bacon.

Osofsky, J. D. (1999). The impact of violence on children. *Future of Children, 9*(3), 33-49.

Peled, E. (1997). Intervention with children of battered women: A review of the current literature. *Children and Youth Services Review, 19*, 277-299.

Pence, E., & Shepard, M. (1999). Developing a coordinated community response. In M. Shepard, & E. Pence (Eds.), *Coordinating community responses to domestic violence: Lessons from Duluth and beyond* (pp. 3-25). Thousand Oaks, CA: Sage.

Peterson, G. W., & Leigh, G. K. (1990). The family and social competence in adolescence. In T. P. Gullota, G. R. Adams, & R. Montemayor (Eds.), *Developing social competency in adolescence* (pp. 97-138). Newbury Park, CA: Sage.

Rosenberg, M. (1989). *Society and the adolescent self-image.* Middletown: Wesleyan University Press.

Schave, D., & Schave, B. (1989). *Early adolescence and the search for self.* New York: Praeger Publications.

Sherer, M., Karniely-Miler, Eisikovits, Z., &, Fishman, G. (2001). *Survey of Israeli youth attitudes–summer 2000.* University of Haifa, Minerva Center for Youth Studies (in Hebrew).

Silva, R. R., Alpert, M., Monuz, D. M., Matzner, F., & Dummit, S. (2000). Stress and vulnerability to posttraumatic stress disorder in children and adolescents. *American Journal of Psychiatry, 157*, 1229-1235.

Silverberg, S. B., & Gondoli, D. M. (1996). Autonomy in adolescence: A contextualized perspective. In G. R. Adams, R. Montemayor, & T. P. Gullota (Eds.), *Psychosocial development during adolescence* (pp.12-61). Thousand Oaks, CA: Sage.

Smooha, S. (1993). Class, ethnic, and national cleavages and democracy in israel. In E. Sprinzak & L. Diamond (Eds.) *Israeli democracy under stress.* (pp. 309-341). Boulder, CO: Lynne Rinner.

Snow, D. A., & Anderson, I. (1987). Identity work among the homeless: The verbal construction and avowal of personal identities. *American Journal of Sociology, 92*, 1336-1371.

Straus, M. A. (1992). Children as witnesses to marital violence: A risk factor for lifelong problems among a nationally representative sample of American men and women. In D. F. Schwartz (Ed.), *Children and violence: Report of the 23rd Ross Roundtable on critical approaches to common pediatric problems* (pp. 98-104). Columbus, OH: Ross Laboratories.

Sugawara, H. M., & MacCallum, R. C. (1993). Effect of estimation method on incremental fit indexes for covariance structure models. *Applied Psychological Measurement, 17*, 365-377.

Thomas, D. L., Gecas, V., Weigert, A., & Rooney, E. (1974). *Family socialization and the adolescent.* Lexington, MA: Lexington Books.

Tomori, M. (1994). Personality characteristics of adolescents with alcoholic parents. *Adolescence, 29* (116), 949-959.

Triandis, H. C., McCusker, C., & Hui, C. H. (1990). Multi-method probes of individualism and collectivism. *Journal of Personality and Social Psychology, 59,* 1006-1020.

Walter, R. J., Trainham, A., & LeDoux, L. (1997, July). *The relationship of parental battering to violent behavior among juvenile first offenders.* Paper presented at The 5th International Family Violence Research Conference, Durham, NH.

Winstok, Z., Eisikovits, Z., & Karniely-Miller, O. (2002). The impact of father-to-mother aggression on the structure and content of adolescents' perceptions of themselves and their parents. Manuscript submitted for publication.

Diversity
of Children's Immediate Coping Responses to Witnessing Domestic Violence

Nicole E. Allen
Angela M. Wolf
Deborah I. Bybee
Cris M. Sullivan

SUMMARY. This study explored the immediate coping strategies children employ (e.g., getting help) in response to witnessing physical and emotional violence against their mothers. Using a clustering technique, children's patterns of coping strategies were examined. While most children shared similar emotional reactions to the abuse against their mothers, their behavioral reactions varied substantially. Four distinct clusters were differentiated by whether or not children (1) became aggressive against the assailant and sought help, (2) became overprotective of their mothers, (3) avoided or ignored the abuse, or (4) had little response at all. An examination of cluster definers suggests that children's responses depend on situational factors rather than child characteristics (e.g., gender). Specifically, children who had little response at all to the

---

Address correspondence to: Nicole E. Allen, 603 East Daniel Street, Champaign, IL 61820.

This research was supported by a grant from the National Center for Injury Prevention and Control of the Centers for Disease Control and Prevention (R49/CCR510531).

[Haworth co-indexing entry note]: "Diversity of Children's Immediate Coping Responses to Witnessing Domestic Violence." Allen, Nicole E. et al. Co-published simultaneously in *Journal of Emotional Abuse* (The Haworth Maltreatment & Trauma Press, an imprint of The Haworth Press, Inc.) Vol. 3, No. 1/2, 2003, pp. 123-147; and: *The Effects of Intimate Partner Violence on Children* (ed: Robert A. Geffner, Robyn Spurling Igelman, and Jennifer Zellner) The Haworth Maltreatment & Trauma Press, an imprint of The Haworth Press, Inc., 2003, pp. 123-147. Single or multiple copies of this article are available for a fee from The Haworth Document Delivery Service [1-800-HAWORTH, 9:00 a.m. - 5:00 p.m. (EST). E-mail address: docdelivery@haworthpress.com].

10.1300J135v03n01_06

abuse had witnessed less physical and emotional abuse than the other children. Children who became aggressive against the assailants were more likely to be living with them than children in other clusters. Virtually no differences were found across groups with regard to the relationship between coping strategy and child well being. *[Article copies available for a fee from The Haworth Document Delivery Service: 1-800-HAWORTH. E-mail address: <docdelivery@haworthpress.com> Website: <http://www.HaworthPress.com>* · © 2003 by The Haworth Press, Inc. All rights reserved.]

KEYWORDS. Children witnessing domestic violence, coping strategies, passive and active coping, problem-focused coping, emotion-focused coping

Historically, the domestic violence literature has paid scant attention to the experiences and needs of children who witness their mothers being abused. Theories regarding these children were initially based on anecdotal reports from clinicians, shelter workers, and retrospective accounts from battered women and their assailants (Carlson, 1984). However, empirical research on children has been growing steadily, raising concerns about the long-term effects of children witnessing and living with domestic abuse (Graham-Bermann & Edleson, 2001; Holden, 1998; Jaffe, Wolfe, & Wilson, 1990; Kolbo, Blakely, & Engleman, 1996; Peled, 1998). It is becoming increasingly clear that even when children are not the direct victims of physical assault, witnessing abuse against their mothers constitutes a form of emotional trauma that warrants further attention. Still notably absent from the body of literature examining the effects of witnessing domestic violence is attention to immediate coping strategies children employ in response to witnessing domestic violence. Immediate coping strategies as examined in this study refer to children's emotional (e.g., fear, anger) and behavioral (e.g., getting help, ignoring the violence) responses during or closely following abusive episodes. Given the role of effective coping as a protective factor for children exposed to stressors (Compas, 1987; Compas, Connor-Smith, Saltzman, Thomsen, & Wadsworth, 2001; Cummings, 1998; Griffith, Dubow, & Ippolito, 2000; see also Kerig, 2003), it is critical that we better understand children's immediate responses to witnessing domestic violence and how these varied responses might relate to their well-being.

Millions of children each year are exposed to their mothers being battered by male partners and ex-partners (Carlson, 1984; Holden, 1998; Straus, 1992), with many directly seeing or hearing the violence. In one of the earlier studies where children themselves were interviewed about the violence they observed, Rosenberg (cited in Rosenberg, 1987) found that although one or both parents might have made attempts to shield the children from the violence, nearly all saw and/or heard the incidents. The types of violence children reported witnessing were: repeated verbal threats of injury; verbal assaults on their mother's character; objects hurled across the room; suicide attempts; beatings; threats with and use of guns and knives; and homicide. Even when parents might have thought their children were asleep through the arguments and beatings, Rosenberg found that the children reported hearing the violence and remained in their bedrooms because they were afraid to leave. Jaffe et al.'s (1990) clinical experience corroborated these findings, indicating that almost all of the children they interviewed could describe detailed accounts of physical and emotional abuse.

A growing body of literature indicates that children who witness abuse against their mothers, even when they are not themselves the targets of violence, are at risk for maladjustment when compared to children that have not been exposed to domestic violence (Rossman, 2001; Tomkins et al., 1994; see also Onyskiw, 2003). Anecdotal and clinical reports indicate that children's emotional and behavioral reactions to witnessing battering can be severe and pervasive, and include somatic complaints, behavioral problems, ambivalent feelings toward the abuser, and/or withdrawal and depression (Barnett, Miller-Perrin, & Perrin, 1997; Christopoulos et al., 1987; Jouriles & Norwood, 1995; Koss et al., 1994; McDonald & Jouriles, 1991; Norris & Kaniasty, 1994).

Not all children, of course, respond in the same way to witnessing abuse against their mothers, and some children appear to be more adversely affected than others (Graham-Bermann, 1998; Hughes, Graham-Bermann, & Gruber, 2001; Jaffe et al., 1990). In fact, children are a very resilient population; it has been estimated that up to 80 percent of children who are exposed to extreme stressors do not sustain developmental damage (Garbarino, Dubrow, Kosteny, & Pardo, 1992; Tomkins et al., 1994). Hughes and colleagues (Hughes et al., 2001; Hughes & Luke, 1998) have conducted the only study to date that examined differential patterns of children's adjustment subsequent to witnessing domestic violence. Looking at children's levels of depression, anxiety, and behavior problems following exposure to violence against their mothers, they found that children could be clustered into five distinct groups. The two largest groups (consisting of 21 and 15 children) appeared relatively resilient while the remaining three (smaller) groups of children appeared to suffer greater emotional and behavioral consequences.

This study suggests it is important to recognize the variability in children's emotional and behavioral responses to witnessing abuse against their mothers, and to view children as active agents operating within complex social systems. Few studies to date, however, have examined the coping strategies children employ in response to witnessing violence against their mothers. Examining such strategies is important given that children's responses to stressors are likely a source of their differential adjustment (Compas, 1987; Sandler, Tein, & West, 1994) and coping strategies appear to serve as either protective or risk factors for an array of behavioral and emotional problems for children (Compas, Malcarne, & Fondacaro, 1988; Ebata & Moos, 1991; see also Kerig, 2003). Anecdotally, we know that some children attempt to intervene to protect their mothers while other children attempt to ignore what is happening (Jaffe et al., 1990). In addition, we know that children who witness abuse against their mothers are likely to exhibit a variety of emotions, including sadness, anxiety and fear (Garcia, O'Hearn, Margolin, & John, 1997; Graham-Bermann, 1996). Interestingly, there is also some evidence that children sometimes choose seemingly opposing strategies to cope with witnessing conflict. For example, O'Brien, Margolin, John, and Krueger (1991) found that children who witnessed abuse against their mothers were more likely to intervene in interparental conflict *and* to use distraction to cope with interparental conflict than comparison children. Taken together, these studies suggest that children employ a variety of methods in response to witnessing violence against their mothers. However, we do not know how many children respond in any given fashion, or whether coping strategies are correlated with child characteristics (e.g., age, gender) or other situational variables (e.g., severity of the violence).

Although there has been little examination of children's coping responses to witnessing abuse against their mothers, there has been research on children's reactions to other extreme stressors that can inform our investigation. Compas et al. (1988) discussed children's responses to stress in terms of problem- and emotion-focused coping strategies. Problem-focused coping is aimed at problem solving or acting in some way to directly alter the level of stress. Emotion-focused coping refers to efforts to manage or ameliorate the emotional distress associated with a problem situation. Compas and colleagues found that problem-focused coping was negatively correlated with both maternal and child reports of emotional and behavioral problems, whereas the use of emotion-focused coping was positively related to emotional and behavioral problems.

In a similar vein, the general literature on coping suggests that individuals who choose "active" coping strategies to deal with stressful events exhibit lower psychological distress than those choosing "passive" coping strategies (Holahan & Moos, 1990, 1991). In the active approach, responses are directed toward the problem, while in the passive or avoidant approach, responses are indirect, including methods that serve to avoid thinking about a stressor (Ebata & Moos, 1991). Similar to Compas et al. (1988), Ebata and Moos (1991) found that adolescents who relied proportionally more on active than passive methods had higher levels of well-being and lower levels of stress.

There is also some evidence that one's choice of coping strategy is related to situational factors. Cummings (1998) stresses that understanding children's coping responses to marital conflict requires an examination of the specific context of exposure, including, for example, the identity of those involved in the conflict and the duration and intensity of the conflict. Furthermore, there is evidence that individuals tend to choose active coping techniques when they perceive they have some control over a stressful situation, and passive, more emotional coping strategies when they feel they do not (Moos & Schaefer, 1993; Valentiner, Holahan, & Moos, 1994). Examining the relationship of situational factors to the use of active or passive coping strategies may be particularly important in the domestic violence context given that some active responses (e.g., attempting to intervene in the abuse) could result in children getting physically injured. In fact, some research suggests that passive methods are not necessarily detrimental when stressors are not easily changed (Altshuler & Ruble, 1989; Ebata & Moos, 1991; Rieder & Cicchetti, 1989). For example, Rieder and Cicchetti (1989) found that when faced with uncontrollable stressors, avoidance and distraction appear to serve as protective responses. Further, passive, emotion focused coping strategies such as acceptance, denial, or distraction can be used to regulate emotional arousal (Kliewer, 1991; Sandler et al., 1994). Coping techniques such as distraction can mitigate the level of frustration and reduce one's negative emotional response (Fabes, Eisenberg, & Eisenbud, 1993; Rothbart, Ziaie, & O'Boyle, 1992).

Overall, little is known about the variety of children's responses that would reduce distress in general (Rossman & Ho, 2000) and even less is known about what coping strategies children employ in response to witnessing abuse against their mothers. Given the potentially unique aspects of responding to witnessing violence against mothers, it is unclear whether passive or active coping strategies are more effective. The current study examined children's immediate emotional and behavioral responses to witnessing violence toward their mothers. Specifically, using a clustering technique, children's *patterns* of reactions and the correlates of these patterns were examined. This study investigated the degree to which children's responses to witnessing violence varied depending on child characteristics (e.g., age, gender) as well as situational factors surrounding the violence (e.g., the frequency and severity of abuse witnessed, the relationship of the child to the assailant, whether the child lived with both the assailant and the mother). In addition, clusters were examined to determine: (1) if different patterns of emotional and behavioral responses to witnessing abuse were associated with differences in the psychological well being of children and (2) whether these differences were consistent with previous research suggesting that children who employed more "active" or "problem-solving" coping strategies (e.g., getting help) would have greater well-being than children who used more "passive" or "emotion-focused" strategies (e.g., ignoring what was happening).

METHOD

Sample

Eighty women and 80 of their children were recruited from a variety of sources, including two domestic violence shelter programs, a community based family services agency, and a Social Services department, all located in a mid-sized urban city. In order to be eligible for the study, women had to have at least one child between the age of 7 and 11 living with them, at least one of their children aged 7-11 was required to be interested in participating, and the mother had to have experienced domestic violence in the prior four months.

If mothers expressed interest in the study, the children aged 7-11 were approached and the study was explained to them. If more than one child aged 7-11 participated, data analyses were conducted on only one child's responses (chosen randomly). Women were paid $15 for the interview, and children were paid $5 (in cash or toys, at their discretion). Interviews were conducted in the community at the families' convenience (primarily in the home), and in separate rooms to ensure privacy and confidentiality of responses. To avoid interviewing families while they were in crisis, women who were recruited from shelter programs were not interviewed until after they had exited the shelter.

Demographics

Seventy-nine percent of the sample was recruited upon exit from domestic violence programs, 4% were recruited from a community organization offering family services, and 18% were recruited from the state department of social services. Forty-nine percent of the mothers were non-Hispanic white, 39% were African American, 5% were Hispanic/Latina, 5% identified as multi-racial, 1% were Asian, and 1% were Native American. Average age was 31 years, with 77% of the sample under 35 years old. Their mean income was $1,200 a month, and 44% of the women were employed. The majority (88%) was receiving some form of governmental assistance. All women had male assailants.

Forty-four percent of the children in the sample were African American, and 40% were non-Hispanic white. Ten percent identified as multi-racial, 5% were Hispanic, and 1% were Asian. The children ranged in age from 6.5 to 11, with the mean at 8.3 (3rd grade). Slightly over half the children in the sample (55%) were girls.

Thirty-seven percent of the assailants were the children's biological fathers ($n = 30$). Forty percent were the children's stepfathers or father figures ($n = 32$), and the remaining 23% were non-father-figures to the children ($n = 18$). Men were classified as stepfathers/father figures if they (a) were legally married to the mother, and/or (b) were reported to play a significant paternal role in the child's life. Non-father-figures were partners or ex-partners who did not play a significant role in the child's life, as determined by the mother and verified by the child. Most children lived with their mothers only (81%), some lived with their mothers and the assailants (14%) and a few lived in other situations (e.g., with another guardian; 2.5%). For two cases living arrangements were unknown.

Five percent of the mothers were currently married to the assailant; 32% were divorced or separated; 9% were cohabitating; 5% were girlfriend/boyfriend, but not living together; 46% were ex-girlfriend/ex-boyfriend; and 3% were dating. Thus, 79% of the women were no longer involved with the men who had abused them. Fourteen percent were living with the men who had abused them, and an additional 7% were involved with the men but were living separately.

Measures

The research utilized preexisting measures in addition to measures created specifically for this study.

Mother's Experience of Abuse

Assailant's Physical Abuse of Mother. A modified version of the Conflict Tactics Scale (CTS; Straus, 1979) was used to assess the assailant's physical abuse of the mother over the prior four months. This scale included seven yes/no items (e.g., "Has he pushed, grabbed, shoved, or slapped you?"). The reliability coefficient for this scale was .62.

Assailant's Emotional Abuse of Mother. A shortened version of the Index of Psychological Abuse (Sullivan, Parisian, & Davidson, 1991) was utilized to assess the assailant's emotional abuse of the mother over the prior four months. Sample items included "How often has he accused you of having other sexual relationships?" and "How often has he threatened to take the children away from you?" Participants responded using a 4-point Likert-type scale (1 = never to 4 = often; α = .90).

Assailant's Injury of Mother. A 12-item scale was utilized to assess the types of injuries mothers received from the assailants over the prior four months (e.g., "Have you ever experienced soreness without bruises?" and "Have you ever experienced internal injuries?"). Participants responded "yes" or "no" to each statement; α = .77.

Assailant's Overall Abuse of Mother. To create a single index of the emotional and physical abuse experienced by the mother over the prior four months, a combined score was created including standardized scores for total physical abuse experienced, total emotional abuse experienced and total injury experienced. This combined scale had a reliability coefficient of .77.

Children's Well-Being

Children's Behavior Problems. A scale was developed specifically for this study utilizing 20 items from the Achenbach Child Behavior Checklist (CBCL; Achenbach & Edelbrock, 1983). Given the length of the interview protocol, this scale was created to keep the interview at a reasonable length. Items were included that would provide a reasonable description of both the aggressive and withdrawal behaviors of children. Only mothers completed this measure. Mothers responded using a Likert-type scale (0 = not at all true to 2 = very true; α = .84).

Children's Depression. The well-established Child Depression Inventory (CDI; Kovacs, 1985) was utilized to address children's depression by their own report ($\alpha = .81$). This scale included twenty-seven items each describing three "feelings or ideas" (e.g., "I do not feel alone," "I feel alone many times," "I feel alone all the time"). For each item, children indicated the statement that best described them over the past two weeks. Each item is scored on a scale of 0 (e.g., "I do not feel alone") to 2 ("I feel alone all the time"). A mean was calculated to reflect the child's overall level of depression.

Children's Self-Perception. To assess children's self-concept and feelings of self-adequacy, Harter's (1985) Self-Perception Profile for Children was utilized. This measure included five specific domain subscales and one global self-worth subscale. Sample items included: "Some kids are pretty slow in finishing their school work, but other kids can do their work quickly" (scholastic competence subscale) and "Some kids would like to have a lot more friends, other kids have as many friends as they want" (social competence subscale). For each item, children were asked, "Which (of these kids) is more like you?" Then children were asked, "Is that sort of true for you or really true for you?" Internal consistencies for these subscales were as follows: scholastic competence, .77; social acceptance, .67; athletic competence, .75; physical appearance, .78; behavioral conduct, .74; and global self-worth, .66.

Witnessing Abuse

The abuse witnessed by children was assessed by both mother and child report of the type of abuse witnessed and the frequency with which witnessing abuse occurred. Mothers' and children's reports of emotional and physical abuse witnessed were significantly correlated.[1]

Mother's Report. Mothers were asked one item regarding ridicule and control (i.e., "How many times has [the child] seen or heard the assailant ridicule, criticize, control, or humiliate you?"), and responded using a 4-point Likert-type scale (1 = never to 4 = often). Mothers were asked two items regarding threats and physical abuse (i.e., "How often has [the child] seen or heard the assailant threaten you?" and "How often has [the child] seen or heard the assailant harm or attempt to harm you?"), and responded using a 6-point Likert-type scale (1 = never to 6 = more than four times per week). Given the desire to examine both the frequency and type of abuse separately, each of these items was examined individually in subsequent analyses.

Child's Report. Children were asked one item capturing how often they heard or saw their mothers emotionally abused (e.g., made fun of and/or called names by the assailant) and responded using a 4-point Likert-type scale (1 = never to 4 = often). Children were also asked two items regarding the degree to which they saw their mothers threatened and/or physically abused by the assailants and responded using a 6-point Likert-type scale (1 = never to 6 = more than four times per week). Given the desire to examine both the frequency and type of abuse separately, each of these items was examined individually in subsequent analyses.

Children's Reactions to Witnessing Violence

Directly following questions about the type and frequency of physical and emotional abuse witnessed, both mothers and children were asked whether the children experienced or engaged in a range of emotional and behavioral responses to witnessing abuse against their mothers (these reactions were not confined to a particular incident). Mothers and children were prompted to reflect on children's reactions *when* they saw or heard abuse. Emotional reactions included being fearful, being angry, and/or being confused. Behavioral reactions included a variety of responses, including getting help, leaving the room, trying to stop what was happening, phoning someone, and pretending to ignore or ignoring what was happening. In addition, mothers were asked if children became overprotective of them, became aggressive toward the assailant and/or got a sibling to help. Children were asked, for each item, whether or not they ever did this when they witnessed abuse (yes/no). Mothers also had the option to indicate that they did not know if their children had a certain reaction. For the purposes of this study, responses of "don't know" were treated as a "no." In some cases the child may have engaged in a particular emotional or behavioral response of which the mother was not aware, but excluding cases in which the mother indicated "don't know" would have resulted in dropping cases from the analyses entirely. Given that mothers used the "don't know" option relatively infrequently, it was more important to retain these cases than to exclude them because of this limitation.[2]

Statistical Analysis

Cluster analysis was used to group children by their pattern of emotional and behavioral responses to abuse against their mothers. The hierarchical agglomerative method of cluster analysis and Ward's method on squared Euclidian distance measure were used. To further refine the groups, a k-means cluster analysis was performed using as start means the cluster centroids and specifying a specific number of clusters from the previous analysis. The purpose of this two-step process was to reduce misclassification due to the sequential nature of the hierarchical agglomerative process. Subsequent analyses included a series of one-way ANOVAs aimed at examining the differentiating characteristics of the four groups and a series of chi-square analyses to examine differences on categorical variables such as gender of the child, relationship to assailant, and with whom the child lived. Mothers' reports of children's reactions were more detailed, given that mothers were asked more questions about children's reactions to witnessing violence (e.g., whether or not the child became aggressive toward the assailant or overprotective of their mother). Therefore, all cluster analyses were based on mother rather than child reports.

RESULTS

A high percentage of children had emotional reactions to witnessing abuse against their mothers: Mothers reported that 81% were fearful, 81% were angry, and 71% were confused. Children reported 82% were fearful, 84% were angry, and 70% were confused. Children's behavioral reactions to witnessing abuse were more variable according to both mother's and children's reports. According to mothers' reports the most common responses included children becoming overprotective of their mothers (71%), leaving the room (61%), or ignoring what was happening (50%). Almost half of the children (44%) became aggressive against the assailant. Similarly, according to children's reports, 67% left the room, 60% ignored what was happening, and 49% tried to stop what was happening. Both mothers' and children's reports indicate that relatively few children sought help from someone other than a sibling (14% and 22%, respectively).[3]

Cluster Analysis

Nine variables representing both emotional and behavioral responses to witnessing abuse were used to generate clusters, including, for example, whether the child was fearful or angry, tried to stop what was happening, and/or became aggressive toward the assailant. Variables regarding whether the child got a sibling to help or tried to call someone on the phone were not included in determining the clusters because not all participants had telephones or siblings and the inclusion of these reactions would have resulted in the exclusion of some cases.

Using the hierarchical agglomerative method of cluster analysis and Ward's method on the Squared Euclidian distance measure, both three and four cluster solutions were generated. Ultimately, the four-group solution was chosen because meaningful significant differences were found between all four groups. That is, these groups were significantly statistically different and the patterns of difference that emerged from the data corresponded meaningfully with previous literature on active and passive coping strategies. K-means cluster analysis was performed to further refine these groups and resulted in the movement of ten individuals.

The final four groups were distinct in their combinations of both emotional and behavioral reactions to witnessing abuse. For the most part, however, the four groups did not differ dramatically regarding children's *emotional* reactions to violence. For example, the majority of children in each group exhibited fear, anger, and confusion. Only one group differed significantly from the others, with fewer children experiencing these emotions. There were distinct differences across all four groups, however, in their behavioral reactions.

The first group, labeled *Aggressive/Helpseeking*, included 17 children. This group was characterized by 100% of children reacting aggressively toward the assailant. Also, over three-quarters (76%) of the children did something to try to stop what was happening. Almost half (47%) of the children in this group attempted to seek help (the highest percentage of children in any group), and 88% left the room during the incident. Interestingly, this group had the lowest percentage of children who reacted with overprotectiveness of their mothers (53%). Regarding emotional reactions, 100% of the children in this group exhibited fear, 94% were confused, and 76% exhibited anger. This group also had a significant number of children (53%) who ignored or pretended to ignore what was happening at least some of the time.

The second group, *Overprotective*, also included 17 children. This group was similar in some ways to the *Aggressive* group. Over three-quarters (76%) of the children in this group reacted with aggressive behavior toward the assailant. In addition, over three-quarters (82%) of the children did something to try to stop what was happening.

However, only 12% of the children in this group actively sought help from someone other than a sibling, and only 12% of the children left the room during the incident. Virtually no children in this group ignored or pretended to ignore what was happening (6%). While the *Aggressive* group had the lowest percentage of children exhibiting overprotectiveness toward their mothers, the *Overprotective* group had the highest, with 94% of the children exhibiting this behavior. Similar to the *Aggressive* group, this group had a high percentage of children exhibiting emotional reactions to witnessing violence: 100% were angry, 88% became fearful and 53% were confused.

The third and largest group, *Avoidant/Ignoring*, included 25 children. Children ignoring or pretending to ignore what was happening characterized this group (100%). A high percentage of the children exhibited emotional reactions to witnessing violence: 92% were angry, 84% were confused and 76% were fearful. Eighty-four percent of the children left the room. However, this group had fewer children who were attempting to stop what was happening (24%), no children who attempted to get help, and few children who became aggressive toward the assailant (16%).

The fourth group, *Less Responsive*, included 19 children and was characterized by a smaller percentage of children exhibiting either emotional or behavioral reactions to violence. Fewer children were fearful, angry, or confused (63%, 53%, 53% respectively). Regarding behavioral reactions, none of the children attempted to try to stop what was happening, only 5% got help from someone, and none of the children became aggressive toward the assailant. In addition, 21% of the children in this group ignored or pretended to ignore what was happening, about half (47%) left the room at some point during an incident, and over half (58%) became overprotective of their mothers. See Table 1 for a summary of children's reactions across the four clusters.

Examining Cluster Definers

Situational Factors

Some of the differences between the four groups can be explained by a more detailed examination of the circumstances of the violence the children witnessed. Factors examined in this study included: (1) the amount of abuse mothers were experiencing, and (2) the type and amount of violence witnessed by the children.

TABLE 1. Children's Emotional and Behavioral Responses to Witnessing Violence Against Their Mothers by Cluster Membership

Children's Responses to Witnessing Abuse	Aggressive $N = 17$	Overprotective $N = 17$	Avoidant/ Ignoring $N = 25$	Less Responsive $N = 19$
Became Fearful	100%	88%	76%	63%
Became Angry	76%	100%	92%	53%
Became Confused	94%	53%	84%	53%
Became Aggressive Toward Assailant	100%	76%	16%	0%
Tried to Stop Violence	76%	82%	24%	0%
Became Overprotective of Mom	53%	94%	76%	58%
Left Room	88%	12%	84%	47%
Got Someone Else to Help	47%	12%	0%	5%
Ignored/Pretended to Ignore	53%	6%	100%	21%

Mother's Experience of Abuse. Differences were found among the four clusters on the level of violence mothers experienced (F (3,74) = 5.24, $p < .01$) and on the extent of injuries they suffered (F (3,74) = 4.92, $p < .01$). Tukey HSD post hoc tests indicated that mothers of children in the *Aggressive, Overprotective,* and *Avoidant/Ignoring* group experienced more violence than mothers in the *Less Responsive* group. Further, mothers of children in the *Aggressive* and *Avoidant/Ignoring* groups were injured more than mothers of children in the *Less Responsive* group. There were no differences among these groups regarding amount of emotional abuse against mothers.

Type and Amount of Violence Witnessed. Significant differences were also found regarding the types and amount of violence witnessed by the children. Overall, children in the *Aggressive* and the *Avoidant/Ignoring* groups witnessed more emotional and physical abuse when compared to children in the *Less Responsive* group. Specifically, according to mothers' reports, children in the *Aggressive* and the *Avoidant/Ignoring* group (at the trend level) witnessed more emotional abuse (e.g., ridicule and threats) of their mothers than children in the *Less Responsive* group (F (3,74) = 3.64, $p < .01$). In addition, while the overall F for the ANOVA comparing group differences demonstrated only a trend toward significance, post hoc tests revealed that children in the *Aggressive* group may have witnessed more physical harm than children in the

Less Responsive group (F (3,74) = 2.54, p = .06). Findings based on children's reports of witnessing violence reveal a similar pattern. According to children's reports, children in the *Overprotective* group witnessed a greater amount emotional abuse of their mothers than children in the *Less Responsive* group (F (3,72) = 2.84, p = .05; mean difference = .99, p < .05). In addition, a trend emerged suggesting that children in the *Aggressive* group reported witnessing greater physical abuse than children in the *Less Responsive* group (F (3,71) = 2.33, p = .08; mean difference = 1.35, p < .10). No differences were found among the *Aggressive, Overprotective* and *Avoidant/Ignoring* groups with regard to witnessing emotional and physical abuse. See Table 2 for a summary of these findings.

Child Characteristics

There were no differences between groups on the majority of demographic variables (child's race; child's age; whether the assailant was the child's biological father, step-father, or non-father figure; how long the child had known the assailant; or how often the child saw the assailant). However, there was a significant difference across groups regarding with whom the child lived (χ^2 (3, N = 76) = 10.23, p < .05). The *Aggressive* group had the largest portion of children living with both their mother and the assailant (35.3%). The *Less Responsive* and the *Overprotective* groups had a smaller portion of children living with both their mother and the assailant (16% and 13%, respectively). All of the children in the *Avoidant/Ignoring* group lived with their mothers only.

Child Well-Being

For the most part, children and mothers reported relatively high levels of child well-being. Specifically, children scores ranged from a mean of 2.68 (SD = .81; athletic competence subscale) to 3.19 (SD = .68; global self-worth subscale) on the Harter subscales measuring perceived self-competence and self-worth. Scores around 3.00 are considered indicative of average self-competency according to research with middle-school children (Harter, 1985). Similarly, children's average sum depression score was 9.20 (SD = 6.58). This score is similar to the mean score reported by Kovacs (1992) for a normal sample of children 12 and younger (i.e., score = 10.5, SD = 7.3) and well below the cutoff for clinical depression (score = 20 or above). While there was some

TABLE 2. Examining Cluster Differences

Variables	F (d.f.) p-value	Aggressive $N = 17$	Overprotective $N = 17$	Avoidant/ Ignoring $N = 25$	Less Emotional/ Less Responsive $N = 19$
		Cluster Means			
Harter Athletic Competence (child report)[1] (scale, 1 - 4)	2.36 (3,74) .079	2.3a	3.0b	2.6ab	2.9ab
Mother's Injury by Assailant (mother report) (0 = no, 1 = yes)	4.92 (3,74) .004	.42a	.33ab	.37a	.18b
Mother's Physical Abuse by Assailant (mother report) (0 = no, 1 = yes)	5.24 (3,74) .002	.71a	.66a	.69a	.45b
Child Witnessing Ridicule (mother report)[2] (1 = never, 4 = a lot)	3.64 (3,74) .017	3.6a	3.4ab	3.4a	2.7b
Child Witnessing Threats (mother report)[3] (1 = never, 6 = more than 4 times/week)	4.37 (3,74) .007	3.9a	3.1ab	3.3a	2.3b
Child Witnessing Physical Harm (mother report) (1 = never, 6 = more than 4 times/week)	2.54 (3,74) .063	3.1a	2.7ab	2.7ab	1.9b
Child Witnessing Ridicule (child report) (1 = never, 4 = a lot)	2.84 (3,72) .044	3.2ab	3.4a	2.8ab	2.4b
Child Witnessing Physical Harm (child report)[4] (1 = never, 6 = more than 4 times/week)	2.33 (3,71) .081	3.2a	2.9ab	2.3ab	1.8b

Note. Values that do not share at least one letter in the subscript are different from one another at the $p < .05$ level unless otherwise indicated (i.e., some group differences emerged at the trend level, $p < .10$, as noted); [1]Groups 1 and 2 are only marginally significantly different ($p < .10$); [2]Groups 3 and 4 are only marginally significantly different ($p < .10$); [3]Groups 3 and 4 are only marginally significantly different ($p < .10$); [4]Groups 1 and 4 are only marginally significantly different ($p < .10$).

variation in children's well-being, no between-group differences existed regarding children's experience of depression, internalizing or externalizing behaviors, or self-perception. One trend did suggest that children in the *Overprotective* group felt more athletically competent than children in the *Aggressive* group (F (3,74) = 2.36, $p < .08$).

DISCUSSION

The findings from this study demonstrate the need to consider children's unique responses to witnessing violence against their mothers and to begin to more thoroughly examine their coping strategies. Distinct patterns of children's immediate responses to witnessing violence did emerge. While children's emotional responses to witnessing abuse were similar, their behavioral responses differed substantially and characterized differences across clusters. These patterns were consistent with previous general research on coping, suggesting that some children employ more active strategies (the *Aggressive* and *Overprotective* groups) while others employ more passive strategies (the *Avoidant/Ignoring* and *Less Responsive* groups). This study also suggests that children's responses depend on situational factors (e.g., amount of abuse witnessed). However, virtually no differences were found across groups with regard to the relationship between coping strategy and child well-being. Interestingly, there is also some evidence that children used combined approaches (i.e., both active and passive strategies).

While the literature on coping strategies suggests that, in general, individuals who choose "active" coping strategies to deal with stressful events exhibit lower psychological distress than those choosing "passive" coping strategies (Holahan & Moos, 1990, 1991) such differences did not emerge in this study. Children's behavioral responses being more "active" and "problem-focused" as demonstrated by the *Aggressive* and *Overprotective* groups were not associated with greater well-being when compared to the more "passive" coping of children in the *Avoidant/Ignoring* or *Less Responsive* groups. This result reflects the contradictory findings in previous research, with some finding that "active" strategies were associated with reduced psychological stress (Holahan & Moos, 1990, 1991) and others suggesting that "passive" or avoidant and distraction strategies may be more adaptive (Altshuler & Ruble, 1989; Ebata & Moos, 1991; Rieder & Cicchetti, 1989), especially when dealing with stressors outside of one's control.

The lack of differences regarding well-being between groups using predominantly active strategies versus passive may be due, in part, to children rarely employing only passive or active strategies, but a combination of both. For example, while 75% of the children in the *Aggressive* group tried to stop the violence during at least one incident in the previous four months, 53% of the children in this group also ignored or pretended to ignore what was happening at least some of the time. Further research is needed to examine under what conditions active versus passive strategies are more functional for children witnessing domestic violence.

This study provides preliminary evidence that children's immediate coping strategies may depend more on situational variables (e.g., the frequency and type of abuse they are witnessing) than individual factors. However, it also raises many questions. Interestingly, the *Aggressive, Overprotective,* and *Avoidant/Ignoring* groups did not differ significantly with regard to the amount of abuse their mothers experienced nor the amount they witnessed. One situational factor did distinguish these groups—with whom the child lived. Children in the *Avoidant/Ignoring* group lived with their mothers only, while children in the *Aggressive* group were more likely to live with both their mother and the assailant. It is possible that some children resort to aggression against assailants when they are more familiar with them (from living together). Or, children may believe the assailant is less likely to leave the home if he lives there, and this might lead some children to actively fight the assailant to get him to stop the abuse. More research is needed to better explicate this relationship.

Situational factors also seemed to explain why the *Less Responsive* group responded the way they did. Mothers of the children in this group were less likely to be assaulted when compared with the other groups and children witnessed less emotional and physical abuse when compared to children in the *Aggressive* group. Children witnessing less frequent or less severe violence against their mothers may not respond as actively or emotionally as children witnessing higher levels of abuse (Peled, 1998).

This study has some important implications for intervention with children who witness domestic violence. Most notably, given that children have such varied responses even when witnessing the same amount of violence, it is critical that interventions not focus on a single approach when teaching children about responding to violence against their mothers. The finding that some children use a combination of strategies suggests that they may tailor their approach depending on their circumstances. Thus, interventions with children should be built upon those strategies that emerge 'naturally' for them. For some children this may emphasize more passive approaches (e.g., hiding in their room) while for others this may emphasize more proactive active coping strategies (e.g., getting help) or a combination of both.

Second, children may need support in making judgments about which strategies are most effective and safe. This is especially important given that a fairly substantial percentage of children are employing coping strategies that could be potentially dangerous (such as intervening to stop the abuse and becoming aggressive toward the assailant). This emphasizes the need to intervene with children to support them in engaging in proactive and safe behaviors when faced with witnessing violence (Peled & Davis, 1995). This is particularly challenging within a domestic violence context; active coping strategies could be dangerous (e.g., getting help or phoning 911) and passive coping strategies (e.g., hiding) could be safer for some children in some situations. Even some seemingly safe active strategies, like leaving the room or getting help, can be dangerous when these actions might involve the child being closer to the violence or when the action could further inflame the assailant. Thus, when building on children's natural responses to witnessing violence, it is important not only to emphasize a particular coping strategy (e.g., getting help, leaving the room), but when that strategy is safe and when it could be potentially harmful.

Finally, it is important to note that the amount of emotional abuse witnessed by children also differentiated the *Less Responsive* group from the *Aggressive/Helpseeking*, *Overprotective*, and *Avoidant/Ignoring* groups. Children are forced not only to respond to witnessing physical abuse, but also the emotional abuse of their mothers, and interventions need to focus on supporting children in coping effectively with this as well.

This study has several limitations that provide direction for future research. Mothers and children were asked to recall children's responses to witnessing domestic violence, but they were not asked to focus on a particular abusive event. This raises a couple of concerns. First, given the nature of the retrospective data collection approach, there is a risk of memory bias. It is possible that some immediate coping responses were missed or not recalled or recalled incorrectly. This may have been exacerbated by the fact that mothers and children were not focusing on a specific event, but rather on a period of time during which abuse occurred. Second, it is possible that children's combined coping strategies did not reflect their responses to a single abusive incident, but rather their collective responses across abusive incidents. Thus, it may be that in some instances children had more passive responses and in others more active. Future research is needed that includes multiple measures of children's coping, and that gathers data both on children's responses to *a single* abusive incident as well as *across* incidents.

Analyses for this study utilized data gathered from mothers because it was more detailed regarding children's behavioral responses (i.e., children were not asked if they became overprotective of their mothers or aggressive toward the assailant). However, it is important to note that for a number of immediate coping strategies, agreement was limited. Using mothers' reports may have resulted in our underreporting passive coping strategies that are inherently more internal experiences (e.g., becoming confused or ignoring or pretending to ignore the abuse). Mothers may have indicated they did not know if the child was engaged in a particular response or may have misjudged their children's responses to witnessing abuse. Further, in the midst of an assault mothers may not be well-positioned to take note of their child's specific actions. It is also possible that mothers and children used different abusive events as reference points when responding to these questions. In future research every effort should be made to assess the full range of emotional and behavioral responses based on children's reports and to incorporate open-ended questions so that children can provide greater detail regarding their specific responses. Still, it is important to consider that mothers' reports may be more accurate than children's. A number of the children were quite young (aged 6 and 7) and may have had less reliable recollections of specific actions (e.g., leaving the room). It is also interesting to note that contrary to previous research suggesting that mothers may underreport or underestimate the amount of violence their children witness (e.g., Sternberg, 1993), a considerable number of mothers in this study reported children witnessing violence when the child did not. Children may have been reluctant to reveal the abuse they had witnessed. Thus, while the findings from this study should be considered preliminary, mothers' reports provide a valuable source of information regarding children's reactions. Future research should take care in gathering detailed data from multiple informants to understand how children are responding to the emotional and physical abuse they witness.

Finally, differences did not emerge regarding the relationship between coping strategies and children's well-being. This lack of differences should be considered preliminary. First, it is important to note that with a larger sample and increased statistical power, between group differences regarding children's well-being may have emerged. It is possible that the clusters were not sufficiently large to detect between group differences. Second, children's current well-being as measured during the interview may not reflect their well-being closer to the incident(s) they are referencing or reflect their future well-being. Third, the relationship between children's immediate responses to witnessing domestic violence and their well-being needs to be examined longitudinally. It is possible that children's coping responses change over time and research on children's responses to other stressors indicates that children's coping responses seem to vary with children's development (Eisenberg, Fabes, & Guthrie, 1997). Longitudinal analyses would also allow for a more sophisticated examination of the relationship of coping to children's well-being over time, especially as it affects their development.

In order to inform interventions with children who are witnessing abuse against their mothers, more work needs to be conducted regarding children's immediate coping responses to witnessing violence. Specifically, future work should examine other variables that may differentiate children's responses, such as the number of years children have been exposed to the abuse, cultural variability, and their attitudes toward violence themselves. In addition, introducing a qualitative approach to inquiry could provide a more contextual understanding of when and how children respond to abuse against their mothers and how the strategies they employ evolve over time. For example, studies are needed that examine the consequence of children's actions, and how those consequences affected children's subsequent responses. If a child called the police, for example, and was then assaulted, one might expect that child to desist from calling for help in the future. If, on the other hand, this action resulted in the assailant fleeing the house, the child might continue using proactive responses when witness to domestic violence.

In conclusion, this study suggests that children respond to witnessing abuse against their mothers in a variety of ways, employing both passive and active coping strategies. Children's responses depend more on situational factors (e.g., amount of abuse witnessed) than on individual factors and no differences were found across groups between coping strategy and child well-being. These findings suggest that there is not necessarily a *single* coping strategy related to children's well-being, and that interventions with children must attend to their unique circumstances.

NOTES

1. Mother and child reports of witnessing emotional and physical abuse were significant with the exception of the frequency of threats which emerged as a trend (for frequency of ridicule $r = .26$, $p < .05$; frequency of threat $r = .20$, $p < .10$; frequency of physical harm $r = .27$, $p < .05$). Interestingly, only 67 of 80 children reported witnessing emotional or physical abuse while 78 of 80 mothers reported that children witnessed. Children may have been reluctant to report the abuse to the interviewer and/or mothers may have overestimated the amount of violence their children see and hear.

2. A relatively small number of mothers used the "don't know" option for the following emotional and behavioral responses: became confused about what to do (6), became angry (4), became overprotective (2), tried to stop the abuse (1), left the room (1), pretended to ignore or ignored abuse (1), and tried to phone someone (1).

3. These percentages are based on the total number of mothers ($n = 78$) and children ($n = 67$) who reported that children witnessed emotional or physical abuse.

REFERENCES

Achenbach, T., & Edelbrock, C. S. (1983). *Manual for the child behavior checklist and revised child behavior profile*. Burlington: University of Vermont.

Altshuler, J. L., & Ruble, D. N. (1989). Developmental changes in children's awareness of strategies for coping with uncontrollable stress. *Child Development, 60,* 1337-1349.

Barnett, O. W., Miller-Perrin, C. L., & Perrin, R. D. (1997). *Family violence across the lifespan*. Thousand Oaks, CA: Sage.

Carlson, B. E. (1984). Children's observations of interpersonal violence. In A. R. Roberts (Ed.), *Battered women and their families* (pp. 147-167). New York: Springer.

Christopoulos, C., Cohn, D. A., Shaw, D. S., Joyce, S., Sullivan-Hanson, J., Kraft, S. P., & Emery, R. E. (1987). Children of abused women: Adjustment at time of shelter residence. *Journal of Marriage and the Family, 49,* 611-619.

Compas, B. E. (1987). Coping with stress during childhood and adolescence. *Psychological Bulletin, 101,* 393-403.

Compas, B. E., Malcarne, V. L., & Fondacaro, K. M. (1988). Coping with stressful events in older children and young adolescents. *Journal of Consulting and Clinical Psychology, 56*(3), 405-411.

Compas, B. E., Connor-Smith, J. K., Saltzman, H., Thomsen, A. H., & Wadsworth, M. E. (2001). Coping with stress during childhood and adolescence: Problems, progress, and potential in theory and research. *Psychological Bulletin, 127*(1), 87-127.

Cummings, E. M. (1998). Children exposed to marital conflict and violence: Conceptual and theoretical directions. In G. W. Holden, R. Geffner, & E. N. Jouriles (Eds.), *Children exposed to marital violence: Theory, research, and applied issues* (pp. 55-93). Washington, DC: American Psychological Association.

Ebata, A. T., & Moos, R. H. (1991). Coping and adjustment in distressed and healthy adolescence. *Journal of Research on Adolescence, 4,* 99-125.

Eisenberg, N., Fabes, R. A., & Guthrie, I. K. (1997). Coping with stress. The roles of regulation and development. In S. A. Wolchik and I. N. Sandler (Eds.), *Handbook of children's coping: Linking theory and intervention* (pp. 41-70). New York, NY: Plenum Press.

Fabes, R. A., Eisenberg, N., & Eisenbud, L. (1993). Physiological and behavior correlates of children's reactions to others in distress. *Developmental Psychology, 29,* 655-663.

Garbarino, J., Dubrow, N., Kostelny, K., & Pardo, C. (1992). *Children in danger. Coping with the consequences of community violence*. San Francisco, CA: Jossey-Bass, Inc.

Garcia-O'Hearn, H., Margolin, G., & John, R. S. (1997). Mothers' and fathers' reports of children's reactions to naturalistic marital conflict. *Journal of the American Academy of Child and Adolescent Psychiatry, 36*(10), 1366-1373.

Graham-Bermann, S. A. (1996). Family worries: The assessment of interpersonal anxiety in children from violent and nonviolent families. *Journal of Clinical Child Psychology, 25,* 280-287.

Graham-Bermann, S. A. (1998). The impact of woman abuse on children's social development: Research and theoretical perspectives. In G. W. Holden, R. Geffner, & E. N. Jouriles (Eds.), *Children exposed to marital violence: Theory, research, and applied issues* (pp. 21-54). Washington, DC: American Psychological Association.

Graham-Bermann, S. A., & Edleson, J. L. (2001). Introduction. In S. A. Graham-Bermann & J. L. Edleson (Eds.), *Domestic violence in the lives of children: The future of research, intervention, and social policy* (pp. 3-10). Washington, DC: American Psychological Association.

Griffith, M. A., Dubow, E. F., & Ippolito, M. F. (2000). Developmental and cross-situational differences in adolescents' coping strategies. *Journal of Youth and Adolescence, 29*(2), 183-204.

Harter, S. (1985). *Manual for the Self-Perception Profile for Children.* University of Denver.

Holahan, C. J., & Moos, R. H. (1990). Life stressors, resistance factors, and improved psychological functioning: An extension of the stress resistance paradigm. *Journal of Personality and Social Psychology, 58*(5), 909-917.

Holahan, C. J., & Moos, R. H. (1991). Life stressors, personal and social resources, and depression: A 4-year structural model. *Journal of Abnormal Psychology, 100*(1), 31-38.

Holden, G. W. (1998). Introduction: The development of research into another consequence of family violence. In G. W. Holden, R. Geffner, & E. N. Jouriles (Eds.), *Children exposed to marital violence: Theory, research, and applied issues* (pp. 1-18). Washington, DC: American Psychological Association.

Hughes, H. M., Graham-Bermann, S. A., & Gruber, G. (2001). Resilience in children exposed to domestic violence. In S. A. Graham-Bermann & J. L. Edleson (Eds.), *Domestic violence in the lives of children: The future of research, intervention, and social policy* (pp. 67-90). Washington, DC: American Psychological Association.

Hughes, H. M., & Luke, D. A. (1998). Heterogeneity in adjustment among children of battered women. In G. W. Holden, R. Geffner, & E. N. Jouriles (Eds.), *Children exposed to marital violence. Theory, research, and applied issues.* Washington, DC: American Psychological Association.

Jaffe, P., Wolfe, D. A., & Wilson, S. (1990). *Children of battered women.* Newbury Park, CA: Sage.

Jouriles, E. N., & Norwood, W. D. (1995). Physical aggression toward boys and girls in families characterized by the battering of women. *Journal of Family Violence, 9,* 69-78.

Kerig, P. (2003). In search of protective processes for children exposed to interparental violence. *Journal of Emotional Abuse, 3*(3/4), 148-181.

Kliewer, W. (1991). Coping in middle childhood: Relations to competence, type A behavior, monitoring, blunting, and locus of control. *Developmental Psychology, 27,* 689-697.

Kolbo, J. R., Blakely, E., & Engleman, D. (1996). Children who witness domestic violence: A review of empirical literature. *Journal of Interpersonal Violence, 11,* 281-293.

Koss, M. P., Goodman, L. A., Browne, A., Fitzgerald, L. F., Keita, G. P., & Russo, N. F. (1994). *No safe haven: Male violence against women at home, at work, and in the community.* Washington, DC: American Psychological Association.

Kovacs, M. (1985). The children's depression inventory. *Psychopharmacology Bulletin, 21,* 995-999.

Kovacs, M. (1992). *Children's Depression Inventory.* North Tonawanda, NY: Multi-Health Systems, Inc.

McCloskey, L. A., Figueredo, A. J., & Koss, M. P. (1995). The effects of systemic family violence on children's mental health. *Child Development, 66,* 1239-1261.

McDonald, R., & Jouriles, E. N. (1991). Marital aggression and child behavior problems: Research findings, mechanisms, and intervention strategies. *Behavior Therapist, 14,* 189-192.

Moos, R. H., & Schaefer, J. A. (1993). Coping resources and processes: Current concepts and measures. In L. Goldberger & S. Breznitz (Eds), *Handbook of stress: Theoretical and clinical aspects* (2nd ed., pp. 234-257). New York: Free Press.

Norris, F. H., & Kaniasty, K. (1994). Psychological distress following criminal victimization in the general population: Cross-sectional, longitudinal, and prospective analyses. *Journal of Consulting and Clinical Psychology, 62,* 111-123.

O'Brien, M., Margolin, G., John, R. S., & Krueger, L. Mothers' and sons' cognitive and emotional reactions to simulated marital and family conflict. *Journal of Consulting & Clinical Psychology, 59*(5), 692-703.

Onyskiw, J. E. (2003). Domestic violence and children's adjustment: A review of research. *Journal of Emotional Abuse, 3*(1/2), 11-45.

Peled, E. (1998). The experience of living with violence for preadolescent children of battered women. *Youth and Society, 29,* 395-430.

Peled, E., & Davis, D. (1995). *Groupwork with children of battered women.* Thousand Oaks, CA: Sage.

Rieder, C., & Cicchetti, D. (1989). Organizational perspective on cognitive control functioning and cognitive-affective balance in maltreated children. *Developmental Psychology, 25,* 382-393.

Rosenberg, M. S. (1987). Children of battered women: The effects of witnessing violence on their social problem-solving abilities. *Behavior Therapist, 10* (4), 85-89.

Rossman, B. B. R. (2001). Longer term effects of children's exposure to domestic violence. In S. A. Graham-Bermann & J. L. Edleson (Eds.), *Domestic violence in the lives of children: The future of research, intervention, and social policy* (pp. 35-66). Washington, DC: American Psychological Association.

Rossman, B. B. R., & Ho, J. (2000). Posttraumatic response and children exposed to parental violence. In R. A. Geffner, P. G. Jaffe, & M. Suderman (Eds.), *Children exposed to domestic violence: Current issues in research, intervention, prevention and policy development* (pp. 85-106). Binghamton, NY: The Haworth Press, Inc.

Rothbart, M. K., Ziaie, H., O'Boyle, C. G., & Cherie G. (1992). Self-regulation and emotion in infancy. In N. Eisenberg & R. A. Fabes (Eds.), *New direction in child development: The development of self-regulation and emotion* (pp. 7-24). San Francisco: Jossey-Bass.

Sandler, I. N., Tein, J.Y., & West, S. G. (1994). Coping, stress, and the psychological symptoms of children of divorce: A cross-sectional and longitudinal study. *Child Development, 65*, 1744-1763.

Sternberg, K. J., Lamb, M. E., Greenbaum, C., Cicchetti, D., Dawud, S., Cortes, R. M., Krispin, O., & Lorey, F. (1993). Effects of domestic violence on children's behavior problems and depression. *Developmental Psychology, 29*, 44-52.

Straus, M. A. (1979). Measuring intrafamily conflict and violence: The conflict tactics scale. *Journal of Marriage and the Family, 41*, 75-88.

Straus, M. A. (1992). Children as witnesses to marital violence: A risk factor for life long problems among a nationally representative sample of American men and women. In D. F. Schwarz (Ed.), *Children and violence* (Report of the 23rd Ross Roundtable on Critical Approaches to Common Pediatric Problems). Columbus, OH: Ross Laboratories.

Sullivan, C. M., Parisian, J. A., & Davidson, W. S. (1991). *Index of Psychological Abuse: Development of a measure.* Poster presentation at the American Psychological Association. San Francisco, CA. August.

Tomkins, A. J., Mohamed, S., Steinman, M., Macolini, R. M., Kenning, M. K., & Afrank, J. (1994). The plight of children who witness woman battering: Psychological knowledge and policy implications. *Law & Psychology Review, 18*(Spr), 137-187.

Valentiner, D. P., Holahan, C. J., & Moos, R. H. (1994). Social support, appraisals of event controllability, and coping: An integrative model. *Journal of Personality and Social Psychology, 66*(6), 1094-1102.

PREVENTION AND INTERVENTION FOR CHILDREN EXPOSED TO INTIMATE PARTNER VIOLENCE

In Search of Protective Processes for Children Exposed to Interparental Violence

Patricia K. Kerig

SUMMARY. Although clinicians have been called upon to develop empirically based interventions for children, the field of family violence has

Address correspondence to: Patricia K. Kerig, PhD, Department of Psychology, University of North Carolina at Chapel Hill, CB #3270 Davie Hall, Chapel Hill, NC 27599-3270 (E-mail: kerigpk@unc.edu).

Portions of this work were funded by the Social Sciences and Humanities Research Council of Canada (Grant # 410-94-1547) and a University Research Council Grant from the University of North Carolina at Chapel Hill.

This paper is based on an invited address presented at the Fifth International Conference on Family Violence, September 2000, San Diego, CA.

[Haworth co-indexing entry note]: "In Search of Protective Processes for Children Exposed to Interparental Violence." Kerig, Patricia K. Co-published simultaneously in *Journal of Emotional Abuse* (The Haworth Maltreatment & Trauma Press, an imprint of The Haworth Press, Inc.) Vol. 3, No. 3/4, 2003, pp. 149-181; and: *The Effects of Intimate Partner Violence on Children* (ed: Robert A. Geffner, Robyn Spurling Igelman, and Jennifer Zellner) The Haworth Maltreatment & Trauma Press, an imprint of The Haworth Press, Inc., 2003, pp. 149-181. Single or multiple copies of this article are available for a fee from The Haworth Document Delivery Service [1-800-HAWORTH, 9:00 a.m. - 5:00 p.m. (EST). E-mail address: docdelivery@haworthpress.com].

only just begun to answer the call. The purpose of the present paper is to integrate theory, research, and clinical work in order to create an intervention model that is empirically informed and empirically testable. To this aim, literature is reviewed that sheds light on risk and resilience in children exposed to interparental violence. Attention is given to the risk outcomes associated with exposure to violence, the mechanisms by which those negative effects come about, the protective processes that can buffer children from risk, and the methods available for studying those processes. *[Article copies available for a fee from The Haworth Document Delivery Service: 1-800-HAWORTH. E-mail address: <docdelivery@haworthpress.com> Website: <http://www.HaworthPress.com> © 2003 by The Haworth Press, Inc. All rights reserved.]*

KEYWORDS. Child witnesses, family violence, interparental conflict, resilience, treatment

At eight years of age, Gemma was a bright and vivacious child, full of humor and hijinks. She was also hearing-impaired and had a fascination with underwater worlds, as silent as her own. What brought Gemma to psychotherapy was her oppositionality with teachers, aggressiveness toward classmates, and lack of tolerance for frustration, including the kind I introduced in therapy when I wanted to talk about feelings instead of playing. However, Gemma had a very effective coping strategy for my intrusions: She simply turned off her hearing aid and looked away. Although Gemma was referred to treatment because of aggressive behavior, in her play she seemed to identify with the victims of aggression rather than its perpetrators. For example, life was not always good for the beautiful mermaids that inhabited her fantasy world. An abrupt change in Gemma's play was ushered in one day with the scenario she drew in Figure 1, accompanied by Gemma's vivid enactment of the terror and helplessness to which her mermaid was subjected. Only afterwards did I uncover the origin of this theme in her play, when Gemma recalled a time that her mother's boyfriend became extremely violent, beating the mother while Gemma clung to her in terror. Her mother managed to push Gemma into the bathroom and shut the door, and for the next several minutes Gemma felt through the door the impact of her mother's body being repeatedly thrown against it. Over the course of treatment, Gemma was able to work through her fears, develop strategies with which to calm herself, and find safe ha-

vens in her internal and external worlds. As her fears subsided, her aggressiveness reduced and she began to have a more positive and hopeful outlook.

Gemma's story is one that illustrates a number of concepts. First, it provides an example of the significant and diverse effects on children of exposure to violence. Secondly, her story suggests that children can be helped to be resilient in the face of even such overwhelming stress as exposure to their mothers' abuse. Knowledge of the processes by which resilience comes about is particularly valuable. Such knowledge can lead directly to the development of interventions that will foster the strengths and competencies needed to overcome "hard growing" (Radke-Yarrow & Sherman, 1990). The purpose of the present paper is to contribute to an understanding of how resilience in children exposed to violence occurs and how it might be promoted. This work-in-progress strives to point the way toward the development of an intervention model, navigating by means of theory, research and clinical experience.

FIGURE 1

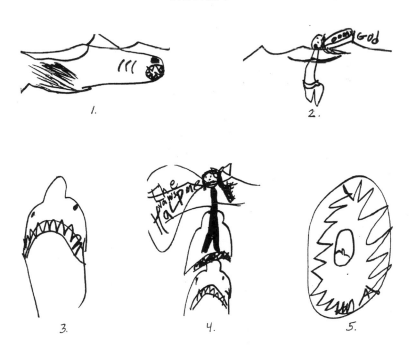

DEFINING RESILIENCE

The concept of resilience arose from the discovery that, among children growing up in conditions of family adversity, poverty, and violence, a small but significant number demonstrated good functioning despite exposure to those risks (Garmezy, 1974; Masten & Coatsworth, 1998). However, there are a number of questions unanswered in the study of resilience, and the concept itself has undergone a process of development (see Luthar, Cicchetti, & Becker, 2000).

Resilience versus Invulnerability. Early formulations referred to children who functioned well despite adversity as "invulnerable" (Anthony & Cohler, 1987). However, the term implies an imperviousness to harm that does not characterize these children accurately. For example, Luthar, Doernberger, and Zigler (1993) point out that, although resilient children may appear to be functioning well, there are subtle ways in which they show the legacy of their painful childhoods. Luthar and her colleagues found that, while resilient individuals were less likely to behave in ways that labeled them as troublesome to others, they still showed signs of being inwardly troubled. For example, 85 percent experienced symptoms of internalized distress such as worry, anxiety, and sadness. Similarly, Werner's (1994) longitudinal study of resilience showed that many adults who overcame adversity nonetheless suffered stress-related health problems and feelings of personal unhappiness.

These studies indicate that resilience is relative, not absolute. Resilient children are not impervious to harm, even if they are better able to overcome adversity than other children. Recognition of the limitations of "invulnerability" also mitigates against concerns that resilience research will minimize the seriousness of risk factors such as family violence, blame the victim, or perpetuate the "Horatio Alger" myth that individual willpower conquers all (Garmezy, 1994). While there are competencies that protect children from the negative impact of violence, and resilience research can help to identify those, there are no children so armor-plated that we need not be concerned about them.

Protective Factors. A second approach to the study of resilience involves identifying the characteristics of children who cope well with stress. For example, investigators have identified a number of variables associated with resilience, including intelligence, social class, gender, easy temperament, physical attractiveness, and sociability (see Masten & Coatsworth, 1998; Wenar & Kerig, 2000). Some of these variables have to do with inherent characteristics of the child, such as physical appearance and gender, or with child and family variables that are difficult to change, such as intelligence and social class. However, resilience "is not a static trait" (Cicchetti & Garmezy, 1993, p. 499) and "cannot be seen as a fixed attribute of the individual" (Rutter, 1990, p. 184). Rather, resilience is a dynamic process (Egeland, Carlson, & Sroufe, 1993), to which a list of protective factors cannot do justice. "Resilience is not something some children 'have a lot of.' It develops" (Sroufe, 1997, p. 256). In the developmental psychopathology view, therefore, resilience emerges as a product of complex transactions between the child and the environment.

Protective Mechanisms. Rutter (1990) offers a third approach to the study of resilience, one that arises from a developmental psychopathology perspective. Rutter argues that we need to focus attention on what *accounts* for the power of protective factors; that is, what is it about intelligence or easy temperament that protects against psychopathology? It is often the case that protective factors are construed as the opposite of risk factors (Wenar & Kerig, 2000). However, for Rutter, protection is more than the absence of risk. Rutter takes a dynamic, transactional view of the processes by which protective variables operate. He conceptualizes these as *protective mechanisms*, and he identifies four of them on the basis of research and theory.

The first of Rutter's protective mechanisms is termed *reduction of risk impact*, which refers to factors that buffer the child from exposure to risk. It cannot be stated strongly enough that the most effective protection will be afforded by preventing children from experiencing violence in their homes, thereby removing the source of risk. Efforts to change the behavior of abusive men are of the utmost importance. However, many factors, including economic, cultural, familial, and psychological pressures, conspire to prevent battered women from calling their abuse to the attention of authorities and thus many violent men will not be referred for treatment. When family violence does takes place, parents can at least minimize the extent to which children witness their conflicts and take care to remind children that they are not to blame for their parents' marital problems (Cummings, Ballard, El-Sheikh, & Lake, 1991; Grych & Fincham, 1993).

Secondly, factors that promote constructive *coping and self-efficacy* can protect children. According to Rutter, children who have a sense of themselves as effective copers are less likely to become overwhelmed by distress and are more likely to approach future life challenges with an optimistic and constructive outlook. For example, children who believe that they can remain calm when their parents argue are better able to cope with the stress of exposure to violence (Kerig, Fedorowicz, Brown, Patenaude, & Warren, 1998; Rossman & Rosenberg, 1992). However, the question remains as how it is that resilient children come to view themselves in positive and efficacious terms. "That is, we need to ask why and how some individuals manage to maintain high self-esteem and self-efficacy in spite of facing the same adversities that lead other people to give up and lose hope" (Rutter, 1990, p. 183). The origins of these protective mechanisms, Rutter suggests, lie in the transactions between children and their social environments.

In this regard, the third protective mechanism involves *reduction of negative chain reactions*, many of which occur in the family context. For example, a large literature has shown that there are a variety of ways in which marital conflicts can "spill over" onto parent-child relationships (Kerig, Cowan, & Cowan, 1993). In the case of domestic violence, a particular worry is that children will not only witness violence but will become the victims of it–the "double whammy," as Hughes, Parkinson, and Vargo (1989) termed it. The transactional nature of the spill-over of violence is suggested by Jouriles and Norwood (1995), who found that boys growing up in violent families were more likely than other children to be maltreated. These investigators speculate that boys, because they react to family conflict with problem behavior, are more likely become the targets of parental anger. Processes that interrupt these negative cycles can buffer children from the negative effects of marital conflict.

Rutter's fourth protective mechanism is termed *opening of opportunities*. Development involves many turning points that offer a chance to reduce the impact of risk factors, and the resilient child is the one who takes advantage of these. "Protection does not reside in the psychological chemistry of the moment but in the ways in which people deal with life changes and in what they do about their stressful or disadvantaging circumstances. Particular attention needs to be paid to the mechanisms operating at key turning points in people's lives, when a risk trajectory may be redirected onto a more adaptive path" (p. 210). For example, Rutter (1990) points out that some children close themselves off from opportunities for personal growth, such as by dropping out of school, or fail to avail themselves of the positive relationships that are available in their environments, such as by rejecting the overtures of a caring neighbor. In the case of family violence, it is important that children not develop the expectation that violence is a normal and inevitable part of relationships and thus be hindered from forming healthy kinds of intimacy in their lives. Protection can occur when children are exposed to models of constructive conflict resolution, nonviolence, and mutually respectful relationships between men and women, models that may be available in the extended family, the school, the community, the women's shelter, or their relationship with their mothers.

There are a number of benefits of Rutter's model of resilience. Because it is process-oriented, this model directs our attention to the mechanisms underlying the positive effects of protective factors. These mechanisms are more accessible to change than are static personal characteristics, and point us toward ways in which we might intervene. Therefore, in order to develop interventions for children exposed to violence, we need to identify the processes that will mitigate its negative effects (see Winstok & Eisikovits, 2003).

CHANGE PROCESSES
AND THE PROCESS OF EMPIRICAL VALIDATION

Ultimately, efforts to identify protective processes will allow us to develop treatments that are not only informed by theory, but are amenable to empirical validation. Clinicians have been called upon to develop empirically supported interventions (Task Force on Promotion and Dissemination of Psychological Procedures, 1995; Chambless & Ollendick, 2001) but the call has been answered rarely in the field of family violence. For example, the National Council of Juvenile and Family Court Judges (1998) recently published a review of 29 promising interventions for children exposed to violence, only two of which included evaluations more rigorous than informal self-studies and client satisfaction ratings. Similarly, Rossman, Hughes, and Rosenberg's (2000) recent careful review uncovers more descriptive than empirical work on interventions for battered women and their children. Highly regarded programs that provide the basis for most interventions in this area, including Jaffe and colleagues (Jaffe, Wilson, & Wolfe, 1986, 1988; Jaffe, Wolfe, & Wilson, 1990; Loosley, Bentley, Rabenstein, & Sudermann, 1997) and Peled, Edleson and their colleagues (Grusznski, Brink, & Edleson, 1988; Peled & Davis, 1994; Peled & Edleson, 1995) so far have been subjected to only limited evaluation.

Although the efficacy of some interventions has been more stringently tested, with positive results (e.g., Graham-Berman, 1998; Jouriles, McDonald, Stephens, Norwood, Spiller, & Ware, 1998), to date none fully meet the APA Task Force's (1995) criteria. In particular, rarely has a comparison treatment or control group been included, and almost all intervention programs have been evaluated in a single study. Even where replication has been attempted, different patterns of results have been found. For example, Jaffe et al. (1988) found that their intervention was successful in improving children's safety planning and perceptions of their mothers, with no changes in behavioral symptoms or attitudes toward anger and violence. In contrast, Wagar and Rodway's (1995) control-group replication found improvements only in attitudes toward anger and responsibility for violence. More work remains to be done to resolve these discrepancies, but the efforts are necessary and worthwhile. Despite the controversies about the standards for empirical validation established by the Task Force (Chambless & Ollendick, 2001), and the challenges of meeting them in the "real world" (Weisz & Hawley, 1998), it is not only of practical importance to demonstrate the efficacy of interventions, it is ethically mandated for psychologists to use techniques for which there is evidence of effectiveness (American Psychological Association, 1992).

Further, Kazdin (1997) argues that, to truly test an intervention's effectiveness, we need to demonstrate not only that the treatment brings about change but also that the factors targeted by the treatment are what indeed account for change. Shirk and Russell (1996) refer to the effective ingredients of treatment as *change processes*. The relevant change processes to be addressed by treatment are derived from theoretical formulations regarding the underlying *pathogenic processes* that cause the disorder. In sum, guided by this model, the task of developing an intervention requires that we explicate our theories of psychopathology, resilience, and change. In turn, the task of validating an intervention requires that we find means of operationalizing and measuring the change processes that presumably underlie the effectiveness of the treatment. In order to accomplish these goals for children exposed to interparental violence, therefore, four questions need to be addressed: (1) what are the likely risk outcomes for children exposed to violence; (2) what processes account for the effects of those outcomes; (3) which protective processes might mitigate against the risks; and (4) how can we measure those protective processes?

RISK OUTCOMES FOR CHILDREN EXPOSED TO VIOLENCE

Risk research can help us to identify the kinds of adjustment problems to which children exposed to violence are most vulnerable and which might, therefore, be priorities for intervention. These encompass the entire spectrum of internalizing and externalizing symptoms: *depression*, including sadness, shame, self-deprecation, hopelessness, and helplessness; *anxiety*, including distress over the violence, worry about themselves and their family; and *aggression* and oppositionality toward parents, teachers, and peers (for recent reviews, see Geffner et al., 2000; Holden et al., 1998; Osofsky & Scheeringa, 1997; and Rossman et al., 2000). In addition, the overwhelming emotions and unregulated distress accompanying exposure to violence may lead to symptoms of *posttraumatic stress disorder*, such as hyperarousal, avoidance, and numbing (Graham-Bermann & Levendosky, 1998a; Kerig, Fedorowicz, Brown, & Warren, 2000; Rossman & Ho, 2000). Feelings of personal vulnerability and negative expectations about the future also are predicted by exposure to violence (Schwab-Stone, Ayers, Kasprow, Voyce, Barone, Shriver, & Weissberg, 1995).

Further, over the long term, there is evidence for the *intergenerational transmission of violence*. Children may grow up to become the next generation of abusers and victims when they carry the violent lessons they learned at home into later relationships. For example, Wolfe, Wekerle, Reitzel-Jaffe, and Lefebvre (1998) found that adolescents from violent homes were more likely to become involved in violent dating relationships. Mechanisms that might explain this intergenerational transmission are sex-role stereotypes and the acceptance of violence against women (Grusznski et al., 1988; Jaffe et al., 1986). Children exposed to models of violence against women are more likely than other children to believe that violence against women is justified. For example, children exposed to violence–especially boys–are more likely to endorse statements indicating less egalitarian sex-role attitudes, such as that men should always be in charge and that it is "okay" for a man to hit a woman who defies his authority (Jaffe et al., 1986; Kerig, 1999a).

RISK PROCESSES FOR CHILDREN EXPOSED TO VIOLENCE

Having identified the particular adjustment problems for which children exposed to violence are vulnerable, our next task is to discover how these effects come about. Taking a page from Rutter's (1990) book, we can look not just for risk factors, but *risk processes*, the mechanisms by which these negative effects take place. A review of the available research suggests four that emerge as particularly important for children's development, not because they are the only factors that can be identified, but because they represent processes that can be changed, thus lending themselves to the development of interventions. *Triangulation in Interparental Conflict.* A number of studies have shown that children's anxiety is greatest when they are exposed to interparental violence in which they are directly implicated or involved (Grych, Fincham, Jouriles, & McDonald, 2001). This can occur in a number of ways. For example, children may directly *witness* the violence (Porter & O'Leary, 1980) or the child may provide the *topic* about which parents argue (Jouriles, Murphy, Farris, Smith, Richters, & Waters, 1991). Family systemic processes, such as *triangulation* (Kerig, 1995; Minuchin, 1974), also inveigle children inappropriately in the marital relationship. Triangulation can occur at parents' initiation, such as when a parent confides in the child about marital problems or encourages the child to take sides in the argument (Kerig, 1996), but children also may volunteer for this role in an attempt to solve their family's problems (Johnston, Gonzales, & Campbell, 1987; Kerig, 2001b). Of particular concern are children who attempt to cope with the problem by physically *intervening* in their parents' conflicts (Kerig, 1999b; also see Allen, Wolf, Bybee, & Sullivan, 2003, for a discussion of children's immediate coping responses to witnessing domestic violence). A child who becomes an actor in the conflict may be placing him/herself in danger if those conflicts are violent ones. Yet, provoked by anxiety, altruism, or anger, children may be only too willing to put themselves in harm's way by intervening in the violence (Christopoulos, Cohn, Shaw, Joyce, Sullivan-Hanson, Kraft, & Emery, 1987; Gordis, Margolin, & John, 1995; Johnston, Campbell, & Mayes, 1985; Kerig et al., 1998). Research indicates that older children are particularly at risk for intervening (Cummings et al., 1991; Davies et al., 1996; Kerig, 1999b) and adolescent boys are especially likely to feel that they are responsible for taking direct action and protecting their mothers (Jaffe, Wolfe, & Wilson, 1990; Kerig, 1999a; Laumakis, Margolin, & John, 1998).

Negative Appraisals. Grych and Fincham (1990) propose that children's appraisals are powerful predictors of their reactions and adjustment to interparental conflict. Grych and Fincham view children as active problem-solvers, who strive to understand the reasons for their parents' marital problems and the role that children might play in solving them. When their parents argue, children attempt to evaluate what is happening (the *properties* of the conflict), how serious it is (*threat*), and whether they have done something to cause it (*self-blame*). In addition, Rossman and Rosenberg (1992) contribute appraisals of *perceived control*, children's belief they can actually stop their parents from quarreling. School-aged children may have unrealistic appraisals of control over their parents' conflicts, leading to feelings of guilt that they did not do something to stop the violence (Osofsky & Scheeringa, 1997), whereas a dilemma for younger children may be the interaction of self-blame and low control: the perception that they are responsible for causing the violence but can do nothing about it (Kerig, 1998a).

Consistent with Grych and Fincham's model (1990), children exposed to violence perceive their parents' conflicts as having more negative properties, feel more threatened, and engage in more self-blame than other children (Kerig et al., 1998). Research has also demonstrated that appraisals mediate the relationship between exposure to violence and children's adjustment, particularly in regard to anxiety and depression (Grych et al., 2001). There may be some gender differences in the pattern of effects; for example, perceived threat has been found to mediate the relationship between exposure to violence and boys' internalizing while appraisals of self blame mediate the relationship between violence and girls' internalizing (Cummings et al., 1994; Kerig, 1998a). Further contributing to a sense of hopelessness are negative appraisals children make, not only of themselves, but of their families–the sense of *shame* about coming from a violent home, and the feelings of isolation that ensue (Grusznski et al., 1988). Further, under conditions of traumatic exposure, preschool children particularly are prone to making distorted appraisals and experiencing cognitive confusions (Kerig et al., 2000; Pynoos, 1993). Often these misperceptions involve disturbing images that can be traumatizing in and of themselves and generate additional distress, further inhibiting children's ability to reason about and work through the trauma (Ribbe, Lipovsky, & Freedy, 1995).

Emotional Insecurity. In contrast to Grych and Fincham's (1990) focus on cognitions, other theorists have focused on children's emotions. Davies and Cummings (1994; Cummings, 1998) argue that conflict and violence in the home affect children through threatening their *emotional security*. Emotional security is disrupted by *unregulated distress*, when children experience overwhelming emotions without the capacity to manage them. Unregulated distress also is a significant contributor to the development of posttraumatic stress disorder (Pynoos, Steinberg, & Wriath, 1995). The chronic experience of intense negative emotions interferes with the development of emotion regulation, interfering with the abilities to identify feelings in early childhood, elaborate on affective expression in the latency years, and understand emotions and their consequences in adolescence (Pynoos, 1993). Further, as Pynoos

(1993) observes, children chronically exposed to violence may gravitate toward dangerous situations and relationships in which the experience of heightened emotional arousal feels ego syntonic. On the other hand, children who have experienced unregulated distress often exhibit avoidant behaviors that can interfere with the development of autonomy. Avoidant coping with stress can foreclose opportunities for growth, such as by inhibiting the development of relationships with multiple caregivers in preschool, academic mastery in the school-age years, and prosocial peer relations in adolescence.

Emotional insecurity also leads children to develop *insecure representations of family relationships*, when marital problems threaten children with family dissolution and the loss of their secure base. While fears of the loss of attachment figures are particularly salient for young children, emotional insecurity appears to motivate older children to actively cope with the problem by *intervening* in their parents' arguments, further increasing the risk of maladjustment (Davies & Cummings, 1998). Thus, emotional insecurity places children at risk for maladaptive coping, whether in the form of pathological avoidance or over-involvement in their parents' quarrels. Moreover, internal working models of relationships act as schemas by which children derive expectations of the trustworthiness of others and the care-worthiness of themselves. Insecure representations of self and other can lead children to approach new relationships in negative or ineffective ways, predisposing children in yet another way toward engaging in victimizing or victimization (Wekerle & Wolfe, 1998; West & George, 1999).

Parent-Child Transactions. As noted above, marital violence can spill over onto children in a variety of ways. Spillover may occur directly, such as when child witnesses are also the targets of *maltreatment*. While the majority of child maltreatment in violent families is accounted for by fathers (O'Keefe, 1995), distressed mothers too may become perpetrators (see Edleson, 1999). Maltreated witnesses are the children most negatively affected by violence in the family (Hughes et al., 1989; O'Keefe, 1995), with wide-ranging effects on adjustment, including depression, anxiety, and aggression (O'Keefe, 1994). Very young children and adolescents are most at risk for the spillover of abuse (National Center on Child Abuse and Neglect, 1995) and boys may be particularly vulnerable due to their propensity to react to violence in the home with misbehavior (Jouriles & Norwood, 1995).

Other mechanisms of spillover are indirect, affecting children through their impact on *parenting* (Levendosky & Graham-Bermann,

2000). For example, maternal stress has emerged as a mediator of the impact of violence on children, affecting mothers' parenting and emotional availability (O'Keefe, 1994; Wolfe, Jaffe, & Zak, 1985; see also Kalil, Tolman, Rosen, & Gruber, 2003). In addition, Graham-Bermann (1996) described "family worries" as sources of stress for children exposed to violence. Children who are concerned about their mother's well-being also must worry about whether they themselves will be "okay." Maternal distress, therefore, can negatively affect parenting and is a source of anxiety and insecurity for children of battered women (Osofsky, 1995). Adolescent girls may be particularly likely to take on the role of caregiver to their emotionally stressed mothers, which may cause them to look highly competent in the short term but which, in the long term, is a developmentally inappropriate burden (Jaffe et al., 1990; Kerig, 1999a).

On the other side of the transaction, children from violent homes engage in *challenging behaviors* including aggression, oppositionality, increased dependency, and the loss of developmental attainments, which can tax the resources of their parents. Particularly disconcerting is that some children of battered women direct aggression toward their mothers. For example, Graham-Bermann and Levendosky (1998b) found that children exposed to violence engaged in more arguing and negative exchanges with their mothers than did other children. Further, some children engage in distorted attributions in which they *blame the mother* for the violence and criticize her for disrupting the family by bringing them to the shelter. Underlying motivations for this may be children's need to retain an attachment to the abuser (Blizard & Bluhm, 1994) or their need to protect themselves from perceived threat by identifying with the aggressor. However, the experience of having anger and blame laid at her door is very painful for the mother, further adding to her distress and undermining her parenting confidence.

Moreover, some battered women report feeling inhibited about disciplining their children, not wanting to be harsh or negative to children who already have been exposed to so much stress. This is borne out by research. Holden and his colleagues (Holden & Ritchie, 1991; Holden, Stein, Ritchie, Harris, & Jouriles, 1998) find that it is *parenting consistency*, the providing of firmness and structure, that is disrupted when mothers are under the traumatic stress of battering. Lack of consistent structure can further contribute to aggression and oppositional behavior in children (Baumrind, 1994), setting in motion one of Rutter's negative chain reactions.

PROTECTIVE PROCESSES
FOR CHILDREN EXPOSED TO VIOLENCE

Based on the above risk processes, there are a number of *protective processes* that are particularly salient for children exposed to violence. These represent possible targets for intervention, each of which would be touched on, ideally, in a multi-faceted intervention.

Constructive Coping. Children's strategies for coping with interparental conflict may be sources of either risk or resilience (Grych & Fincham, 1993; Kerig, 1999). However, one of the limitations of coping research is that the typologies used most widely, such as the emotion-focused versus problem-focused distinction, are very broad and do not make discriminations that are important in the context of family violence (Kerig, 2001a). For example, problem-focused coping may lead children to attempt to take action by entering into the argument as a participant, whether directly or indirectly (Davies, Myers, & Cummings, 1996; Grych & Fincham, 1993). It is when children are triangulated in this way that they are most at risk for becoming the targets of their parents' anger (Kerig, Brown, & Patenaude, 2001). However, little attention has been paid to identifying ways in which children might avoid entanglement in their parents' marital issues (Kerig, 1999b). *Detriangulation* refers to strategies children use to escape involvement in their parents' arguments by disentangling themselves physically, cognitively, and/or emotionally (see Table 1). Younger children may be characterized by a combination of perceived responsibility for solving their parents' problems but inability to do so, leading to forms of cognitive involvement such as "worried avoidance" (O'Brien, Badahur, Gee, Balto, & Erber, 1997) with its concomitant feelings of helplessness and failure. With older children, in turn, it is important to be sensitive to more subtle forms of emotional involvement, such as caregiving and role-reversal, particularly for girls (Kerig, 1999b).

Despite the fact that some forms of problem-focused coping are maladaptive, such as triangulation, there are potentially *constructive active coping* strategies children might use to respond to interparental violence, such as going to a safe place, calling 911, or turning to a third party for assistance. Such "safety planning" is targeted consistently by treatments for children exposed to violence (Grusznski et al., 1988; Jaffe et al., 1986; Loosely et al., 1997; Peled & Davis, 1995; Rossman, 2000). Coaching children in constructive active coping may increase not only their ability to detriangulate and their appraisals of self-efficacy (see Table 2), but also their receptivity to the intervention.

TABLE 1. Child Intervening in Interparental Conflict Scale (Kerig, 1994)

Triangulation: "I went in and yelled at Dad, 'Stop picking on Mom!'"

Mediation: "I suggested they take turns using the car."

Interruption: "I went in the room and asked them to please stop fighting."

Indirect-Misbehavior: "I went in the next room and knocked over the rack of CDs."

Indirect-Prosocial Behavior: "I cleaned up the house so Mom and Dad wouldn't be so stressed."

Emotional Involvement/Caregiving: "Afterward, Mom was crying so I gave her a hug."

Cognitive Involvement/Information-seeking: "Afterward I asked, were you fighting about me?"

Constructive Actions/Help-Seeking: "I called 911." "I called my uncle and asked him for help."

Passive Noninvolvement: "I just stood there."

Detriangulation: "I knew they'd work it out better if I stayed out of it." "I asked them not to make me take sides."

When children are distressed, it is hard for them to feel comforted by the idea of "just doing nothing," and this is particularly true for older boys (Kerig et al., 1998; Kerig, 1999). Therefore, children benefit from having a repertoire of positive actions to perform, rather than a list of "don'ts."

Lastly, even when there is nothing children can do to actually solve their parents' marital problems, there are coping strategies children can use to stay calm, quell their anxiety, and prevent themselves from being overwhelmed by distress. Therefore, children can benefit from learning *emotion-focused coping* strategies when their parents argue. Examples of emotion-focused coping are provided in the many measures of coping used with children (see Kerig, 2001a), including spending time with friends, listening to music, or writing in a diary. Studies have confirmed that, in contrast to problem-focused coping, emotion-focused coping can buffer children from the negative effects of interparental conflict (Kerig, 1997a; O'Brien et al., 1997) and violence (Kerig et al., 1998).

Emotional Security. Given that the unregulated stress evoked by interparental violence is a particular risk for the development of emotional insecurity, a subtype of emotion-focused coping called *emotion regulation* can act as an important buffer against anxiety and perceived helplessness. The goal of emotion regulation is to help children calm themselves and reduce their feelings of distress. Emotion regulation involves simple cognitive-behavioral strategies that can be taught directly

TABLE 2. Perceived Coping Efficacy Scale Sample Items (Children's Coping Questionnaire; Fedorowicz & Kerig, 1995)

"Think about all the things you do when this problem happens. How much do they help?"

"Think about the things you do to change the situation when this problem happens. How much do they help?"

"Think about all the things you do change the way you feel when this problem happens. How much do they help?"

---

to even young children (Fedorowicz & Kerig, 1995; see Table 3). As children learn how to prevent themselves from being overwhelmed by distress, they will gain a sense of competence and internal security. Affect regulation also is a key element in interventions designed to help children with symptoms of posttraumatic stress, allowing them to engage in the kind of therapeutic exposure necessary for integration and mastery of traumatic experiences (Kerig et al., 2000; Silvern, Karyl, & Landis, 1995).

Children's emotional insecurity also will be reduced to the extent that they make positive attributions about their mothers. In particular, children will benefit from having confidence in their mothers' capacity to protect them and care for them. Gemma is a good example: Despite her terror about the violence in her home, she perceived her mother as her protector and found reassurance in that fact. Thus, a secure attachment to her mother acted as a buffer against the development of negative schemas of self and other and enabled her to engage in caring relationships with adults and peers. *Perceived maternal efficacy* can be measured by eliciting children's positive appraisals of the mother and her ability to provide them with instrumental and emotional support (Kerig, 1997b; see Table 4).

Positive Appraisals. Given the harmful role of negative appraisals in children's reactions to interparental conflict, it is surprising that little attention has been given to positive appraisals that might buffer them from the effects of family violence (Kerig, 1998b). One such positive appraisal is *perceived coping efficacy* (see Table 2). As Rutter notes, belief that they can cope effectively leads children to develop a sense confidence that helps them to rise above adversity. Research has confirmed that perceived coping efficacy buffers children from the stress of exposure to interparental conflict (El-Sheikh & Cummings, 1992; Kerig, 1997a). Perceived coping efficacy also can be increased when children learn that there are constructive strategies they can perform (Rossman, 2000).

TABLE 3. Affect Regulation Scale Sample Items (Children's Coping Question-naire; Fedorowicz & Kerig, 1995)

"Count to ten."
"Take a deep breath."
"Tell myself it will be over soon."

TABLE 4. Perceived Maternal Efficacy Scale Sample Items (Kerig, 1997b)

"If something bad happens, my Mom will take care of me."
"My Mom makes sure I'm safe."
"If I'm scared, my Mom can help my scared feelings go away."

Another positive appraisal involves *absolution from self-blame*. It is often difficult to shift children from attributions of self-blame, even when such appraisals involve cognitive distortions. Children tend to reason in an egocentric fashion, seeing themselves as causal to what is happening around them. Further, Janoff-Bulman (1979) speculated that self-blame can serve an adaptive function, allowing one to achieve a sense of control over an uncontrollable stressor. Nonetheless, self-blame for violence is a negative and distorted attribution, leading to depression and helplessness in battered women (O'Neill & Kerig, 2000) and their children (Kerig, 1998a). Children can be helped to absolve themselves of blame through direct work countering their distorted cognitions (Grusznski et al., 1988; Jaffe et al., 1986; Peled & Edleson, 1995). In addition, as Cummings et al. (1991) have found, parents can help by explicitly stating that children are not responsible for causing or solving the violence. The effectiveness of these interventions can be assessed by changes in perceived blame on measures of children's appraisals about interparental conflict (e.g., Grych, Seid, & Fincham, 1992).

Finally, in order to rid themselves of a sense of stigma and shame, children of violence need to find ways to make *affirmations of self and family*. Given that self-esteem and perceived competence moderate the effects of exposure to violence (O'Keefe, 1994), interventions quite rightly focus on helping children to recognize their own worth (e.g., Peled & Davis, 1995; Rossman, 2000). For example, Grusznski et al. (1988) enhance self-esteem directly, by encouraging children to make self-affirmations, and indirectly, by teaching parents to have appropriate expectations for their children's development. In addition, children need to be helped to find family strengths and qualities in which they can feel pride (Kerig, 1999; Loosely et al., 1997). Changes in self-esteem can be measured by using one of the many standard measures available, while perceptions of family strengths might be assessed through adaptations of instruments developed by Stark, Humphrey, Crook, and Lewis (1990) and, for younger children, Measelle, Ablow, Cowan, and Cowan (1998).

Alternatives to Violence. If children are to keep open opportunities for engaging in healthy relationships with others, they need alternatives to violence as a way of solving interpersonal problems. Countering children's acceptance of violence is both important and challenging, given that the inability to imagine a brighter future is common among children exposed to trauma (Pynoos & Nader, 1993). Consequently, much attention is paid in most intervention programs to changing children's beliefs that violence is normal and expectable, and teaching children prosocial interpersonal problem-solving strategies (Grusznski et al., 1988; Jaffe et al., 1986; Peled & Edleson, 1995). In this way, the intergenerational transmission of violence can be disrupted. Further, interventions must go beyond the individual child and family in order to foster nonviolent attitudes and behavior in the child's school and larger social environment (Osofsky, 1995). Peer group interventions have proven to be powerful tools in the prevention of interpersonal violence in children (Lochman & Lenhart, 1993) and adolescents (Wolfe, Wekerle, Reitzel-Jaffe, Grasley, Pittman, & MacEachran, 1997). Change in children's propensity for aggression can be measured by a number of well-established scales assessing prosocial conflict resolution strategies, including some that are sensitive to gender differences in the ways that children react to conflict (e.g., Crick & Grotpeter, 1995).

Positive Parent-Child Relationships. Consistent with other research on resilience (Masten & Coatsworth, 1998; Rutter, 1990), O'Keefe (1994) finds that positive parent-child relationships provide the single best buffer against the effects of exposure to violence. The quality of parent-child relationships can be enhanced by interventions targeted at children, mothers, and the interactions between them (see Carter, Kay, George, & King, 2003). Interventions with children can address distorted appraisals of maternal blame for the violence, thus *absolving mother of blame*. In turn, interventions with mothers can be focused on decreasing the likelihood that parental distress will spill over onto mother-child relationships. An essential starting point is the *reduction of maternal distress*, for which the provision of emotional and instrumental support to mothers is essential (Jouriles et al., 1998; Sullivan &

Bybee, 1999). Parenting consistency can be targeted by fostering the development of effective parenting skills (Jouriles et al., 1998), particularly *authoritativeness*. Authoritative parenting is characterized by high levels of both warmth and structure, and is associated with the best developmental outcomes for children, serving to reduce the likelihood of both internalizing and externalizing problems (Baumrind, 1994). Parents who have a repertoire of effective strategies for coping with child behavior problems also are less likely to resort to inappropriate or abusive parenting strategies. Although self-report measures are available, observational coding has proved to be an effective way of assessing parenting skills in studies of battered women and their children (Holden et al., 1998; Jouriles et al., 1998; Levendosky & Graham-Bermann, 1997).

Another focus of intervention with mothers is to help them to maintain clear *boundaries* with their children. For example, Kerig (in press) developed a model of the various ways in which the generational and emotional boundaries between parents and children might break down and, with her colleagues, constructed measures to assess various dimensions of boundary dissolution from parents' and children's perspectives (Brown & Kerig, 1998; Kerig, 2001c; Rowa, Kerig, & Geller, 2001). These include *role reversal*, when a parent turns to a child for emotional support; *enmeshment*, when parents do not acknowledge the separate selfhood of the child; *overprotectiveness/psychological control*, when parents fail to grant the child appropriate levels of autonomy; and *spousification*, when a parent attributes to the child negative qualities of the spouse. However, consistent with the idea that resilience is more than the absence of risk (Rutter, 1990), this measure also taps positive dimensions of boundary maintenance. The *protection from dissolution* subscale assesses the ways in which mothers can protect their children from the negative effects of their personal or marital distress (Kerig, 2001c; see Table 5).

Child-focused and parent-focused treatments can enhance the quality of parent-child relationships, but, to be most effective, interventions must directly address the interactions between parent and child. Parent-child therapy can increase relational warmth, mutuality, empathy, and attachment security (Jouriles et al., 1998; Loosley et al., 1997). For example Rabenstein and Lehman (2000) describe mother-child groups that enable mothers and children to learn from and support one another as they engage in recovery from family violence. Even when the goals of intervention are to make changes within the child, such as those di-

TABLE 5. Protection from Spillover Subscale Sample Items (Revised Parent-Child Boundaries Scale; Kerig, 2001c)

"I try hard to protect my child from the stresses I'm going through."
"I make every effort to 'be there' for my child even when I'm distracted by worries."
"If my child tries to get involved in my troubles, I make clear that is not her/his job."

rected toward children's appraisals, coping strategies, and working models of relationships, effectiveness can be enhanced by the enlistment of mothers as "co-therapists" in the process (Briesmeister & Schaefer, 1998). Mothers who are knowledgeable and active participants in their children's therapy can better reinforce and facilitate change, as has been found in investigations of treatments for many risk outcomes associated with violence exposure, including anxiety (Howard, Chu, Krain, Marrs-Garcia, & Kendall, 2000), depression (Stark et al., 1996), aggression (Webster-Stratton & Hammond, 1997), and PTSD (Pynoos & Nader, 1993). As Pynoos (1993) notes, parental responsiveness is essential to the success of children's attempts to cognitively and emotionally reprocess traumatic experiences and reappraise them in adaptive ways. Traumatized mothers will need support in order to allow them to engage in such work, given that it will require them to be re-exposed to traumatic cues, as well (Kerig et al., 2000; Pynoos, 1993).

Positive Transactions. Taken together, a primary goal of these interventions is to reduce the likelihood of negative chain reactions between mothers and children. When children have constructive coping strategies at their disposal, they are less likely to fall back on maladaptive tactics such as triangulation and aggression. Further, there are fewer opportunities for the spillover of marital aggression to occur when children refrain from intervening in interparental conflicts and when parents reinforce the boundaries between marital and child relationships. As mothers' ability to provide consistent and responsive parenting is enhanced, they will be better able to set firm limits while still meeting children's needs for comforting and support. Ultimately, these protective processes will spark a set of positive transactions, as mothers and children interact with one another in more adaptive and more mutually supportive ways. Although a myriad of self-report measures are available for assessing the quality of parent-child relationships from the perspective of both child and parent, direct observation can provide the richest and most informative data (Kerig, 2001).

DEVELOPMENTAL ISSUES

While developmental differences are noted frequently in the review of risk and protective mechanisms presented above, age has been addressed inconsistently in interventions developed for children exposed to violence. Some programs for children of battered women exclusively focus on one developmental stage, such as middle childhood (e.g., Graham-Bermann, 1998; Jaffe et al., 1986; Roseby & Johnston, 1997; Rossman, 2000), early childhood (e.g., Jouriles et al., 1998), or adolescence (Wolfe et al., 1997). Others include children ranging in age from 4 to 13, separated into groups on the basis of age so that interventions can be presented at the appropriate cognitive level (e.g., Grusznski et al., 1988; Peled & Edleson, 1985). Only a few detail how they tailor treatment to the developmental status of the participants, such as by providing hands-on materials for younger children (e.g., Ragg & Webb, 1992; Rossman, 2000) or including discussions of sexuality for adolescents (e.g., Alessi & Hearn, 1998). While developmental issues have been relatively neglected in this literature, guidelines for developmentally sensitive treatments have been developed for specific risk outcomes associated with violence exposure, such as PTSD (Berliner, 1997; Kerig et al., 2000; Pynoos & Nader, 1993).

However, attention to children's age is not sufficient. Consideration must also be given to the developmental processes underlying children's reactions to family violence (Cummings, 1998; Kerig & Fedorowicz, 1999). As Jaffe et al. (1986) state: "In designing intervention strategies for children who are victims of family violence, one must adopt a developmental perspective on cognitive and behavioral factors that are related to the etiology of family violence, as well as those factors that may be important to helping children to recover from the turmoil" (p. 360). From a developmental psychopathology perspective, interventions need to attend to the *stage salient issues* (Cicchetti, Toth, Bush, & Gillespie, 1988) or *developmental tasks* (Waters & Sroufe, 1983; Forehand & Wierson, 1993) that might be disrupted by exposure to violence: for example, attachment in the preschool years, self-efficacy in middle childhood, and intimacy in adolescence (see Cicchetti &

Lynch, 1995; Osofsky & Scheeringa, 1997; Pynoos, Steinberg, & Wriath, 1995). Pynoos (1993) offers a particularly rich developmental account of the effects of trauma on emerging psychological processes, including emotion regulation, the self system, ego defenses, internal working models of relationships, interpersonal trust, and future orientation.

An additional age-related complication for intervention research is the fact that most of the child-report measures of key constructs, such as appraisals, symptoms, and parent-child relationships, are designed for children school-aged and older. Younger children may lack the cognitive and linguistic sophistication to reliably report on stressful events and their reactions to them (Pynoos, 1993), at least on paper and pencil measures. However, children preschool-age or younger are disproportionately represented among those exposed to violence (Fantuzzo, Boruch, Beriana, Atkins, & Marcus, 1997). Therefore, it is important to develop interventions that are appropriate for preschoolers, as well as to design developmentally appropriate measures of outcomes and change processes so as to validate those interventions. Promising new techniques for interviewing preschoolers exposed to violence are emerging, which utilize creative strategies such as story telling and puppet play procedures (e.g., Grych & Wachsmuth-Shlaefer, 2001).

REFINING RESILIENCE

On a final note, there is another conundrum in the resilience literature that suggests we need to be more thoughtful about the outcome measures we choose. There is, as yet, no generally accepted definition of resiliency nor is there a standard method of "diagnosing" it (Masten et al., 1999). It was noted above that a narrow focus on externalized manifestations of maladjustment might blind us to the internalized distress of seemingly resilient children. We also need to look beneath children's overt misbehavior in order to be sensitive to potential sources of strength and resilience underneath. For example, Richters and Cicchetti (1993) are concerned about the ease with which diagnostic labels such as Conduct Disorder are applied to children. They point out that some of the best-loved characters in fiction, such as Tom Sawyer and Huckleberry Finn–and even such real-life characters as their creator, Mark Twain–would not fit the picture of the "invulnerable" child. However, some of the characteristics that marked Tom Sawyer and Mark Twain as troublesome youth–"oppositionality, defiance, sense of irony, and 'mischeevousness' " (p. 25)–were also the characteristics that helped them to rise above adversity. Again, Gemma is a case in point. She was not particularly compliant with adults and got into many scrapes with her peers, and she certainly benefited from finding more appropriate ways to resolve interpersonal conflicts. However, these problem behaviors were also linked to some of the personal qualities that served her well: Gemma was feisty, strong-willed, and quick to defend herself against any perceived violations of her rights. In short, she was no one's victim.

Thus, research on resilience needs to consider another point, one originally made by Anna Freud (1965): There is a difference between the child who is disturbed and the child who is disturbing to others. Clearly there are children with behavior problems who are emotionally troubled and whose misbehavior presages more trouble to come. However, as Richters and Cicchetti (1993) argue, it is equally important not to pathologize a child because of characteristics–such as non-conformity, independent-mindedness, and an impish sense of humor–that could be sources of resilience over the long term. Therefore, it will behoove us to pay more attention to our outcome measures. In particular, resilience research needs to go beyond measuring children's misbehavior on the Child Behavior Checklist (Achenbach, 1991) and to develop ways of assessing adaptation using the richer, process-oriented, integrative framework of developmental psychopathology (Cicchetti & Garmezy, 1993).

CONCLUSION

While not an exhaustive model by any means, this paper has made an effort to use the leads provided by the research literature, as well as theory and clinical observations, in order to identify the protective processes that have the greatest potential to make a difference for children exposed to domestic violence. This model suggests that the most effective interventions will need to be multifaceted, multimodal, and multisystemic in order address the needs of children and their mothers and to support the relationships between them (see Table 6). Essentially, it is our goal to turn images like the first set of Gemma's drawings (see Figure 1) into images such as the drawing she presented to me on our termination day (see Figure 2).

TABLE 6. Risks, Risk Processes, Protective Processes, and Change Processes for Children Exposed to Interparental Violence

Risk outcome	Risk process	Protective process	Change process
Depression	Child involvement	Detriangulation	Boundary maintenance
	Self blame, helplessness	Positive appraisals	Absolution from blame
	Stigma, hopelessness	Affirmations of family	Identification of family strengths
Anxiety	Emotional insecurity	Perceived coping efficacy	Constructive coping
	Perceived threat	Maternal well-being	Maternal social support
	Maternal distress	Perceived maternal efficacy	Maternal empowerment
PTSD	Unregulated distress	Emotion regulation	Affect regulation skills
	Denial and numbing	Mastery, affect expression	Therapeutic re-exposure
Aggression	Disrupted parenting	Parenting effectiveness	Authoritative parenting
Intergenerational	Identification with aggressor	Alternatives to violence	Interpersonal problem-solving skills
Transmission of violence	Maternal blame	Positive appraisals of mother	Empathic mutuality
	Spill-over	Positive mother-child relations	Boundary maintenance

FIGURE 2

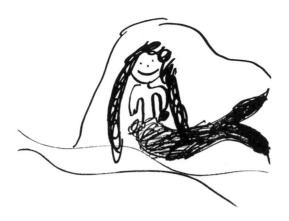

REFERENCES

Achenbach, T. M. (1991). *Manual for the Child Behavior Checklist/4-18 and 1991 Profile*. Burlington, VT: University of Vermont Department of Psychiatry.

Allen, N. E., Wolf, A. M., Bybee, D. I., & Sullivan, C. M. (2003). Diversity of children's immediate coping responses to witnessing domestic violence. *Journal of Emotional Abuse*, *3*(1/2), 123-147.

American Psychological Association. (1992). Ethical principles of psychologists and code of conduct. *American Psychologist*, *47*, 1597-1611.

Anthony, E. J., & Cohler, B. J. (1987). *The invulnerable child*. New York: Guilford.

Baumrind, D. (1994). The social context of child maltreatment. *Family Relations*, *43*, 360-368.

Berliner, L. (1997). Intervention with children who experience trauma. In D. Cicchetti & S. L. Toth (Eds.), *Developmental perspectives on trauma: Theory, research, and intervention* (pp. 491-514). Rochester, NY: University of Rochester Press.

Blizard, R. A., & Bluhm, A. M. (1994). Attachment to the abuser: Integrating object-relations and trauma theories in treatment of abuse survivors. *Psychotherapy*, *31*, 383-390.

Briesmeister, J. M., & Schaefer, C. E. (Eds.). (1998). *Handbook of parent training: Parents as co-therapists for children's behavior problems*. New York: Wiley.

Brown, C. A., & Kerig, P. K. (1998, August). *Parent-child boundaries as mediators of the effects of maternal distress on children's adjustment*. Poster presented at the annual meeting of the American Psychological Association, San Francisco.

Carter, L., Kay, S. J., George, J. L., & King, P. (2003). Treating children exposed to domestic violence. *Journal of Emotional Abuse*, *3*(3/4), 183-202.

Chambless, D. L., & Ollendick, T. H. (2001). Empirically supported psychological interventions: Controversies and evidence. *Annual Review of Psychology*, *52*, 685-716.

Christopoulos, C., Cohn, D. A., Shaw, D. S., Joyce, S., Sullivan-Hanson, J., Kraft, S. P., & Emery, R. E. (1987). Children of abused women: I. Adjustment at the time of shelter residence. *Journal of Marriage and the Family*, *49*, 611-619.

Cicchetti, D., & Garmezy, N. (1993). Prospects and promises in the study of resilience. *Development and Psychopathology, 5,* 497-502.

Cicchetti, D., & Lynch, M. (1995). Failures in the expectable environment and their impact on individual development: The case of child maltreatment. In D. Cicchetti & D. J. Cohen (Eds.), *Developmental psychopathology: Vol. 2. Risk, disorder, and adaptation* (32-71). New York: Wiley.

Cicchetti, D., Toth, S. L., Bush, M. A., & Gillespie, J. F. (1988). Stage-salient issues: A transactional model of intervention. In E. D. Nannis & P. A. Cowan (Eds.), *Developmental psychopathology and its treatment* (pp. 123-146). San Francisco: Jossey-Bass.

Crick, N. R., & Grotpeter, J. K. (1995). Relational aggression, gender, and social-psychological adjustment. *Child Development, 66,* 710-722.

Cummings, E. M. (1998). Children exposed to marital conflict and violence: Conceptual and theoretical directions. In G. W. Holden, R. A. Geffner, & E. N. Jouriles (Eds.), *Children exposed to marital violence: Theory, research and applied issues* (pp. 55-93). Washington, DC: American Psychological Association.

Cummings, E. M., Ballard, M., El-Sheikh, & Lake, M. (1991). Resolution and child's responses to interadult anger. *Developmental Psychology, 27,* 462-470.

Davies, P. T., & Cummings, E. M. (1994). Marital conflict and child adjustment: An emotional security hypothesis. *Psychological Bulletin, 116,* 387-411.

Davies, P. T., & Cummings, E. M. (1998). Exploring children's emotional security as a mediator of the link between marital relations and child adjustment. *Child Development, 69,* 124-139.

Davies, P. T., Myers, R. L., & Cummings, E. M. (1996). Responses of children and adolescents to marital conflict scenarios as a function of the emotionality of conflict endings. *Merrill-Palmer Quarterly, 42,* 1-21.

Edleson, J. L. (1999). Interventions and issues in the co-occurrence of child abuse and domestic violence [Special issue]. *Child Maltreatment, 4(2),* 91-182.

Egeland, B., Carlson, E., & Sroufe, L. A. (1993). Resilience as process. *Development and Psychopathology, 5,* 517-528.

El-Sheikh, M., & Cummings, E. M. (1992). Availability of control and preschoolers' responses to interadult anger. *International Journal of Behavioral Development, 15,* 207-226.

Fantuzzo, J. W., Boruch, R., Beriana, A., Atkins, M., & Marcus, S. (1997). Domestic violence and children: Prevalence and risk in five major US cities. *Journal of the American Academy of Child and Adolescent Psychiatry, 36,* 116-122.

Fedorowicz, A. E., & Kerig, P. K. (1995). *Children's Coping Questionnaire.* Unpublished measure, Simon Fraser University.

Forehand, R., & Wierson, M. (1993). The role of developmental factors in planning behavioral interventions for children: Disruptive behavior as an example. *Behavior Therapy, 24,* 117-141.

Freud, A. (1965). *Normality and pathology in childhood: Assessment of development.* New York: International Universities Press.

Garmezy, N. (1974). The study of competence in children at risk for severe psychopathology. In E. J. Anthony & C. Koupernik (Eds.), *The child in his family* (pp. 77-98). New York: Wiley.

Garmezy, N. (1994). Reflections and commentary on risk, resilience, and development. In R. J. Haggerty, L. R. Sherrod, N. Garmezy, & M. Rutter (Eds.), *Stress, risk, and resilience in children and adolescents: Processes, mechanisms, and interventions* (pp. 1-18). Cambridge: Cambridge University Press.

Geffner, R., Jaffe, P. G., & Sudermann, M. (Eds.). (2000). *Children exposed to domestic violence: Current issues in research, intervention, prevention, and policy development.* New York: The Haworth Press, Inc.

Gordis, E. B., Margolin, G., & John, R. S. (1997). Marital aggression, observed parental hostility, and child behavior during triadic family interaction. *Journal of Family Psychology, 11,* 76-89.

Graham-Bermann, S. A. (1996). Family worries: The assessment of interpersonal anxiety of children in families with domestic violence. *Journal of Clinical Child Psychology, 25,* 280-287.

Graham-Bermann, S. A. (1998, October). *An evaluation of "Kids' Club."* Paper presented at the Fourth International Conference on Children Exposed to Family Violence, San Diego.

Graham-Bermann, S. A., & Levendosky, A. A. (1998a). Traumatic stress symptoms in children of battered women. *Journal of Interpersonal Violence, 13,* 111-138.

Graham-Bermann, S. A., & Levendosky, A. (1998b). The social functioning of preschool-age children whose mothers are emotionally and physically abused. *Journal of Emotional Abuse, 1,* 57-82.

Grych, J. H., & Wachsmuth-Shlaefer, T. (2001, April). Representations of relationships: Integrating cognitive and attachment perspectives on the sequelae of interpersonal conflict. In E. M. Cummings (Chair), *Marital conflict and child functioning: New directions toward process-oriented research.* Society for Research in Child Development, Minneapolis.

Grych, J. H., & Fincham, F. D. (1990). Marital conflict and children's adjustment: A cognitive-contextual framework. *Psychological Bulletin, 108,* 267-290.

Grych, J. H., & Fincham, F. D. (1993). Children's appraisals of interparental conflict: Initial investigations of the cognitive-contextual framework. *Child Development, 64,* 215-230.

Grych, J. H., Fincham, F. D., Jouriles, E. N., & McDonald, R. (2001). Interparental conflict and child adjustment: Testing the mediational role of appraisals in the cognitive-contextual framework. *Child Development, 71,* 1648-1661.

Grych, J. H., Seid, M., & Fincham, F. D. (1992). Assessing marital conflict from the child's perspective: The Children's Perception of Interparental Conflict Scale. *Child Development, 63,* 558-572.

Holden, G. W., Geffner, R. A., & Jouriles, E. N. (Eds.). (1998). *Children exposed to marital violence: Theory, research, and intervention.* Washington, DC: American Psychological Association.

Holden, G. W., & Ritchie, K. L. (1991). Linking extreme marital discord, child rearing, and child behavior problems: Evidence from battered women. *Child Development, 62,* 311-327.

Holden, G. W., Stein, J. D., Ritchie, K. L., Harris, S. O., & Jouriles, E. N. (1998). The parenting behaviors and beliefs of battered women. In G. W. Holden, R. A. Geffner, & E. N. Jouriles (Eds.), *Children exposed to marital violence: Theory, research, and intervention* (pp. 289-334). Washington, DC: American Psychological Association.

Howard, B., Chu, B., Krain, A. L., Marrs-Garcia, A. L., & Kendall, P. C. (2000). *Cognitive-behavioral family therapy for anxious children: Therapist manual.* Ardmore, PA: Workbook Publishing.

Hughes, H. M., Parkinson, D., & Vargo, M. (1989). Witnessing spouse abuse and experiencing physical abuse: A "double whammy"? *Journal of Family Violence, 4,* 197-209.

Janoff-Bulman, R. (1979). Characterological versus behavioral self-blame: Inquiries into depression and rape. *American Psychologist,* 1798-1809.

Jaffe, P., Wilson, S., & Wolfe, D. (1986). Promoting changes in attitudes and understanding of conflict resolution among child witnesses of family violence. *Canadian Journal of Behavioural Science, 18,* 356-366.

Jaffe, P. G., Wolfe, D. A., & Wilson, S. K. (1990). *Children of battered women.* Newbury Park: Sage.

Johnston, J. R., Campbell, L. E., & Mayes, S. S. (1985). Latency children in post-separation and divorce disputes. *Journal of the American Academy of Child Psychiatry, 24,* 563-574.

Johnston, J. R., Gonzales, R., & Campbell, L. E. (1987). Ongoing postdivorce conflict and child disturbance. *Journal of Abnormal Child Psychology, 15,* 493-509.

Jouriles, E. N., McDonald, R., Stephens, N., Norwood, W., Spiller, L. C., & Ware, H. S. (1998). Breaking the cycle of violence: Helping families departing from battered women's shelters. In G. W. Holden, R. A. Geffner, & E. N. Jouriles (Eds.), *Children exposed to marital violence: Theory, research, and applied issues* (pp. 337-370). Washington, DC: American Psychological Association.

Jouriles, E. N., Murphy, C. M., Farris, A. M., Smith, D. A., Richters, J. E., & Waters, E. (1991). Marital adjustment, parental disagreements about child rearing, and behavior problems in boys: Increasing the specificity of marital assessment. *Child Development, 62,* 1424-1433.

Jouriles, E. N., & Norwood, W. D. (1995). Physical aggression toward boys and girls in families characterized by the battering of women. *Journal of Family Psychology, 9,* 69-78.

Kalil, A., Tolman, R., Rosen, D., & Gruber, G. (2003). Domestic violence and children's behavior in low-income families. *Journal of Emotional Abuse, 3*(1/2), 75-101.

Kazdin, A. E. (1997). A model for developing effective treatments: Progression and interplay of theory, research, and practice. *Journal of Clinical Child Psychology, 26,* 114-129.

Kazdin, A. E., & Weisz, J. R. (1998). Identifying and developing empirically supported child and adolescent treatments. *Journal of Consulting and Clinical Psychology, 66,* 19-36.

Kerig, P. K. (1994). *Measures for the study of children's coping with interparental conflict.* Unpublished measures, Simon Fraser University.

Kerig, P. K. (1995). Triangles in the family circle: Effects of family structure on marriage, parenting, and child adjustment. *Journal of Family Psychology, 9,* 28-43.

Kerig, P. K. (1996). Assessing the links between marital conflict and child development: The Conflicts and Problem-Solving Scales. *Journal of Family Psychology, 10,* 454-473.

Kerig, P. K. (1997a, April). Gender and children's coping efforts as moderators of the effects of interparental conflict on adjustment. In K. M. Lindahl & L. F. Katz (Chairs), *Marital conflict and children's adjustment: Risk and protective mechanisms in family subsystems.* Symposium presented at the biennial meeting of the Society for Research in Child Development, Washington, DC.

Kerig, P. K. (1997b). *Perceived Maternal Efficacy scale.* Unpublished measure, Department of Psychology, Simon Fraser University.

Kerig, P. K. (1998a). Gender and appraisals as mediators of adjustment in children exposed to interparental violence. *Journal of Family Violence, 15,* 345-363.

Kerig, P. K. (1998b). Moderators and mediators of the effects of interparental conflict on child adjustment. *Journal of Abnormal Child Psychology, 26,* 199-212.

Kerig, P. K. (1999a). Gender issues in the effects of exposure to violence on children. *Journal of Emotional Abuse, 1,* 87-105.

Kerig, P. K. (1999b, April). "Put a sock in it!" Predictors and consequences of children's interventions into interparental conflict. Paper presented in G. Harold (Chair), *Gender-differentiated processing of family conflict.* Symposium presented at the biennial meeting of the Society for Research in Child Development, Albuquerque, NM.

Kerig, P. K. (2001a). Coping with interparental conflict. In J. H. Grych & F. D. Fincham (Eds.), *Interparental conflict and child development* (pp. 213-245). Cambridge: Cambridge University Press.

Kerig, P. K. (2001b). Conceptual issues in family observational research. In P. K. Kerig & K. M. Lindahl (Eds.), *Family observational coding systems: Resources for systemic research* (pp. 1-22). Hillsdale, NJ: Erlbaum.

Kerig, P. K. (2001c). *Revised Parent-Child Boundaries Scale.* Unpublished measure, University of North Carolina at Chapel Hill.

Kerig, P. K. (in press). Boundary dissolution. In J. Ponzetti, R. Hamon, Y. Kellar-Guenther, P. K. Kerig, R. Raeann, T. Scales, & J. White (Eds.), *International encyclopedia of marriage and family relationships.* New York: Macmillan.

Kerig, P. K., Brown, C., & Patenaude, R. (2001, April). Ties that bind: Coparenting, parent-child relations, and triangulation in postdivorce interparental conflicts. In M. El-Sheikh (Chair), *Marital conflict and child outcome: Processes, risk variables, and protective factors.* Society for Research in Child Development, Minneapolis.

Kerig, P. K., Cowan, P. A., & Cowan, C. P. (1993). Marital quality and gender differences in parent-child interaction. *Developmental Psychology, 29,* 931-939.

Kerig, P. K., & Fedorowicz, A. E. (1999). Assessing maltreatment in children of battered women: Methodological and ethical issues. *Child Maltreatment, 4,* 103-115.

Kerig, P. K., Fedorowicz, A. E., Brown, C. A., Patenaude, R. L., & Warren, M. (1998). When warriors are worriers: Gender, appraisals, and children's strategies for coping with interparental violence. *Journal of Emotional Abuse, 1,* 89-114.

Kerig, P. K., Fedorowicz, A. E., Brown, C. A., & Warren, M. (2000). PTSD in children exposed to violence: Assessment and intervention. In R. Geffner, P. Jaffe, & M. Sudermann (Eds.), *Children exposed to domestic violence: Current issues in research, intervention, prevention, and policy development* (p. 161-184). Binghamton, NY: The Haworth Press, Inc.

Kruttschnitt, C., & Dornfeld, M. (1993). Exposure to family violence: A partial explanation for initial and subsequent levels of delinquency? *Criminal Behaviour and Mental Health, 3,* 63-75.

Levendosky, A. A., & Graham-Bermann, S. A. (2000). Trauma and parenting in battered women: An addition to an ecological model of parenting. In R. A. Geffner, P. G. Jaffe, & M. Sudermann (Eds.), *Children exposed to domestic violence: Current issues in research, intervention, prevention, and policy development* (pp. 25-35). New York: The Haworth Press, Inc.

Lochman, J. E., & Lenhart, L. A. (1993). Anger coping intervention for aggressive children: Conceptual models and outcome effects. *Clinical Psychology Review, 13*, 785-805.

Loosely, S., Bentley, L., Rabenstein, S., & Sudermann, M. (1997). *Group treatment for children who witness woman abuse.* London, ON: Community Group Treatment Program.

Luthar, S. S., Cicchetti, D., & Becker, B. (2000). The construct of resilience: A critical evaluation and guidelines for future work. *Child Development, 71*, 543-562.

Luthar, S. S., Doernberger, C. H., & Zigler, E. (1993). Resilience is not a unidimensional construct: Insights from a prospective study of inner-city adolescents. *Development and Psychopathology, 5*, 703-717.

Masten, A. S., & Coatsworth, J. D. (1998). The development of competence in favorable and unfavorable environments. *American Psychologist, 53*, 205-220.

Masten, A. S., Hubbard, J. J., Gest, S. D., Tellegen, A., Garmezy, N., & Ramirez, M. L. (1999). Competence in the context of adversity: Pathways to resilience and maladaptation from childhood to late adolescence. *Development and Psychopathology, 11*, 143-169.

Measelle, J. R., Ablow, J. C., Cowan, P. A., & Cowan, C. P. (1998). Assessing young children's views of their academic, social, and emotional lives: An evaluation of the self-perception scales of the Berkeley Puppet Interview. *Child Development, 69*, 1556-1576.

Minuchin, S. (1974). *Families and family therapy.* Cambridge, MA: Harvard University Press.

National Center on Child Abuse and Neglect. (1995). *Child maltreatment 1993: Reports from the states to the National Center on Child Abuse and Neglect (Contract Number ACF-105-91-1802).* Washington, DC: US Government Printing Office.

National Council of Juvenile and Family Court Judges. (1998). *Family violence: Emerging programs.* Reno, NV: Author.

O'Brien, M., Bahadur, M. A., Gee, C., Balto, K., & Erber, S. (1997). Child exposure to marital conflict and child coping responses as predictors of child adjustment. *Cognitive Therapy and Research, 21*, 39-59.

O'Keefe, M. (1994). Linking marital violence, mother-child/father-child aggression, and child behavior problems. *Journal of Family Violence, 9*, 63-78.

O'Keefe, M. (1995). Predictors of child abuse in maritally violent families. *Journal of Family Violence, 10*, 3-25.

O'Neill, M., & Kerig, P. K. (2000). Attributions of self-blame and perceived control as moderators of adjustment in battered women. *Journal of Interpersonal Violence, 15*, 1036-1049.

Osofsky, J. D. (1995). Children who witness domestic violence: The invisible victims. *Social Policy Report: Society for Research in Child Development, 9(3)*, 1-36.

Osofsky, J. D., & Scheeringa, M. S. (1997). Community and domestic violence exposure: Effects on development and psychopathology. In D. Cicchetti & S. L. Toth (Eds.), *Developmental perspectives on trauma: Theory, research, and intervention* (p. 180). Rochester: University of Rochester Press.

Peled, E., & Davis, D. (Eds.). (1994). *Groupwork with children of battered women: A practitioner's manual.* Thousand Oaks, CA: Sage.

Peled, E., & Edleson, J. L. (1995). Process and outcome in small groups for children of battered women. In E. Peled, P. G. Jaffe, & J. L. Edleson (Eds.), *Ending the cycle of violence: Community responses to children of battered women* (pp. 77-96). Thousand Oaks, CA: Sage.

Porter, B., & O'Leary, K. D. (1980). Marital discord and childhood behavior problems. *Journal of Abnormal Child Psychology, 8*, 287-295.

Pynoos, R. S. (1993). Traumatic stress and developmental psychopathology in children and adolescents. In J. Oldham, M. Riba, & A. Tasman (Eds.), *American Psychiatric Press Review of Psychiatry, Vol. 12* (pp. 205-238). Washington, DC: American Psychiatric Press.

Pynoos, R. S., & Nader, K. (1993). Issues in the treatment of posttraumatic stress in children and adolescents. In J. P. Wilson & B. Raphael (Eds.), *International handbook of traumatic stress syndromes* (pp. 535-549). New York: Plenum.

Pynoos, R. S., Steinberg, A. M., & Wriath, R. (1995). A developmental model of childhood traumatic stress. In D. Cicchetti & D. J. Cohen (Eds.) *Developmental psychopathology. Vol. II: Risk, disorder, and adaptation* (pp. 72-95). New York: Wiley.

Rabenstein, S., & Lehmann, P. (2000). Mothers and children together: A family group treatment approach. In R. Geffner, P. G. Jaffe, & M. Sudermann (Eds.), *Children exposed to woman abuse: Current issues in research, intervention, prevention, and policy development*. New York: The Haworth Press, Inc.

Radke-Yarrow, M., & Sherman, T. (1990). Hard growing: Children who survive. In J. Rolf, A. S. Masten, D. Cicchetti, K. H. Nuechterlein, & S. Weintraub (Eds.), *Risk and protective factors in the development of psychopathology* (pp. 97-119). Cambridge: Cambridge University Press.

Ragg, D. M., & Webb, C. (1992). Group treatment for the preschool child witness of spouse abuse. *Journal of Child and Youth Care, 7*, 1-19.

Ribbe, D. P., Lipovsky, J. A., & Freedy, J. R. (1995). Post-traumatic stress disorder. In A. R. Eisen, C. A. Kearney, & C. E. Schaefer (Eds.), *Clinical handbook of anxiety disorder in children and adolescents* (pp. 315-356). Northvale, NJ: Jason Aronson.

Richters, J. E., & Cicchetti, D. (1993). Mark Twain meets DSM-III-R: Conduct disorder, development, and the concept of harmful dysfunction. *Development and Psychopathology, 5*, 5-30.

Roseby, V., & Johnston, J. R. (1997). *High-conflict, violent, and separating families: A group treatment manual for school age children*. New York: Free Press.

Rossman, B. B. R. (2000, September). Mother-child interaction activities in interventions for exposed children. Presentation at the Fourth International Conference on Family Violence, San Diego, CA.

Rossman, B. B. R., & Ho, J. (2000). Posttraumatic response and children exposed to parental violence. In R. Geffner, P. Jaffe, & M. Sudermann (Eds.), *Children exposed to domestic violence: Research, intervention, prevention, and policy implications* (pp. 85-106). NY: The Haworth Press, Inc.

Rossman, B. B. R., Hughes, H. M., & Rosenberg, M. S. (1999). *Children and interparental violence: The impact of exposure*. New York: Brunner/Mazel.

Rossman, B. B. R., & Rosenberg, M. S. (1992). Family stress and functioning in children: The moderating effects of children's beliefs about their control over parental conflict. *Journal of Child Psychology and Psychiatry, 33*, 699-715.

Rowa, K., Kerig, P. K., & Geller, J. (2001). The family and anorexia nervosa: Examining parent-child boundary problems. *European Eating Disorders Review, 9,* 97-114.

Rutter, M. (1990). Psychosocial resilience and protective mechanisms. In J. Rolf, A. S. Masten, D. Cicchetti, K. H. Nuechterlein, & S. Weintraub (Eds.), *Risk and protective factors in the development of psychopathology* (pp. 181-214). Cambridge: Cambridge University Press.

Schwab-Stone, M. E., Ayers, T. S., Kasprow, W., Voyce, C., Barone, C., Shriver, T., & Weissberg, R. P. (1995). No safe haven: A study of violence exposure in an urban community. *Journal of the American Academy of Child and Adolescent Psychiatry, 34,* 1343-1352.

Shirk, S. R., & Russell, R. L. (1996). *Change processes in child psychotherapy: Revitalizing treatment and research.* New York: Guilford.

Silvern, L., Karyl, J., & Landis, T. Y. (1995). Individual psychotherapy for the traumatized children of abused women. In E. Peled, P. G. Jaffe, & J. L. Edleson (Eds.), *Ending the cycle of violence: Community responses to children of battered women* (pp. 43-76). Thousand Oaks, CA: Sage.

Sroufe, L. A. (1997). Psychopathology as an outcome of development. *Development and Psychopathology, 9,* 251-268.

Stark, K. D., Kendall, P. C., McCarthy, M., Stafford, M., Barron, R., & Thomeer, M. (1996). *Taking action: A workbook for overcoming depression.* Ardmore, PA: Workbook Publishing.

Stark, K. D., Humphrey, L. L., Laurent, J. L., Livingston, R., & Christopher, J. C. (1993). Cognitive, behavioral, and family factors in the differentiation of depressive and anxiety disorders during childhood. *Journal of Consulting and Clinical Psychology, 61,* 878-886.

Sullivan, C. M., & Bybee, D. I. (1999). Reducing violence using community-based advocacy for women with abusive partners. *Journal of Consulting and Clinical Psychology, 67,* 43-53.

Task Force on Promotion and Dissemination of Psychological Procedures, American Psychological Association. (1995). Training in and dissemination of empirically-validated psychological treatments: Report and recommendations. *Clinical Psychologist, 48,* 3-23.

Wagar, J. M., & Rodway, M. R. (1995). An evaluation of a group treatment approach for children who have witnessed wife abuse. *Journal of Family Violence, 10,* 295-307.

Waters, E., & Sroufe, L. A. (1983). Social competence as a developmental construct. *Developmental Review, 3,* 79-97.

Webster-Stratton, C., & Hammond, M. (1997). Treating children with early-onset conduct problems: A comparison of child and parent training interventions. *Journal of Consulting and Clinical Psychology, 65,* 93-109.

Wekerle, C., & Wolfe, D. A. (1998). The role of child maltreatment and attachment style in adolescent relationship violence. *Development-and-Psychopathology, 10,* 571-586.

Weisz, J. R., & Hawley, K. M. (1998). Finding, evaluating, refining, and applying empirically supported treatments for children and adolescents. *Journal of Clinical Child Psychology, 27,* 206-216.

Wenar, C., & Kerig, P. K. (2000). *Developmental psychopathology: From infancy through adolescence* (4th ed.) New York McGraw-Hill.

Werner, E. E. (1994). Overcoming the odds. *Developmental and Behavioral Pediatrics, 15*, 131-136.

West, M., & George, C. (1999). Abuse and violence in intimate adult relationships: New perspectives from attachment theory. *Attachment-and-Human-Development, 12*, 137-156.

Wilson, S. K., Cameron, S., Jaffe, P. G., & Wolfe, D. (1986). *Manual for a group program for children exposed to wife abuse.* London, ON: London Family Court Clinic.

Winstok, Z., & Eisikovits, Z. (2003). Divorcing the parents: The impact of adolescents' exposure to father-to-mother aggression on their perceptions of affinity with their parents. *Journal of Emotional Abuse, 3*(1/2), 103-121.

Wolfe, D. A., Jaffe, P., & Zak, L. (1985). Children of battered women: The relation of child behaviour to family violence and maternal stress. *Journal of Consulting and Clinical Psychology, 53*, 657-665.

Wolfe, D. A., Wekerle, C., Reitzel-Jaffe, D., & Lefebvre, L. (1998). Factors associated with abusive relationships among maltreated and nonmaltreated youth. *Development and Psychopathology, 10*, 61-85.

Wolfe, D. A., Wekerle, C., Reitzel-Jaffe, D., Grasley, C., Pittman, A. L., & MacEachran, A. (1997). Interrupting the cycle of violence: Empowering youth to promote healthy relationships. In D. A. Wolfe, R. J. McMahon, & R. D. Peters (Eds.), *Child abuse: New directions in prevention and treatment across the life span.* Thousand Oaks, CA: Sage.

Treating Children
Exposed to Domestic Violence

Laurel Carter
Steven J. Kay
Jacqueline L. George
Pamela King

SUMMARY. It has been estimated that 3 to 10 million children are exposed to domestic violence between their parents each year. Research has clearly shown that children who live in homes where domestic violence exists are at risk for a wide variety of problems. The objectives of this pilot program were: (1) to provide treatment to children who have been exposed to domestic violence; (2) to provide treatment to their parents; (3) to measure the effectiveness of that treatment; and (4) to develop interagency treatment protocols that other agencies could replicate. This study supports the importance of treatment for children who experience family violence and their parent(s). Following treatment, children exposed to domestic violence demonstrated a decrease in behavior problems, an increase in their abilities to recognize and discuss abuse, and an ability to utilize a safety plan. Parents reported less stress following treatment. *[Article copies available for a fee from The Haworth Document Delivery Service: 1-800-HAWORTH. E-mail address:*

Address correspondence to: Laurel Carter, MS, LMFT, 167 East 200 North, Logan, UT 84321 (E-mail: laurelc@mtwest.net).

A special thanks to Brian Thorn for his work in getting this project started.

[Haworth co-indexing entry note]: "Treating Children Exposed to Domestic Violence." Carter, Laurel et al. Co-published simultaneously in *Journal of Emotional Abuse* (The Haworth Maltreatment & Trauma Press, an imprint of The Haworth Press, Inc.) Vol. 3, No. 3/4, 2003, pp. 183-202; and: *The Effects of Intimate Partner Violence on Children* (ed: Robert A. Geffner, Robyn Spurling Igelman, and Jennifer Zellner) The Haworth Maltreatment & Trauma Press, an imprint of The Haworth Press, Inc., 2003, pp. 183-202. Single or multiple copies of this article are available for a fee from The Haworth Document Delivery Service [1-800-HAWORTH, 9:00 a.m. - 5:00 p.m. (EST). E-mail address: docdelivery@haworthpress.com].

KEYWORDS. Child witness, treatment, domestic violence, intimate partner abuse

It has been estimated that 3 to 10 million children are exposed to domestic violence between their parents each year (Straus, 1992). Research has clearly shown that children who live in homes where domestic violence exists are at risk for a wide variety of problems (see Geffner, Jaffe, & Sudermann, 2000, for a recent review, as well as other articles in this volume for recent research). Studies have found that in any given group of children exposed to domestic violence, approximately 40% have problems severe enough to warrant clinical intervention (Holden, 1998; McDonald & Jouriles, 1991). Children exposed to domestic violence are at high risk for exhibiting behavioral and adjustment problems, and are also at high risk for impaired development.

BEHAVIORAL AND ADJUSTMENT PROBLEMS

Many investigations have found that children exhibit "externalizing" behaviors such as noncompliance, hostility, and aggression, as well as "internalizing" problems such as depression and anxiety when marital violence is part of their family experience (Holden, 1998; Jouriles, Norwood, McDonald, Vincent, & Mahoney, 1996; Kashani & Allan, 1998). Evidence also indicates that long-term exposure to marital violence in childhood is associated with low self-esteem, depression, and various trauma-related symptoms (Silvern et al., 1995). Graham-Bermann and Levendosky (1998) found that in a sample of 64 children exposed to domestic violence, most displayed trauma related symptoms, including intrusive and unwanted remembering of the violence, traumatic avoidance, and traumatic arousal symptoms, such as exaggerated startle responses. Research has also found that children exposed to domestic violence experience trauma symptoms such as dissociation, traumatic memories, intrusive play, and a general vulnerability to stress (Graham-Bermann, 1998). Other research has highlighted the intense fears and worries children exposed to domestic violence experience regarding the vulnerability of the victim and the child's siblings, and about the harmful behavior of the perpetrator (Graham-Bermann, 1996).

Other behavioral, health, school, and social interaction problems identified in the literature include: substance abuse, poor academic performance, truancy, poor problem-solving skills, deficits in social skills, social alienation, low empathy, early antisocial behavior, and acceptance of violence in relationships (Holden, 1998). A comparison of delinquent and non-delinquent youth found a history of family violence or abuse is the most significant difference between the two groups (Miller, 1989). Other studies have also found an association of delinquency and exposure to domestic violence (Koss, Goodman, Browne, Fitzgerald, Keita, & Russo, 1994; Wolfe, 1994).

ELEVATED RISK FOR IMPAIRED DEVELOPMENT

There is also evidence in the scientific literature that a high percentage of children exposed to marital violence experience serious developmental impairment (Davis, 1988; Graham-Bermann, 1998). When exposed to family violence, children have adjustment difficulties similar in severity to child abuse victims (Jaffe, Wolfe, & Wilson, 1990). Typically, these children experience neglect, abandonment, threats, and acts of abuse (emotional or physical) at the hands of one or both parents. They are more likely than other children to be the recipients of inadequate and abusive parenting during crucial and vulnerable stages, which predisposes them to a myriad of developmental obstacles. Exposure to domestic violence may have immediate and/or long-term effects leading to the development of problems in adulthood.

The social, emotional, cognitive, and physical limitations which often result from this environmental impoverishment and exposure to family violence may seriously handicap a child's ability to acquire the attitudes, skills and insights necessary for future functioning as an adequate spouse and parent. Social effects may include problems with developing a capacity for empathy, which provides the foundation on which strong interpersonal bonds are formed (Rosenberg, 1984). Additionally, children exposed to family violence demonstrate increased aggression, coupled with inadequate anger management and conflict resolution skills. These factors make healthy peer relationships problematic, with both the same and the opposite sex peers. Dodge and Tomlin (1987) found that aggression and antisocial behavior in early childhood is the primary factor underlying social rejection.

Recent research is clear in its findings that exposure to domestic violence affects children's emotional functioning (Henning, Leitenbergh, Coffey, Turner, & Bennett, 1996). Children exposed to domestic violence exhibit emotional characteristics that are parallel to those exhibited by other victims of violence: anxiety, guilt, shame, lack of trust, diminished self-esteem, helplessness, and hopelessness. A combination of loss of control and the loss of positive adult figures with whom to identify results in well-developed defense mechanisms (Henning et al., 1996). These defenses, while potentially useful as crisis management techniques for traumatized children, often become dysfunctional traits in adulthood.

Information processing deficits in traumatized children have been well-documented (Dodge & Price, 1994). Children exposed to domestic violence may acquire unconventional belief systems or world views in which anger and violence are synonymous, and violence is the norm. Clearly, children exposed to domestic violence readily learn aggression tactics (Graham-Bermann, 1998). Further, traumatic parental bonding may dictate that children equate caring with abuse, and possession or control with love. Perpetuation of harmful stereotypes through social learning and identification with parental roles may equate being male with hurting women and femaleness with vulnerability to men. These children may also believe that dominance and submission are inherent in all relationships (Elbow, 1982).

In addition to the effects of exposure to domestic violence upon childhood development, parental stress resulting from domestic violence has been found to have a potential independent effect on child adjustment. Levendosky and Graham-Bermann (1998) found that parenting stress resulting from domestic violence moderated the overall effects of domestic violence exposure for some children, a finding that supports the inclusion of addressing parental stress in treating children exposed to domestic violence.

In the last 20 years, many intervention programs for children of batterers have been developed and studied (Graham-Bermann & Edleson, 2001). Most of these programs involve 60 to 90 minute group sessions that meet anywhere from 6 to 12 weeks, and have a highly structured curriculum with specific goals and objectives (Peled & Edleson, 1995). These programs have targeted a wide range of treatment issues, including child anxiety, family attitudes, coping skills, behavioral difficulties, peer relations, and self esteem among others (Graham-Bermann, 1999).

One statewide survey of female residents in Utah found 25% of respondents had been exposed to domestic violence as a child, and 7.1% currently have children who witness or hear physical abuse (Jones & Associates, 1997). In 1998, the State of Utah appropriated funds for a pilot study to provide specialized treatment services for children exposed to domestic violence, including supplementary services for their parents. The state requested agencies in one rural and two urban areas. Family Institute of Northern Utah in Logan (rural), Cornerstone Counseling Center in Salt Lake City (urban), and Weber Human Services in Ogden (urban), were the agencies chosen to participate in the project. The objectives of this pilot program were: (1) to provide treatment to children who had been exposed to domestic violence; (2) to provide treatment to their parents (mostly mothers, a few fathers with specific circumstances); (3) to measure the effectiveness of that treatment; and (4) to develop interagency treatment protocols that other agencies could replicate.

METHOD

Participants

One hundred ninety-two children and 64 parents participated in the program during the two years of this study. The children ranged in age from 4-18, the average age being 9. The majority of children lived in divorced or separated families (66%), followed by intact families (16%), cohabitating families (9%), and single mom families (9%). Twenty-five percent of the mothers had no high school diploma; 33% had a high school diploma; 36% had some college and 6% were college graduates. Fifty-one percent of the families had annual income levels less than $12,000, 37% had incomes of $12,000-$24,000, and the remaining 12% had annual incomes above $24,000. Seventy-five percent of the children were White, 18% were Hispanic, 3% were Black Americans, 3% were Native Americans, and 1% were Pacific Islander. Ninety-seven percent of the perpetrators were male and 27% of them lived in the home with the child. Most of the perpetrators were the child's biological parent (76%), while the others were the partner of the child's parent (12%) or stepparent (11%). Only 36% of the male perpetrators were in, or had been in, a domestic violence treatment program.

The 192 children and their parent(s) entered the program in one of three ways: as the children of perpetrators or victims in our domestic violence treatment programs, through community agency referrals, or as self-referred clients. Before children entered treatment, a risk assessment was conducted to determine the appropriateness of this child being in the program. For a child to be approved, the offending parent had to be out of the home or have either completed, or be in the process of completing, a state licensed adult domestic violence treatment program.

The parent included in treatment was typically the mother. However, there were 12 men throughout the two years who were included in the parenting group. Eight of the fathers who had successfully completed a domestic violence treatment program were included. Four current male partners (non-offenders) of the women who were included in parenting in the home were also included. Three of the mothers in the group were offenders.

Treatment

Children and their parents attended individual, group, and family therapy services; the central component was group treatment. Children and adults benefit from group treatment because it reduces perceptions of isolation and the feeling that their family is the only one with problems of violence. The children were grouped by age and grade in school. The three groups were: (1) younger elementary children, (2) older elementary and middle school-aged children, and (3) teenagers. The groups were kept small, averaging 6-9 participants. Groups were co-facilitated by licensed therapists and advanced practicum students from Utah State University Psychology and Marriage and Family Therapy Programs. Group facilitator to child ratios averaged 1:3. If possible, male-female leader teams were utilized. The closed-ended children's group ran for 11 (Ogden site) or 12 (Logan and Salt Lake sites) weeks. Each group lasted for 1.5 hours and included check-in, group sharing, psycho-educational activity, play therapy, and snack. The treatment goals for the children were to:

1. Provide intervention to build safety planning skills, self-esteem, developmentally appropriate ways of expressing feelings, pro-social skills, conflict resolution skills, parent-child relationship skills, and to identify and strengthen support systems; and
2. Provide an atmosphere conducive to self-disclosure and therapeutic interventions to heal trauma responses.

The three sites agreed on 14 objectives that would guide treatment and provide consistency between the sites. The objectives were:

1. Child will talk about/discuss domestic violence incident(s) with parent;
2. Child will tell parent how he/she feels emotionally;
3. When angry, child will state he/she is angry;
4. When angry, child will not become aggressive;
5. Child knows what physical abuse is;
6. Child knows what sexual abuse is;
7. Child knows what emotional abuse is;
8. Child asks questions when confused about family issues;
9. Child knows about the privacy of his/her body and his/her right to protect that privacy;
10. Child knows what the word aggressive means;
11. Child knows what the word assertive means;
12. Child has a safety plan in the event of a DV incident in the house;
13. In the event of a DV incident at home, child can dial 911 for his/her safety; and
14. Child knows whom to call (family member or friend) in the event he/she feels unsafe or afraid at home.

The parent group, facilitated by a licensed therapist, paralleled the children's treatment group. Parents addressed the same topics that the children addressed in their groups, with a discussion on how to encourage their child to be nonviolent, express emotions, and feel safe at home. Additionally, the parent group included information on child development, effects of family violence on children, and parenting skills. It also served to provide support for parents and their families.

Group treatment was preceded by two to four individual appointments for the purposes of assessment, treatment planning and data collection. Each child had a primary therapist who tracked progress throughout the group and followed up on any critical issues that surfaced in group. Family therapy was offered after the course of group treatment when appropriate, and when safety allowed, in order to address family relationship issues.

We introduced the concept of a safety plan for both victims and perpetrators during the early phase of treatment. If the adult victim had used the services of a women's shelter, we supported the development and implementation of her safety plan. If we discovered that there was ongoing or recent violence, appropriate reports to the Division of Child and Family Services and/or law enforcement were made. Safety was assessed with input from the mother and the child as a regular and ongoing part of the assessment and treatment process on a weekly basis. Regular agency and interagency case staffings assisted in the ongoing process of monitoring safety within the family.

Measures

Youth Outcome Questionnaire (YOQ). The YOQ (Burlingham, Wells, & Lambert, 1996) is a parent-report measure of treatment progress for children ages 4-17 receiving psychological treatment. It is specifically constructed to assess the occurrence of behavior change. Parents complete the questionnaire at intake and then at regular intervals throughout treatment. The YOQ has 64 items that comprise six separate subscales including: (1) intrapersonal distress, (2) somatic symptoms, (3) interpersonal relations, (4) critical items, (5) social problems, and (6) behavioral dysfunction. The cutoff score determining a "normal" range of behavior was devised by comparing community and clinical samples (Burlingham et al.). The cutoff scores are as follows: total = 46, intrapersonal distress = 16.4, somatic symptoms = 5, interpersonal relations = 4.4, critical items = 5, social problems = 3, and behavioral dysfunction = 12.

Objectives Checklist. The Objectives Checklist (Thorne, 1998) is a 14-item parent report measure of the child's ability to express emotions, define abuse, discuss violence, express anger appropriately, and create a safety plan. This measure was developed specifically for this treatment program to assess the program's 14 treatment objectives. The objectives can be grouped into six categories: (1) expressing emotions, (2) defining abuse, (3) discussing violence in the family, (4) expressing anger appropriately, and (5) creating a safety plan. Each objective was scored on a 4-point Likert scale (e.g., Child has a safety plan in the event of a DV incident in the house: 1-not true, 2-sometimes true, 3-usually true, 4-always true).

Social Skills Rating System (SSRS). The parent version of the SSRS (Gresham & Elliot, 1990) assesses the frequency and importance of behaviors influencing a child's development of social competence and adaptive functioning. The measure emphasizes prosocial skills and also includes potential problem behaviors. The 36-item measure is answered on a 3-point scale: 1-never, 2-sometimes, 3-very often.

Parenting Stress Index/Short Form (PSI/SF). The PSI/SF (Abidin, 1995) is a parent measure that assesses the amount of stress in the parent-child system. The parent responds to 36 items by circling SA-Strongly Agree, A-Agree, NS-Not Sure, D-Disagree, or SD-Strongly Disagree. There are three subscales. The Parental Distress subscale determines the distress a parent is experiencing in their role as a parent. The Parent-Child Dysfunctional Interaction subscale focuses on the parent's perception that their child does not meet parental expectations, and has non-reinforcing interactions with the child. The Difficult Child subscale focuses on the basic behavioral characteristics of the child such as temperament and learned patterns of behavior. The normal range for scores is within the 15th to 80th percentiles. High scores are considered to be scores at or above the 85th percentile. The cutoff score to determine clinically significant levels of total stress is 90 (at or above the 90th percentile).

Trauma Symptom Checklist for Children (TSCC-A). The TSCC-A (Briere, 1996) is a self-report measure of posttraumatic distress and related psychological symptoms. It is designed for use with children who have experienced or witnessed traumatic events. The 44-item version has two validity scales (Underresponse and Hyperresponse) and six clinical scales (Anxiety, Depression, Anger, Posttraumatic Stress, Dissociation).

Piers-Harris Children's Self-Concept Scale. The Piers-Harris (Piers, 1984) is an 80-item self-report questionnaire designed to assess how children feel about themselves. Items are scored in either a positive or negative direction; higher scores indicate a positive self-evaluation, and lower scores indicate negative self-evaluation.

Family Worries Scale (FWS). The FWS (Graham-Bermann, 1999) is a 20-item self-report measure of worries and concerns that children have about people in their families. The child rates their concerns about family members' vulnerability to harm and potential to harm on a 4-point Likert scale.

Family Stereotypes Card Sort (FSCS). The FSCS (Graham-Bermann & Brescoll, 2000) is a 40-item Likert scale self-report measure of child's ratings of stereotyped beliefs about power and violence in the family. Four subscales include Male Power, Female Power, Violence Privilege, and Family Autonomy.

Procedure

Three sites participated in the project. The Family Institute of Northern Utah, Cornerstone Counseling Center, and Weber Human Services coordinated program treatment protocols and evaluation design. The procedures, assessment instruments, and treatment objectives were developed collectively and followed by each site. A number of resources were consulted in developing the treatment program, including: *The Kid's Club: An Intervention Group for Children Exposed to Domestic Violence* (Graham-Bermann, 1992), *Groupwork With Children of Battered Women* (Peled & Davis, 1995), and *Group Treatment for Children Who Witness Woman Abuse* (Loosely, 1997).

In the first year of the project, the YOQ, Objectives Checklist, SSRS, PSI/SF, TSCC-A, and Piers-Harris Children's Self-Concept Scale were used. During the second year of the project we added the FWS (Graham-Bermann, 1996) and the FSCS (Graham-Bermann & Brescoll, 2000). The number of measures we could require clients to fill out was limited; therefore, we did not use the SSRS, TSCC-A, or the Piers-Harris to assess progress in the second year. Thus, sample sizes differ for each measure depending upon if the measure was used for one year or two years (sample sizes are reported for each measure in their corresponding tables described below). We had at least one year of complete Time 1 and Time 2 data for each measure.

Data were collected before treatment began (Time 1), and approximately 12 weeks later upon completion of treatment (Time 2), with the exception of the YOQ which was collected at three different points in time. The child and the parent completed their respective measures at each point in time. The mother was the parent who completed the parent measures 98% of the time.

RESULTS

For each measure, statistical analyses were performed to identify change over time by comparing an individual's pre-treatment scores with their post-treatment scores. As the YOQ is designed to measure treatment progress, three points of data were gathered: Time 1a (pre-treatment), Time 1b (six weeks into treatment), and Time 2 (post-treatment). The mean scores at Time 1 for intrapersonal distress, somatic symptoms, interpersonal relations, social problems, behavioral dysfunction, and critical items (e.g., suicide, eating disorders, delusions) were all above the cutoff score. The tests of trends in YOQ scores using the repeated measures MANOVA procedure were consistent and positive. Across all scales of the YOQ, the linear trends over time were statistically significant ($p < .001$). Additionally, changes between Time 1a and Time 1b and between Time 1b and Time 2 were tested using a difference contrast test. All YOQ scores over all times were statistically significant. In other words, there were significant changes in scores six weeks into treatment and again following treatment. At Time 2, following treatment, parents reported statistically significant drops in their child's intrapersonal distress, somatic symptoms, interpersonal relations, social problems, behavioral dysfunction, and critical items (see Table 1). However, although scores significantly dropped between Time 1 and Time 2, the means of the total score, intrapersonal distress, interpersonal relations, and critical items subscales at Time 2 remained clinically significant (i.e., above the cutoff scores for clinical significance).

Paired *t*-tests were performed on each variable from the following measures, comparing an individual's Time 1 (pre-treatment) scores to Time 2 (post-treatment) scores to identify change. Prior to treatment, parents reported social skills within the average range for their children on the SSRS. There were no significant changes in social skills following treatment. However, parents reported significantly fewer behavior problems in their children following treatment as measured by the SSRS (see Table 2).

The mothers of these children were highly stressed prior to treatment. The Time 1 Total Stress mean score for these mothers was clinically significant at 90. The Parent-Child Dysfunctional Interaction and Difficult Child subscale mean scores at Time 1 were at the 85th percentile and The Parental Distress subscale mean scores were at the 90th percentile. At Time 2, following treatment, the Total Parent Stress, Parent-Child Dysfunctional Interaction, and Difficult Child subscale score means significantly dropped to the 80th percentile. The Parental Distress mean score, which is the parents' stress in their role as a parent as a function of personal factors, significantly dropped to the 55th percentile (see Table 3).

Prior to treatment, parents identified how much knowledge they perceived their children to have about violence, abuse, and safety behaviors on the Objectives Checklist. Parents rated their child on a Likert scale for each objective. Following treatment, parents reported they thought their children knew significantly more about these topics than before treatment (see Table 4).

Children did not report clinical levels of anger, anxiety, depression, dissociation or posttraumatic stress on the TSCC-A at Time 1, and there were no statistically significant changes in scores from Time 1 to Time 2. There is an underresponse scale in the TSCC-A that reflects the extent to which the child denies behaviors, thoughts, or feelings that most oth-

TABLE 1. Youth Outcome Questionnaire (N = 132)

Scale	Time 1a	Time 1b	Time 2	F-value
	M (SD)	M (SD)	M (SD)	(1,131)
Intrapersonal distress	21.2 (11.4)	17.8 (10.2)	15.2 (10.2)	40.8**
Somatic symptoms	6.0 (5.0)	5.2 (4.3)	4.3 (4.4)	22.7**
Interpersonal relations	8.0 (7.3)	6.3 (6.2)	5.4 (6.2)	17.7**
Social problems	5.0 (4.8)	3.6 (3.8)	3.4 (4.0)	25.0**
Behavioral dysfunction	14.4 (8.7)	13.2 (8.1)	11.8 (7.9)	15.3**
Critical items	6.8 (5.0)	5.5 (4.1)	4.8 (3.9)	24.9**
Total	60.3 (34.2)	51.3 (30.3)	44.8 (30.5)	33.4**

** p < .001

TABLE 2. Social Skills Rating System (N = 41)

Scale	Time 1	Time 2	Difference
	M (SD)	M (SD)	(40)
Social Skills	95.6 (19.6)	96.8 (20.6)	t = −.43
Behavior Problems	111.3 (14.3)	102.1 (15.6)	t = 3.43**

Standard scores (Mean of 100, standard deviation of 15)
*p < .05 ** p < .01

ers would respond at some level (e.g., daydreaming). Seventeen percent of the children had underresponse scores so high that they were considered invalid. These scores were not included in the final analysis. The means and standard deviations for Times 1 and 2 are presented in Table 5.

Children reported self-concept levels close to the mean score of 50 (*M* = 53.4, *SD* = 11.6) on the Piers-Harris Self-Concept Scale at Time 1, with no significant change at Time 2 (*M* = 55.5, *SD* = 12.1). At Time 2, 15% reported total self-concept scores 1.5 standard deviations above the mean. Scores this high may reflect a strong need to present oneself in a conventional or favorable light (Piers, 1984).

On the FWS, children reported they were worried about themselves and their moms being hurt, and also worried about their dads hurting

TABLE 3. Parenting Stress Index Raw Scores with Percentiles (N = 102)

	Time 1		Time 2		Difference
	M (SD)	%tile	*M (SD)*	%tile	(101)
Parent-Child Interaction	26.3 (8.2)	85th	24.6 (7.4)	80th	*t* = 2.88**
Difficult Child	33.8 (10.3)	85th	31.0 (9.3)	80th	*t* = 4.01**
Parental Distress	29.0 (7.4)	90th	26.1(7.8)	55th	*t* = 4.56**
Total Parent Stress	90.0 (23.3)	90th	82.3 (21.0)	80th	*t* = 4.91**

* *p* < .05 ** *p* < .01

TABLE 4. Objectives Checklist (N = 162)

	Time 1	Time 2	Difference
	M (SD)	*M (SD)*	(161)
1. Discusses DV incident with parent.	2.4 (1.6)	2.8 (.9)	*t* = −3.91**
2. Tells parent how feels emotionally.	2.6 (.9)	3.0 (.9)	*t* = −4.57**
3. When angry, will state he/she is angry.	2.7 (.9)	2.9 (.9)	*t* = −1.96*
4. When angry, will not become aggressive.	2.4 (1.1)	2.7 (.9)	*t* = −2.01*
5. Knows what physical abuse is.	3.2 (1.0)	3.6 (.7)	*t* = −4.29**
6. Knows what sexual abuse is.	2.9 (1.1)	3.4 (.9)	*t* = −4.87**
7. Knows what emotional abuse is.	2.2 (1.1)	3.1 (.9)	*t* = −6.99**
8. Asks questions when confused.	2.5 (.9)	3.0 (.9)	*t* = −4.14**
9. Knows right to protect privacy of body.	3.6 (.7)	3.7 (.6)	*t* = −1.04
10. Knows what aggressive means.	2.1 (1.0)	2.9 (1.0)	*t* = −6.63**
11. Knows what assertive means.	1.6 (.9)	2.4 (.9)	*t* = −7.42**
12. Has a safety plan in the event of DV.	2.2 (1.0)	3.2 (1.0)	*t* = −7.24**
13. In event of DV, can dial 911.	3.2 (1.1)	3.6 (.8)	*t* = −3.95**
14. Knows who to call if event feels unsafe.	3.1 (1.1)	3.5 (.9)	*t* = −3.44**
Total	2.7 (.7)	3.0 (.5)	*t* = −8.53**

p < .05 **p* < .01

TABLE 5. Trauma Sympton Checklist (TSCC-A) Scores (N = 53)

Scale	Time 1	Time 2	Difference
	M (SD)	M (SD)	(52)
Anger	49.8 (9.4)	47.8 (10.1)	$t = 1.67$
Anxiety	50.8 (11.8)	49.8 (13.6)	$t = .62$
Depression	51.9 (11.5)	49.6 (12.3)	$t = 1.52$
Dissociation	50.6 (11.3)	49.1 (11.6)	$t = 1.39$
PTSD	50.7 (11.8)	48.8 (11.3)	$t = 1.16$

someone. They rated their moms as being most vulnerable to harm and their fathers as most likely to be harmful. Following treatment, children reported having significantly fewer worries about their moms and themselves being vulnerable to injury. They perceived their fathers, their mothers and themselves as less likely to cause harm (see Table 6).

On the FSCS, children attributed similar amounts of power to men and women at Time 1. They attributed significantly less power to both men and women at Time 2, and thought their family members had less of a right to be violent. Beliefs about family rights to privacy and autonomy did not change (see Table 7).

DISCUSSION

The results of this study are suggestive of positive results following treatment for children of domestic violence across a broad range of violence issues. In addition, significant, positive changes were indicated for both the children and their parents at the end of treatment. Mothers initially reported difficulties with their children in the areas of intrapersonal distress, somatic symptoms, interpersonal relations, and social problems. Over the course of treatment parents reported significant change regarding their children in each of these areas. These findings are consistent with the research of Kashani and Allan (1998) concerning externalized and internalized problems of children who experience family violence, and with Dodge and Tomlin (1987) concerning the importance of positive interpersonal relationships.

TABLE 6. Family Worries (N = 33)

	VULNERABILITY			HARM		
	Time 1	Time 2	Difference	Time 1	Time 2	Difference
	M (SD)	M (SD)	(32)	M (SD)	M (SD)	(32)
Mom	2.5 (.7)	2.2 (.7)	t = 2.66*	2.1 (.7)	1.8 (.5)	t = 3.42**
Dad	2.1 (.7)	1.8 (.7)	t = 2.37*	2.3 (.7)	2.0 (.8)	t = 2.64*
Self	2.2 (.7)	1.93 (.7)	t = 2.63*	2.1 (.6)	1.8 (.5)	t = 3.21**

* $p < .05$ ** $p < .01$

TABLE 7. Family Stereotypes Card Sort (N = 36)

	Time 1	Time 2	Difference
	M (SD)	M (SD)	(35)
Male Power	2.0 (.64)	1.7 (.51)	t = 2.40*
Female Power	2.0 (.59)	1.8 (.63)	t = 2.47*
Violence Privilege	1.6 (.65)	1.3 (.41)	t = 2.03*
Family Autonomy	2.6 (.75)	2.6 (.88)	t = −.27

* $p < .05$

The targeted objectives specified on the Objectives Inventory can be grouped into the following six categories: (1) expressing emotions, (2) defining abuse, (3) discussing violence in the family, (4) expressing anger appropriately, and (5) creating a safety plan. Parents reported a significant increase in their children's knowledge of and ability to act positively within each of these domains.

With such strong research findings that exposure to family violence negatively impacts children's emotional functioning (Henning et al., 1996; see also Kalil, Tolman, Rosen, & Gruber, 2003; Onyskiw, 2003) it would appear obvious that a child's self image would thus be negatively impacted by the experiences of family violence. However, on the self-report scales utilized in this research, children indicated average levels of self-concept, and they did not report clinical levels of internalized emotional difficulties. This view differed widely from parental and therapist reports of behavior. It is possible that the children did not perceive or experience these problems; however, it is more likely that they felt the need to look good and protect the family. High self-concept scores can indicate a very positive self-concept or a strong need to present oneself in a conventional or favorable light (Piers, 1984). It is also possible that some children were in denial or had repressed the memories of the traumatic events. Avoidance of revealing information regarding traumatic events appears to be a core response to trauma (Carlson, 1997). Children who tend to underrespond to questions about their thoughts, feelings, and behaviors are likely to be especially defensive, avoidant, or oppositional regarding test-taking (Briere, 1996). Briere has also indicated that it is not uncommon for children to mark zeros on a symptom checklist measure rather than refuse to complete the measure altogether. It is also possible that the child self-report measures used were not sufficient to detect the particular issues facing these children exposed to domestic violence.

The children in treatment were worried about family members being harmed or causing harm. This is consistent with the findings of Graham-Bermann (1996). At the conclusion of treatment, children reported they were less worried about themselves and their mothers being harmed. They also felt less worried about their moms, their dads, and themselves harming someone else. It is possible the group discussions facilitated more confidence in their choices and abilities to use methods other than violence to solve problems. The children also changed some of their attitudes about family stereotypes, particularly with regard to how much power men and women have in the home and their right to be violent.

Mothers reported being less stressed following treatment. Levendosky and Graham-Bermann (1998) documented the moderating effects a parent may have on children who are exposed to violence, thus verifying the need for lower parental stress. Mothers also reported fewer behavior problems with their children following treatment, which may be related to the decrease in parental stress. A highly stressed parent is less able to respond to a child's emotional or physical needs. As the mother's stress decreases, she can be a more skillful parent, and has a better opportunity to meet her children's developmental needs.

The three agencies working in collaboration on this pilot project created treatment protocols used in each treatment program. This information has been made available to other agencies treating similar populations to duplicate. The agencies have conducted training seminars and shared materials and learning experiences to facilitate other agencies interested in treating children who witness domestic violence. Other agencies are in the process of replicating the treatment and research findings of this project.

Limitations

This study lacks a control group by which to contrast the positive impact that group treatment has with children who experience family violence. While it cannot be viewed as ethical to deny treatment to a child, a control group could be comprised of children on a waiting list, children in another type of treatment, or those children who did not have the opportunity to receive treatment. Without such a control group the true efficacy of the treatment is not as clear.

This study also did not control for the possibility that parents might anticipate positive change in their child as a result of being in treatment. It is possible that the parents expected their children's functioning would improve following treatment and that those expectations affected their perceptions of their child's behavior. It is also possible that the positive changes observed at follow-up may be attributed to factors other than the treatment intervention.

This study did not address the impact of other traumatic events during treatment, such as divorce, death, or parental drug use, on measured treatment outcomes. We consistently found that these families were dealing with numerous other events along with the domestic violence. Major events impact parental and child stress levels and emotional functioning. This may affect the ability to absorb and implement long term what is presented in treatment.

This study was a pilot and therefore, it does not include a long-term follow-up to ascertain the continuation of positive results indicated at the conclusion of treatment. Perhaps the weekly therapy session itself provided the ground upon which children dealt with their emotional and developmental issues. Thus, when treatment ceases, the continued growth of the child may not continue. A follow-up study is essential to validate that what has been gained by the children is not lost with the cessation of treatment.

CONCLUSION

This study provides preliminary evidence for the effectiveness of treatment for children who are exposed to domestic violence and for their parent(s). Following treatment, children who had been exposed to domestic violence demonstrated a decrease in behavior problems, and an increase in their abilities to recognize abuse. They were able to discuss the abuse with a parent, appropriately express their emotions, and utilize a safety plan. Additionally, involvement of the child's mother in treatment may have contributed to a decrease in parental stress, thereby increasing the possibility of positive parenting, emotional growth, and bonding between children and their mothers.

REFERENCES

Abidin, R. R. (1995). *Parenting stress index/Short form*. Odessa, FL: Psychological Assessment Resources, Inc.

Briere, J. (1996). *Trauma symptom checklist for children: Professional manual*. Odessa, FL: Psychological Assessment Resources.

Burlingham, G. M., Wells, M. G., & Lambert, M. J. (1996). *Youth Outcome Questionnaire*. Stevenson, MD: American Professional Credentialing Services.

Carlson, E. B. (1997). *Trauma assessments: A clinicians guide*. New York: Guilford.

Davis, K. E. (1988). Interparental violence: The children as victims. *Issues in Comprehensive Pediatric Nursing, 11*, 291-302.

Dodge, K. A., & Price, J. M. (1994). On the relation between social information processing and socially competent behavior in early school-aged children. *Child Development, 65*, 1385-1897.

Dodge, K. A., & Tomlin, A. M. (1987). Utilization of self-schemas as a mechanism of interpretational bias in aggressive children. *Social Cognition, 5*, 280-300.

Elbow, M. (1982). Children of violent marriages: The forgotten victims. *Social Casework, 63*, 465-471.

Geffner, R. A., Jaffe, P. G., & Sudermann, M. (Eds.). (2000). *Children exposed to domestic violence: Current issues in research, intervention, prevention, and policy development*. New York: The Haworth Press, Inc.

Graham-Bermann, S. A. (1992). *The kid's club: An intervention group for children exposed to domestic violence*. University of Michigan.

Graham-Bermann, S. A. (1996). Family worries: The assessment of interpersonal anxiety in children from violent and nonviolent families. *Journal of Clinical Child Psychology, 25*, 280-287.

Graham-Bermann, S. A. (1998). The impact of woman abuse on children's social development: Research and theoretical perspectives. In G. W. Holden, R. Geffner, & E. N. Jouriles (Eds.), *Children exposed to marital violence: Theory, research, and applied issues* (pp. 21-54). Washington, DC: American Psychological Association.

Graham-Bermann, S. A. (1999). Family worries scale (FWS). In J. Touliatos, B. Perlmutter, & G. Holder (Eds.), *Handbook of Family Measurement Techniques*, Second Edition (Vol. 1), Thousand Oaks, CA: Sage.

Graham-Bermann, S. A., & Brescoll, V. (2000). Gender, power, and violence: Assessing the family stereotypes of the children of batterers. *Journal of Family Psychology, 14*(4), 600-612.

Graham-Bermann, S. A., & Edleson, J. L. (Eds.). (2001). *Domestic violence in the lives of children: The future of research, intervention, and social policy.* Washington, DC: American Psychological Association.

Graham-Bermann, S. A., & Levendosky, A. A. (1998). Traumatic stress symptoms in children of battered women. *Journal of Interpersonal Violence, 13,* 111-128.

Gresham, F. M., & Elliot, S. N. (1990). *Social skills rating system.* Circle Pines, MN: American Guidance Service.

Henning, K., Leitenbergh, H., Coffey, P., Turner, T., & Bennett, R. T. (1996). Long-term psychological and social impact of witnessing physical conflict between parents. *Journal of Interpersonal Violence, 11,* 35-51.

Holden, G. W. (1998). Introduction: The development of research into another consequence of family violence. In G. W. Holden, R. Geffner, & E. N. Jouriles (Eds.), *Children exposed to marital violence: Theory, research, and applied issues* (pp. 1-18). Washington, DC: American Psychological Association.

Jaffe, P. G., Wolfe, D. A., & Wilson, S. K. (1990). *Children of battered women,* Thousand Oaks, CA: Sage.

Jones, D. (1997). *Domestic violence incidence and prevalence study conducted for governor's commission on women and families, April-May, 1997.* Salt Lake City, UT: Dan Jones & Associates.

Jouriles, E. N., Norwood, W. D., McDonald, R., Vincent, J. P., & Mahoney, A. (1996). Physical violence and other forms of marital aggression: Links with children's behavior problems. *Journal of Consulting and Clinical Psychology, 57,* 453-455.

Kalil, A., Tolman, R., Rosen, D., & Gruber, G. (2003). Domestic violence and children's behavior in low-income families. *Journal of Emotional Abuse, 3*(1/2), 75 101.

Kashani, J. H., & Allen, W. D. (1998). *The impact of family violence on children and adolescents.* Thousand Oaks, CA: Sage.

Koss, M. P., Goodman, L. A., Browne, A., Fitzgerald, L. F., Keita, G. P., & Russo, M. F. (1994). *No safe haven: Male violence against women at home, at work, and in the community.* Washington, DC: American Psychological Association.

Levendosky, A. A., & Graham-Bermann, S. A. (1998). The moderating effects of parenting stress on children's adjustment in woman-abusing families. *Journal of Interpersonal Violence, 13,* 383-398.

Loosely, S. (1997). *Group treatment for children who witness woman abuse.* London, Canada: Children's Aid Society of London and Middlesex.

McDonald, R., & Jouriles, E. N. (1991). Marital aggression and child behavior problems: Research findings, mechanisms, and intervention strategies. *Behavior Therapist, 14,* 189-192.

Miller, D. (1989). Family violence and the helping system. In L. Combrinck-Graham (Ed.) *Children in family contexts: Perspectives on treatment* (pp. 413-434). New York: Guilford.

Onyskiw, J. (2003). Domestic violence and children's adjustment: A review of research. *Journal of Emotional Abuse, 3*(1/2), 11-45.

Piers, E. V. (1984). *Piers-Harris children's self-concept scale.* Los Angeles, CA: Western Psychological Services.

Peled, E., & Edleson, J. L. (1995). Process and outcome in small groups for children of battered women. In E. Peled, P. G. Jaffe, & J. L. Edleson (Eds.) *Ending the cycle of violence: Community responses to children of battered women* (pp. 77-96). Thousand Oaks, CA: Sage.

Rosenberg, M. S. (1984). The children of battered women: The effects of witnessing violence on their social problem-solving abilities, *Behavior Therapist, 4*, 85-89.

Silvern, L., Karyl, J., Waedle, L., Hodges, W. E., Starek, J., Heidt, E., & Min, K. (1995). Retrospective reports of parental partner abuse: Relationships to depression, trauma symptoms and self-esteem among college students. *Journal of Family Violence, 10*, 177-202.

Straus, M. A. (1992). Children as witness to marital violence: A risk factor for life long problems among a nationally representative sample of American men and women. In D. F. Schwarz (Ed.), *Children and violence: Report on the Twenty-Third Ross Roundtable on Critical Approaches to Common Pediatric Problems* (pp. 98-109). Columbus, OH: Ross Laboratories.

Thorn, B. (1998). *Objectives checklist.* Salt Lake City, UT: Cornerstone Counseling Center.

Wolfe, D. A. (1994). *Promoting healthy, nonviolent relationships: A group approach with adolescents for the prevention of woman abuse and interpersonal violence.* London, Canada: University of Western Ontario, Department of Psychology.

EFFECTS OF TREATMENT: OUTCOME RESEARCH

Group Interventions for Children At-Risk from Family Abuse and Exposure to Violence: A Report of a Study

Janet R. Johnston

SUMMARY. This paper describes the rationale, content, and preliminary data on outcome effectiveness of a therapeutic curriculum designed

Address correspondence to: Janet R. Johnston, PhD, Administration of Justice Department, San Jose State University, 1 Washington Square, San Jose, CA 95192-0050.

Vivienne Roseby, PhD, is acknowledged and thanked for her thoughtful comments on the theoretical formulation and treatment model described in this paper.

The work described in this paper was supported by grants from the Zellerbach Family Fund, the David and Lucile Packard Foundation, and the Marin Community Foundation.

This paper was presented at the Victimization of Children and Youth: An International Research Conference sponsored by the Family Research Laboratory & Crimes Against Children Research Center, University of New Hampshire, June 25-28, 2000.

[Haworth co-indexing entry note]: "Group Interventions for Children At-Risk from Family Abuse and Exposure to Violence: A Report of a Study." Johnston, Janet R. Co-published simultaneously in *Journal of Emotional Abuse* (The Haworth Maltreatment & Trauma Press, an imprint of The Haworth Press, Inc.) Vol. 3, No. 3/4, 2003, pp. 203-226; and: *The Effects of Intimate Partner Violence on Children* (ed: Robert A. Geffner, Robyn Spurling Igelman, and Jennifer Zellner) The Haworth Maltreatment & Trauma Press, an imprint of The Haworth Press, Inc., 2003, pp. 203-226. Single or multiple copies of this article are available for a fee from The Haworth Document Delivery Service [1-800-HAWORTH, 9:00 a.m. - 5:00 p.m. (EST). E-mail address: docdelivery@haworthpress.com].

http://www.haworthpress.com/store/product.asp?sku=J135
10.1300J135v03n03_03

for groups of children from highly conflicted and violent families, implemented in family agency and school settings. Data for 223 children (ages 5-14 years, most of whom were from single-parent, indigent, ethnic minority families) who participated in the study indicate that the majority had been exposed to multiple types of stressful and traumatic events. These include separation and loss of a parent or caretaker, exposure to spousal and child abuse, neighborhood violence, and having a family member in trouble with the law. The absence of a control group makes it difficult to determine to what extent the positive outcomes can be attributed to the group intervention. However, a pre- and post-assessment of the children's behavioral problems and social competence by clinicians, teachers, and parents showed significant improvement in their functioning over a six-month follow-up. Conclusions are drawn as to the basic elements of group interventions that are ecologically and economically feasible and clinically sound. *[Article copies available for a fee from The Haworth Document Delivery Service: 1-800-HAWORTH. E-mail address: <docdelivery@haworthpress.com> Website: <http://www.HaworthPress.com> © 2003 by The Haworth Press, Inc. All rights reserved.]*

KEYWORDS. Children's groups, treatment, domestic violence, trauma, abuse

Domestic violence does not occur as a singular traumatic life event for children (Fantuzzo & Mohr, 1999; Jaffe, Wolfe, & Wilson, 1990; Osofsky, 1999). Child witnesses to domestic abuse are likely to have a history of multiple stressors that include separation, high-conflict divorce, loss, and disruptions of their care-taking (see DeVoe & Smith, 2003; Shaffer & Bala, 2003). In addition, their parents or caretakers may abuse alcohol and drugs, suffer from emotional distress or psychopathology, and abuse them or their siblings directly. The stress on these families is often compounded by poverty, racial discrimination, ethnic minority status, and language barriers, especially for those who live in poor communities where there is neighborhood violence. Although many domestic violence researchers have acknowledged the multiple victimization of children in these circumstances, most consider family violence as the central defining event. Moreover, domestic violence prevention and intervention efforts for children have largely focused on the abuse itself, which may or may not be what is of central concern to the children and their families (Wolfe & Jaffe, 1999). This paper takes a look at the array of multiple stressors for children and parents in high-risk neighborhoods and presents a group treatment model that addresses their multiple and varied concerns.

EFFECTS ON CHILDREN

A plethora of research findings confirm that exposure to high-conflict and violent family environments is seriously damaging to infants, children, and youth. In fact, to varying degrees, children from violent homes have substantially the same kinds of problems as those who are directly abused by their caretakers (Cummings & Davies, 1994; Davies & Cummings, 1994; Dodge, Bates, & Pettit, 1990; Jaffe et al., 1990). Depending upon the severity, chronicity, and multiplicity of the victimization that often co-occurs in violent families, children can suffer from a range of emotional and behavioral difficulties and developmental distortions. They have problems with behavioral control and emotional regulation (Trickett, 1998). They suffer diminished self-esteem and self-efficacy and experience a fragmented sense of self-continuity and cohesiveness (Harter, 1998). Their capacity to relate to other people can be compromised by their basic distrust and hypervigilance (Roseby, Erdberg, Bardenstein, & Johnston, 1995). Their cognitive capacities are impacted in that they are less able to read social cues accurately, possibly because they do not trust sufficiently to check out the validity of their perceptions with others. Their understanding of social situations is distorted by their tendency to strip down complexity, avoid ambiguity, and, in some cases, to readily attribute hostile intent to others (Dodge et al., 1990; Murray & Son, 1998; Roseby et al., 1995). In effect, these children tend to be overly aggressive and controlling or overly passive and victimized in relations with their peers and to have poor coping skills (Cole-Detke & Kobak, 1998; Rosenberg & Rossman, 1990). The long-term prognosis for the children of violent families is at best guarded: There is evidence that as adults they have problems with anxiety and depression, and tend to make poor choices in selecting mates (Cappell & Heiner, 1990; Carlson, 1990; Forsstrom-Cohen & Rosenbaum, 1985). Compared to those who have no history of violence and abuse in their family of origin, these children as adults, especially the boys, are more likely to repeat the cycle of victimization in the next generation (Kalmuss, 1984; Kaufman & Zigler, 1987; Straus, Gelles, & Steinmetz, 1980; Widom, 1989; Zeanah & Zeanah, 1989).

APPROACHES TO TREATMENT

In the face of the kind of damage that is likely to have affected children from violent environments, it is doubtful that they can recuperate and regain their developmental stride simply by stopping the abuse and ensuring their safety. Remedial interventions need to systematically address children's specific vulnerabilities and deficits and do so by building on those factors that are known to produce resiliency and protect them emotionally (Rutter, 1987). This paper will briefly review current approaches that have been taken in direct prevention and intervention efforts to date with these at-risk children as the context in which to present an alternative model with some data on outcome. This is not intended to be a comprehensive review of all psycho-educational and therapeutic programs that have been developed. Rather, it is confined to a selection of published works that have explicitly documented the intervention model and are good representatives of the general approach being discussed.

Broadly speaking, existing family violence prevention and intervention approaches for children and youth have evolved somewhat independently of one another, partly in response to practitioners with diverse professional backgrounds working with different populations of family violence. There are three major approaches discussed here: (1) psycho-educational group treatment for children and mothers, most often provided by battered women's shelters; (2) post-traumatic stress disorder (PTSD) therapy for acutely traumatized children in hospital and clinic settings; and (3) the model that is presented and illustrated in this paper–developmental psychotherapy for children from chronically conflicted and intermittently violent families in the broader community.

Psycho-Educational Approaches for Children of Family Violence

For the past two decades, battered women's advocates have pioneered ways of helping children who have lived in violent family environments (Hughes, 1982). Group treatment programs have slowly emerged for school-age children transitioning through shelters for battered women at the time their mothers are struggling to leave an abusive partner. These programs are primarily informed by cognitive-behavioral principles, learning theory, and feminist scholarship. The behavioral difficulties in these children and their cognitive beliefs that serve to support them are seen as learned social responses, modeled by their abusive caretakers and peers, conditioned by stimulus cues, and reinforced by the fact that coercive, controlling and aggressive interpersonal behavior is likely to be rewarded. It follows that the intervention of choice is a corrective socialization experience wherein more appropriate social skills and problem-solving are taught, modeled and practiced. The emotional difficulties in these children (anxiety and depression) are viewed as evidence of poor coping skills and self-blaming attitudes that can be addressed by teaching children safety skills and by encouraging them to assign full culpability to the abuser, rather than to themselves or the victim.

Although there are many unpublished manuals and guides available, Peled and Davis (1995) provide one of the few published resources for this kind of work with school-age children. Their practitioner's manual provides a detailed ten-week session-by-session blueprint for a model of intervention. Children are encouraged to break the secret of the family violence and label it as wrong. They are taught how to understand and express their feelings; how to protect themselves in future violent emergencies; how to recover playfulness and the capacity for pleasure; and how to strengthen their self-esteem. Parent educational and support groups for victims of abuse, primarily mothers, are frequent accompaniments to the children's program.

High-risk teenagers who have grown up in violent home environments have been a focus of a related group program (Wolfe, Wkerle, & Scott, 1997; Wolfe et al., 1996). A manual outlines a twelve-session curriculum to help young people understand the abuse of power and control in dating and intimate relationships and the many ways that sexism or male-chauvinism is expressed in families and reinforced through peer pressure. Date rape and dating violence are explicitly addressed. Video segments, case vignettes, exercises, and group discussions are used to raise students' consciousness about the problem and to invite them to choose healthier, egalitarian relationships and practice new relationship skills.

Evaluation research on these kinds of models is in its infancy and the studies that do exist have been plagued by methodological deficiencies, namely small sample sizes, lack of control or comparison groups, no random assignment to conditions, failure to document treatment fidelity, use of non-standardized outcome measures, and lack of longer-term follow-up. However, Graham-Bermann (1999) has reviewed a small but growing body of outcome studies and identified thirteen (most yet unpublished) that meet minimal research design standards. She documented the effectiveness of this general psycho-educational approach, specifically in terms of children's increased knowledge and decreased anxiety, with mixed but generally positive findings with respect to behavior, attitudes and skills. (See also review by Ezell, McDonald, & Jouriles, 2000.)

Post-Traumatic Stress Disorder (PTSD) Therapy

Children who have suffered fairly recent, acute traumatic exposure to episodes of severe domestic violence, such as battering, rape, murder, suicide, abduction, and other critical incidents referred to as Type I trauma (Terr, 1991), have been the focus of PTSD therapy (see MacMillan & Harpur, 2003). This psychiatric approach has been informed by a growing body of research on biochemical and neurological changes that underlie symptoms of PTSD: flashbacks, nightmares, dissociative states, numbness, hyper-alertness, inability to concentrate, and re-enactment. Infants and young children that have been traumatized typically respond organismically with hyper-arousal and dissociation, and interpersonally with disruptions in attachment capacities to caretakers. In the developing brain, such traumatic states organize neural systems and pathways, resulting in relatively enduring traits or behavioral and emotional capacities. Specifically the loss of the ability to regulate the intensity of feeling is viewed as one of the most far-reaching effect of early trauma and neglect (Briere, 1997; van der Kolk, van der Hart & Marmar, 1996). From this perspective, critical incidents of traumatic proportions for children are highly influential in the development of psychopathology (Lewis, Amini & Lannon, 2000).

It has been argued that the therapy of choice in these cases is to facilitate the child's disclosure of the traumatic event (both the memory and the terrifying feelings associated with it) in a safe place. Therapists vary in their techniques, but the general idea is to systematically de-sensitize the child to the overwhelming terror and help him or her express expectable feelings. The therapist can then help the child to cognitively restructure any fixated or erroneous beliefs about his or her helplessness, vulnerability, culpability, and fantasies of rescue and revenge. Finally, some interpretation of the PTSD symptoms usually helps the child understand and manage them better (Silvern, Karyl, & Landis, 1995).

These kinds of mental health services are often sited in hospitals and clinics where social casework services are also provided for the child's family (McAlister Groves, 1999). Pynoos and Eth (1986) have provided an exemplary protocol for interviewing children who have experienced severe forms of acute trauma. Their methods have also been adapted for groups of children and youth that have experienced repeated trauma of this nature, at home and on the street (Murphy, Pynoos, & James, 1997). To our knowledge, there has not yet been published any empirical evaluation of this group approach. However, as researchers and clinicians have come to understand more about PTSD, they increasingly emphasize the need for early identification and timely intervention to prevent the acute symptoms of this disorder from becoming chronic ones. Emergency emotional first aid, triage, referral, and early therapeutic intervention, provided at the scene by police officers and mental health consultants, may be vital for children who are acutely traumatized as victim-witnesses to family violence (NCJFCJ, 1998).

Developmental Psychotherapy for Children of Chronically Conflicted and Violent Families

Studies of children who have experienced more pervasive and ongoing conflict, emotional abuse, and intermittent family violence (referred to as Type II trauma by Terr, 1991) have highlighted the defensive operations that pervasively distort children's social-emotional development (Johnston & Roseby, 1997; Wolfe, 1999). Although this type of trauma may not be as acute as that described above, it is often insidious because of its early onset and chronicity in the child's life. These children have usually forged considerable psychological defenses to regain a sense of control, predictability and safety in the face of intermittent exposure to physical assault, inadequate, neglectful or dangerous parenting, and the myriad of stressful life events that accompany the abuse. The problem is that these defensive strategies become organized as invariant and scripted rules and expectations about the self and others in ways that may be functional within their chaotic families but act as blinders that neutralize, distort, or simply block-out corrective feedback and experience in other settings. Hence these scripts result in entrenched, constricted patterns of feeling, dealing with emotions, perceiving reality, and solving problems that are formidable barriers to effective therapeutic intervention of any persuasion. Moreover, these impoverished scripts about relationships underlie the serious disruption in attachments to primary caretakers amongst infants and toddlers (Lieberman & Van Horn, 1998) and deficits in social awareness and problems in relating to peers amongst the older school-age children (Roseby & Johnston, 1998; Wolfe, 1999).

This understanding of the developmental impact of trauma is the basis of the treatment model that is described in this paper. The central goal of the work is to help the children to make conscious and revise their internal scripts, and the rules and expectations that support them. The model is organized as a structured, activity-based group curriculum with adaptations for different age groups (Roseby & Johnston, 1997; Roseby, Gentner, & Enomoto, 1998). More specifically, initially group exercises are designed to develop children's interpersonal trust and decrease their hypervigilance. Then, through games, drawing and charades, children learn about the gradations and language of feelings that can be articulated, rather than blocked or acted out. The purpose of guided imagery and mask-making is to increase their capacity for empathy by helping them identify distinctions among their own feelings, and boundaries between their own and others' feelings, ideas, motives, and preferences. Psycho-dramatic role-plays that are video recorded are the central tools of the group model and are used to distinguish between first person, second person and third person perspectives of the child's social experience. The goal of role playing is to surface and revise the children's unconscious rules and expectations that govern their scripted and constricted views of themselves and other people. In this endeavor, it is not assumed that being a witness to violence is the central concern for these children. Rather, the children's *own* traumatic memories and stressful experiences generate the themes in the dramatic role-plays and family sculptures that they devise. Further, their hopes and dreams are nurtured by having them revise and replay those critical incidents. Within a context of relative emotional safety, they are encouraged to explore the complexity and nuance of relationships, and to tolerate ambiguity and ambivalence without simplifying and distorting their understanding of and feelings about their social world. It is within the context of these new understandings that children are encouraged to develop a more internalized sense of right and wrong, to restore a consensual moral order, and to practice new interpersonal and problem-solving skills.

This therapeutic group curriculum was first developed for children who are the centerpiece of parental fights in highly conflicted and violent families disputing custody in family court. Concurrent group and individual treatment models were developed for parents and other family members in this setting (Johnston & Campbell, 1988; Johnston & Roseby, 1997; McDonough, Radovanovic, Stein, Sagar, & Hood, unpublished manual). In the study described in this paper, the children's group model was modified and implemented in neighborhood schools and family counseling agencies for ethnically diverse populations of children who have been identified as victims of physical abuse or as victim-witnesses of violence. Concurrently, parents and other caretakers were offered brief psycho-educational group and individual feedback sessions on their children's progress (see Johnston, 1999, for full details). It was hypothesized that children from these environments would have experienced a multiplicity of stressful and traumatic life events. The further and principal hypothesis was that children who received the group intervention would show significant improvement on measures of behavioral problems and social competence over a six-month follow-up period, according to parents', teachers' and clinicians' ratings.

REPORT OF A STUDY

Selection of Sample and Attrition

The group interventions, commonly known as the Children's Wellbeing Groups, were implemented and evaluated in three family service agency sites and five elementary schools in the San Francisco Bay Area. Sites were chosen because of the high-risk neighborhoods they served and because they also offered a range of individual and family therapy, case management, advocacy, and referral services to families. During the time period of the study (1996-1999), a total of 488 children and their parents were served by the project. Approximately 10% of the children received the group intervention twice. Baseline data from at least two of the three sources (clinicians, teachers, and parents) were available for 223 children (from 193 families), 106 girls and 117 boys (aged 5-14 years). This represents 66% of those who were eligible. Six-month follow-up data were sought for only those children for whom baseline data were provided. This yielded clinicians' ratings for 199 (89%), teachers' ratings for 123 (55%), and parents' ratings for 106 (48%) of the children. (Staff in three of the five schools declined to solicit data from parents.)

Eligibility for the Wellbeing Groups included children who had: (1) witnessed violence or had been the object of violence (at home, in the neighborhood, or at school); (2) experienced highly conflictual marriages and litigated divorce (in which parents were hostile, verbally abusive, fearful, and highly distrustful of each other); (3) suffered the precipitous loss of a primary caregiver as a consequence of violence, abuse, or criminal behavior (by death, desertion, incarceration, parental abduction, deportation); and (4) been exposed to abusive and neglectful environments due to parents' or other adults' substance abuse. All types of abuse except direct sexual abuse were included. However, the groups were not regarded as appropriate for severely emotionally disturbed and behaviorally uncontrollable children.

Children were identified through a variety of extant referral networks within the schools and agency sites. Referral sources included judges, mediators, teachers, school counselors, principals, therapists, advocates, and parents or legal guardians. The primary custodial caretaker gave permission for each child's participation and agreed to provide data at intake interviews and about six months later. In addition, parents, guardians and foster parents, grandparents, and other relatives were invited to attend parent groups, held monthly at most sites whereas some of the school sites offered weekly parent support groups. Those adults who had been abusive met in separate groups from their victims.

Group Composition

On average, seven children attended each group series. Each series comprised ten weekly meetings, each 90 minutes long, at the family agency sites. At the school sites, the meetings occurred over one semester, or 15 weeks, of sessions, each almost one hour in duration. The groups were composed of children of similar grade level and same age range (5-7 year-olds; 8-11 year-olds, and 12-14 year-olds). The groups were usually led by two clinicians, one a trained and experienced counselor (who was paid), and one a student counselor (who was unpaid). However, when short-staffed, groups were conducted by only one experienced counselor in some sites. One bilingual/bicultural counselor participated at each school site, where groups were often conducted concurrently in English and Spanish.

Attendance

Attendance at the children's group sessions averaged 85%. The school sites tended to have slightly better attendance (89%) compared to the agency sites (80%). Parent involvement in the program was less than anticipated. Attendance at parent groups varied widely across settings and over time, with about one half of parents participating at least once during the series. Generally, a small group of 4 to 5 parents attended regularly.

Demographic Descriptors

The families were of multi-ethnic origin, the two largest groups being Caucasian (42%) and Hispanic (36%). African-Americans comprised 10% and other racial groups made up 12% of the sample. Socio-economic status of the families was obtained from indirect measures since income data was not available. Three-fourths of parents had obtained no more than a high school education; 42% received government welfare benefits (MediCal), and 23% received Victims of Crime (VOC) funding.

In terms of family composition, there were, on average, 2.4 children per family (range = 1-6). Half the children were the oldest child and one third were the second oldest. They lived in households that on average included 4 members (range: 2-11). The children were predominantly from single parent families (80%). It was equally likely that parents had never married, were separated, or were already divorced. Parents who were currently married and still living together were the minority (20%). Mothers were the primary caretakers of the children in 58% of cases. Foster parents, grandparents, and other relatives cared for 15% of the children. The average age of the children's caretakers across all sites was 38 years (range: 23-74 years).

Stressful Family Life Events

The primary caretaker, at times with the help of the family advocate or counselor, completed the Family Wellbeing Checklist that documents the history of stressful family life events, trauma, and social support experienced during the past six months, and during the lifetime of the child. *Health Problems* included serious acute and chronic injury or physical illness, mental illness, and difficulty obtaining basic health care. A history of Health Problems was reported for 63% of the sample, 49% within the last six months. *Housing Problems* included being evicted or suffering foreclosure, homelessness, and overcrowded, substandard, or unsafe living conditions. A history of Housing Problems was indicated for 39%, 26% within the past six months. *Employment/Financial Problems* included being laid off or fired, difficulty finding work, being deeply in debt, and having costly legal expenses. A history of Employment/Financial problems had been experienced for 68% of the sample, 57% in the past six months.

Children's Exposure to Violence and Crime

The Family Wellbeing Checklist also provided data about these kinds of trauma. *Separation and Loss* included parental separation and divorce, separation of parent and child, migration to another country, loss of a good friend/relative, and death of a close family member. *Neighborhood Violence* involved arguments, threats, or actual violence from neighbors, trouble with gangs, and being the victim of burglary. *Domestic Violence* included frequent household arguments and insults, any physical assault (grabbing, shoving, hitting, kicking, choking, beating up, use of a weapon), and any consequent physical injury. *Parenting Difficulties* included concerns about child neglect, physical and sexual abuse. It also included having a child who was hard to control, who was not warm or close, or who did not respect family values. *Drug/Alcohol Abuse* included concerns about a household member drinking excessively, using illegal drugs, or abusing prescription drugs. *Trouble with the Law* was recorded if anyone in the household had been arrested, incarcerated, or was on probation or parole. *Other Stressful Life Events* was a residual category.

Table 1 ranks the frequency of occurrence of each family trauma or stress experienced by the children. Note that separation and loss was the most frequently recorded event (87%), about two-thirds of which in-

TABLE 1. History of Family Trauma Experienced by Children Ranked by Frequency (n = 180)

	Recent (last 6 months)	Past (prior to 6 months)	Any Problems (during child's life)
Separation & Loss	46%	74%	87%
Domestic Violence	41%	53%	70%
Parenting Difficulties	58%	43%	69%
Other Stressful Life Events	--	--	47%
Trouble with the Law	18%	33%	43%
Drug & Alcohol Abuse	11%	31%	36%
Neighborhood Violence	25%	13%	32%

Note. Missing *n* = 13 families.

volved parental separation and divorce. Domestic violence was reported for 70% of the families. Prevalence of other stressful life events (mostly highly conflicted and litigated custody) and criminal involvement of a household member was 43%-47%. Substance abuse by a household member and neighborhood violence had occurred for about one-third (32%-36%).

With regard to the cumulative nature of stressful events to which these children were exposed, 52% of the children had experienced three of the six types of events that included Separation and Loss, Neighborhood Violence, Domestic Violence, Parenting Difficulties, Drug/Alcohol Abuse, and Trouble with the Law. Another 25% of the children had a history of four of the six events; 17% had experienced five types; and a small proportion (6%) had suffered all six types of events. For only 3% of children who had experienced Domestic Violence was there no other kind of trauma reported. These findings illustrate the multiplicity of traumatic and stressful life events for the majority of the children and amply support the first hypothesis of the study.

Evaluating the Effectiveness of the Group Intervention

Children were assessed at baseline and again at the end of the group intervention by the group clinicians/leaders. They were also assessed at baseline and at a six-month follow-up by parents and teachers using standardized measures of adjustment.

Measures. The outcome measure used by both the teachers and the clinicians was the Teachers Rating Scale (TRS; Hightower et al., 1986). The TRS has two parts. Part I consists of 18 behaviorally oriented items, each rated on a 5-point scale that describes the child's Behavioral Problems including items that measure acting-out, shy-anxious behaviors, and learning problems. (The last group of items was not rated by clinicians.) Part II consists of 20 items assessing the child's Social Competencies, each rated on a 5-point scale, including items measuring frustration tolerance, assertive social skills, task orientation, and peer social skills. Mean scores for both Behavioral Problems and Social Competence were calculated.

Parents completed the Child Behavior Checklist (CBCL; Achenbach & Edelbrock, 1983), a 118-item checklist–each rated on a 3-point scale–yielding a raw score for Total Behavioral Problems. The two sub-scales common to both genders and all ages of children on this measure were also used, namely Internalizing Problems (measuring anxiety, depression, withdrawal, and somatic complaints) and Externalizing Problems (measuring aggression and conduct disorders). Repeated measures t-tests on the available data for these measures were utilized to test the principal hypothesis that children, compared to baseline, would show significant improvement at follow-up.

RESULTS

As shown in Table 2, according to clinicians' ratings on the TRS, children's Behavioral Problems significantly declined and their Social Competence was judged to have significantly increased after the group intervention, compared to baseline. Although boys were perceived to have more behavioral difficulties and to be less socially competent than were girls, both before and after treatment, on the average boys and girls made similar gains in their adjustment over the duration of the group intervention.

Table 3 shows parents' ratings of their children's Total Behavioral Problems, Internalizing Problems, and Externalizing Problems on the CBCL before the group intervention compared to those at a follow-up about six-months later. As with clinicians' ratings, boys tended to be rated as more behaviorally difficult compared to girls, which is in accord with the vast majority of prior research. Most important, as predicted, parents rated their children as having fewer emotional and behavioral difficulties at follow-up compared to baseline. Both boys and girls made substantial gains following their involvement in the project (a 20%-25% improvement).

How do parents' ratings of their children compare with normal children on this standardized measure? It is interesting to report that the average raw scores for Total Behavioral Problems on the CBCL for both girls and boys in this sample lie on the borderline between what is within normal and clinically abnormal ranges of emotional and behavioral disturbance in the broader population of children (Achenbach & Edelbrock, 1983). As shown in Table 4, at baseline 50 (47%) of the children scored in the abnormal range, whereas less than 16% of the total population of children was expected to have scores in this range. It was gratifying to note that, at follow-up, only 27 (25%) of the children scored in the abnormal range on this measure. As shown in Table 4, one-third of the children who were rated as abnormal on this measure at baseline rated as being within the normal range at the follow-up, whereas only 5% changed from normal to abnormal during this time period. These findings are statistically significant.

TABLE 2. Clinicians' Ratings of Children's Behavioral Problems and Social Competence at Baseline and Follow-Up

	Girls (n = 96)	Boys (n = 103)	Total (N = 199)
Behavior Problems			
At baseline	2.68 (.84)	3.05 (.83)	2.87 (.85)
Behavior Problems			
At follow-up	2.11 (.75)	2.36 (.82)	2.24 (.80)
	t = 9.26***	t = 9.54***	t = 13.21***
Social Competence			
At baseline	2.52 (.80)	2.24 (.71)	2.37 (.77)
Social Competence			
At follow-up	3.01 (.78)	2.71 (.75)	2.85 (.78)
	t = −12.01***	t = −12.60***	t = −17.44***

Note. Mean and (sd) for TRS on 5-point scale and paired-difference t tests (one tailed).
*** p < .001

TABLE 3. Parents' Ratings of Children's Behavioral Problems at Baseline and After Group Program

	Girls (n = 50)	Boys (n = 56)	Total (N = 106)
Total Behavior Problems			
At baseline	37.12 (25.09)	41.14 (24.31)	39.25 (24.65)
Total Behavior Problems			
At follow-up	28.26 (23.23)	32.45 (25.80)	30.47 (24.59)
	t − 3.22***	t − 3.32***	t = 4.64***
Internalizing Problems			
At baseline	16.08 (13.15)	15.84 (11.10)	15.95 (12.05)
Internalizing Problems			
At follow-up	11.14 (9.97)	11.95 (11.35)	11.57 (10.68)
	t = 3.30***	t = 3.16***	t = 4.58***
Externalizing Problems			
At baseline	18.52 (12.73)	20.95 (12.96)	19.80 (12.85)
Externalizing Problems			
At follow-up	14.80 (12.98)	16.52 (13.21)	15.71 (13.07)
	t = 2.45**	t = 3.35***	t = 4.11***

Note. Mean and (sd) raw score for CBCL and paired-difference t tests (one tailed).
** p < .01 *** p < .001

TABLE 4. Normal and Abnormal Rates of Behavioral Disturbances in Children Before and After Treatment (from CBCL) (n = 106)

	Before		
After	Normal	Abnormal	Total
Normal	53 (67%)	26 (33%)	79 (75%)
Abnormal	3 (5%)	24 (48%)	27 (56%)
Total	56 (53%)	50 (47%)	106 (100%)

Note. $\chi^2 = 25.3$, $p < .001$.

Table 5 compares teachers' ratings of children's Behavioral Problems and Social Competence at baseline with those at follow-up. According to teachers' perceptions, children's Behavioral Problems showed a significant decrease over this period. Furthermore, teachers' ratings of children's Social Competence significantly increased during that time period for the total sample of children. However, these changes were not as extensive as those recorded by the group clinicians. Sub-analysis of teachers' ratings of children who received the group intervention twice suggests that improvements occur in two stages. In the first stage, the children tend to become both more socially assertive (practicing their new social skills) but also more behaviorally demanding as they express their negative feelings more freely. In the second stage, they seem to settle into more appropriate ways of managing their social relationships, and behavioral problems diminish.

Sub-analysis conducted to see if the results varied depending upon the sites indicated that clinicians' and parents' ratings across all sites showed similar improvement. However, in three of the five schools, the teachers' ratings of improvement were not statistically significant at follow-up. It is important to note that only in school sites were teachers aware that the children were receiving the group treatment. Hence, the results obtained contradict the interpretation that the positive outcomes were only a reflection of expectations of improvement. The most likely explanation for discrepancy in outcomes among school sites is the fact that in the three schools where the teachers' ratings were not significant, the family and group services were in operation for only a six-to-eight-month period. The teachers and school administrators did not understand the purpose of the program, short-staffing limited the

TABLE 5. Teacher Ratings of Children's Behavioral Problems and Social Competence at Baseline and Follow-Up

	Girls (*n* = 58)	Boys (*n* = 65)	Total (*N* = 123)
Behavior Problems			
At baseline	2.31 (.73)	2.89 (.71)	2.62 (.78)
Behavior Problems			
At follow-up	2.03 (.62)	2.76 (.79)	2.41 (.80)
	$t = 3.27***$	$t = 1.98*$	$t = 3.75***$
Social Competence			
At baseline	3.04 (.69)	2.76 (.70)	2.89 (.71)
Social Competence			
At follow-up	3.34 (.80)	2.93 (.68)	3.13 (.76)
	$t = -3.85***$	$t = -2.9**$	$t = -4.8***$

Note. Mean and (*sd*) rating for TRS on 5-point scale and paired-difference *t* tests (one tailed).
*$p < .05$ ** $p < .01$ *** $p < .001$

extent to which families received collateral services, and the group leaders had little or no training.

In sum, the overall findings on all measures were uniformly positive; the effects were modest to substantial in size, and statistically significant. According to clinicians', parents', and teachers' ratings on standardized measures, children who received the group intervention showed significantly fewer behavioral problems. Teachers and clinicians also perceived significantly improved social competence. Boys and girls made similar amounts of improvement.

The Relationship Between Family Trauma and Children's Outcomes

Findings (from exploratory correlational analysis) confirm the kind of family trauma and stressful life events that are more likely to adversely affect children and the contexts in which children are more protected. Children whose development had been disrupted by separation and loss were those more likely to be behaviorally troubled and to have difficulties getting along with their peers. The experience of domestic abuse and exposure to neighborhood violence was less closely related to children's difficulties than was a history of loss. Interestingly, a cumulative history of stressful or traumatic events was more closely related to children's adjustment at the follow-up than to their functioning at baseline, suggesting the more serious impact of chronic stress. This finding also suggests the possibility of latent effects that emerge over time, possibly as a consequence of uncovering traumatic memories within group treatment.

DISCUSSION

This was a preliminary outcome study of a therapeutic curriculum designed for groups of school-age children at-risk from living in highly conflicted and violent homes. The intervention model was designed to respond to the history of multiple traumas and stressful life events that typically co-occur in these children's families, rather than assuming domestic abuse to be the central event. The group program was implemented within several family counseling and school sites in high-risk, multi-ethnic, socio-economically disadvantaged neighborhoods. The findings confirm the hypotheses that these children have suffered multiple and cumulative stress or trauma, and that the group intervention resulted in uniformly more positive outcomes (fewer behavioral problems and increased social competence) at a six-month follow-up, according to clinicians', parents' and teachers' ratings of the children.

Caution needs to be used in interpreting these promising results. On the one hand, it strengthens the evaluation design to gather multiple perspectives on the children's functioning from parents, clinicians and teachers, especially in agency sites where teachers were unaware that the children were receiving the group intervention. This provides more assurance that the improvements reported were real and not the result of observer bias or the expectation that children in treatment would improve. On the other hand, the study design is weakened by the absence of a no-treatment control group. Nor was it feasible to employ a comparison sample of children that received a different kind of treatment (e.g., individual therapy). This makes it impossible to conclude that the positive effects observed were due to the specific model of group intervention, or that these groups are likely to be more effective than other types of interventions (e.g., services provided to the children's families). The only definitive way of determining causal effects is to employ a well-designed experimental study, wherein children and families are randomly assigned to treatment group, comparison group, and no treatment conditions.

A second limitation is the extent of subject attrition–data for about half the total number of children served were not available, a not unusual situation in practice settings where busy clinicians, rather than researchers, are responsible for collecting the data. This makes it difficult to determine the extent to which those families who did provide data are different from those that did not, and the extent to which the findings are generalizable to broader populations.

Despite these limitations, this study offers support for an ecologically appropriate and economically feasible model of intervention for large numbers of high-risk populations of children who are exposed to intimate violence. First, the model addresses the multiple victimization and history of cumulative stressful life events typically experienced by these children, rather than assuming domestic violence is primarily responsible for the children's difficulties. Second, this general trauma approach is more acceptable to parents and to school personnel who must give their permission for children to participate in the program. The stigma of exposing domestic violence and receiving mental health services is less likely to result in resistance to treatment within such "Wellbeing Groups," where the focus is on helping children cope with a diverse array of stressful life events. Third, the group intervention aims to remedy specific developmental deficits in emotional and behavioral regulation, self-esteem, coping, interpersonal judgment, and moral reasoning. This is in contrast to approaches that recommend different interventions for specific behavioral symptoms such as aggression, anxiety, and depression, all of which tend to be highly correlated in these children.

Fourth, the interventions described here are economically feasible. It is estimated that the group program costs only 43% of what a similar number of hours of individual therapy would cost (see Johnston, 1999, for details). That is, on average it costs 12 counselor contact hours for each child seen within groups, whereas children seen individually for a similar length of time would cost 28 counselor-contact hours. In fact, these groups were self-sustaining on a combination of MediCal and VOC funding in schools, both of which were supplemented by low sliding-scale fees in agency settings. There is a critical need to provide low-cost preventive mental health services for broad populations of at-risk children, and it appears that group interventions are the only way in which this can be accomplished.

Fifth and finally, the group interventions described here were adapted to the local cultures and language within multi-ethnic neighborhoods and made easily accessible to poor families. However, they were not sited without giving careful consideration also to providing an array of family support services–individual and family counseling, practical assistance, advocacy, referral, and case management. The findings about the differential impact of the program in new school settings points to the need for careful preparation and training of staff as well as attention to the synergy between classroom teachers, school administrators, and staff in program implementation. Moreover, these group interventions that address children's trauma are not sufficient in themselves. They need to be properly sequenced within a continuum of other kinds of group programs within schools and other neighborhood settings that include socialization groups, divorce adjustment groups, education about domestic violence and substance abuse, gang prevention, mentoring programs, and supportive social and recreational activities.

CONCLUSIONS

The development of interventions for children from violent and abusive homes has been a recent phenomenon in response to the needs of different populations of children of family violence. To some extent, the philosophical differences and diverse professional backgrounds of their respective treatment teams have also influenced the models. Battered women's advocates and feminist theory have strongly influenced the formulation of an approach that is largely psycho-educational in nature. The development of posttraumatic stress disorder syndrome with its attendant physiological correlates has been the theoretical position of a second approach that relies upon a psychiatric or medical model of trauma. The third approach presented here is based primarily on theories of the socio-emotional development of children derived from developmental psychopathology.

In the final analysis, however, making distinctions between theoretical approaches will likely prove less useful than identifying the most effective clinical practices that are contributed by each. Taken together, such practices can form a complementary and inclusive set of core treatment principles, some of which have already been identified by skilled practitioners in the field (Shirk & Eltz, 1998). First, children of serious and chronic family violence have experienced such a profound betrayal of trust that it is often difficult to form a treatment alliance with them. The initial task, then, is to establish a benign sense of safety and order within the treatment context. Second, young children from violent environments feel extremely helpless and dis-empowered. It follows that maximizing a sense of predictability and appropriate control will be important if the children are to relinquish their pervasive hypervigilance.

Third, these children bring a formidable array of psychological defenses that profoundly constricts their affective experience. As a result, their engagement with treatment is likely to be a kind of alienated compliance that lacks authentic emotional response. The conundrum here is that if treatment does evoke affect in these children, and this is particularly likely when uncovering traumatic material, they are vulnerable to becoming flooded and disorganized because they have little practice with assimilating rather than blocking feelings. This suggests that children need to acquire some facility in using language to identify, label, modulate, transform and express a range of emotion. This learned use of emotional language can provide them with the kind of control that helps them to tolerate and learn from affective experience, while mitigating against a flight into defense. Fourth, these rigidly defended children are compromised in their emotional, social and moral development. They need to learn how to solve problems, cope interpersonally and understand and apply age-appropriate standards of right and wrong. Psycho-educational approaches that are designed to teach these essential skills need to do so within a safe and reliable treatment framework that also teaches emotional expression and regulation, and actively addresses the children's underlying defensive scripts. Overall, it seems that the clinical strategies that are embedded in these different theoretical approaches need to be synthesized. This could maximize the possibility that these children will truly assimilate (rather than distort or ignore) the range of information, skills, and experience that they will need to mature into healthy adulthood, and break the intergenerational cycle of violence and victimization.

REFERENCES

Achenbach, T. M., & Edelbrock, C. (1983). *Manual for the child behavior checklist and revised child behavior profile.* Burlington, VT: Queen City Printers.

Briere, J. (1997). Treating adults severely abused as children: The self-trauma model. In D. A. Wolfe, R. J. McMahon & R.deV.Peters (Eds.) *Child abuse: New directions in prevention and treatment across the lifespan,* (pp. 177-204). Thousand Oaks, CA: Sage.

Cappell, C., & Heiner, R. B. (1990). The intergenerational transmission of family aggression. *Journal of Family Violence, 5,* 135-152.

Carlson, B. E. (1990). Adolescent observers of marital violence. *Journal of Family Violence, 5,* 285-299.

Cummings, E. M., & Davies, P. T. (1994). Children and marital conflict: The impact of family dispute and resolution. New York: Guilford.

Cole-Detke, H., & Kobak, R. (1998). The effects of multiple abuse in interpersonal relationships: An attachment perspective. In B. B. Robbie Rossman & M. S. Rosenberg (Eds.), Multiple victimization of children: Conceptual, developmental, research and treatment issues (pp. 189-206). New York: The Haworth Press, Inc.

Davies, P. T., & Cummings, E. M. (1994). Marital conflict and child adjustment: An emotional security hypothesis. Psychological Bulletin, 116, 387-411.

DeVoe, E., & Smith, E. (2003). Don't take my kids: Barriers to service delivery for battered mothers and their young children. Journal of Emotional Abuse, 3(3/4), 277-294.

Dodge, K. A., Bates, J. E., & Pettit, G. S. (1990). Mechanisms in the cycle of violence. Science, 250, 1678-1683.

Ezell, E., McDonald, R., & Jouriles, E. N. (2000). Helping children of battered women: A review of research, sampling of programs, and presentation of project SUPPORT. In J. Vincent & E. Jouriles (Eds.), Domestic violence: Guidelines for research-informed practice. London: Jessica Kingsley Publishers.

Fantuzzo, J. W., & Mohr, W. K. (1999). Prevalence and effects of child exposure to domestic violence. The Future of Children, 9, 21-32.

Forsstrom-Cohen, B., & Rosenbaum, A. (1985). The effects of parental marital violence on young adults: An exploratory investigation. Journal of Marriage & the Family, 47, 467-472.

Graham-Bermann, S. A. (1999). Designing interventions for children exposed to adult domestic violence: Applications of research and theory. In S. A. Graham-Bermann & J. L. Edleson (Eds.), Intimate violence in the lives of children: The future of research, intervention and social policy (pp. 269-306). Washington, DC: American Psychological Association Books.

Harter, S. (1998). The effects of child abuse on the self-system. In B. B. Robbie Rossman & M. S. Rosenberg (Eds.), Multiple victimization of children: Conceptual, developmental, research and treatment issues (pp. 147-170). New York: The Haworth Press, Inc.

Hightower, A. D., Work, W. C., Cowen, E. L., Lotyczewski, B. S., Spinell, A. P., Guare, J. C., & Rohrbeck, C. A. (1986). The teacher-child rating scale: A brief objective measure of elementary children's school problem behaviors and competencies. School Psychology Review, 15, 393-409.

Hughes, H. M. (1982). Brief interventions with children in a battered women's shelter: A model preventive program. Family Relations, 31, 495-502.

Jaffe, P., Wolfe, D. A., & Wilson, S. (1990). Children of battered women. Newbury Park, CA: Sage.

Johnston, J. R. (1999). Final report on group interventions for children and parents at-risk from abuse and violence. Technical Report of the Protecting Children from Conflict Project. P.O. Box 2483, Menlo Park, CA 94026, Ph. (650) 366-3234.

Johnston, J. R., & Campbell, L. E. G. (1988). Impasses of divorce: The dynamics and resolution of family conflict. New York: Free Press.

Johnston, J. R., & Roseby, V. (1997). In the name of the child: A developmental approach to understanding and helping children of conflicted and violent divorce. New York: Free Press.

Kalmuss, D. (1984). The intergenerational transmission of marital aggression. *Journal of Marriage & the Family, 46,* 11-19.

Kaufman, J., & Zigler, E. (1987). Do abused children become abusive parents? *American Journal of Orthopsychiatry, 57,* 186-192.

Lewis, T., Amini, F., & Lannon, R. (2000). *A general theory of love.* New York: Random House.

Lieberman, A. F., & Van Horn, P. (1998). Attachment, trauma, and domestic violence: Implications for child custody. In K. D. Pruett & M. Kline Pruett (Eds.), *Child and Adolescent Psychiatric Clinics of North America: Child Custody, 7,* 423-444. Philadelphia: W.B. Saunders.

MacMillan, K. M., & Harpur, L. L. (2003). An examination of children exposed to marital violence accessing a treatment intervention. *Journal of Emotional Abuse, 3*(3/4), 227-252.

McAlister Groves, B. (1999). Mental health services for children who witness domestic violence. *The Future of Children, 9,* 122-132.

McDonough, H., Radovanovic, H., Stein, L., Sagar, A., & Hood, E. (undated). *For kids' sake: A treatment program for high conflict separated families: Parents' group manual.* Unpublished report by the Family Court Clinic, Clarke Institute of Psychiatry, 250 College St., Toronto, Ontario, M5T 1R8.

Murray, C. C., & Son, L. (1998). The effect of multiple victimization on children's cognition: Variations in response. In B. B. Robbie Rossman & M. S. Rosenberg (Eds.), *Multiple victimization of children: Conceptual, developmental, research and treatment issues* (pp. 131-146). New York: The Haworth Press, Inc.

Murphy, L., Pynoos, R. S., & James, C. B. (1997). The trauma/grief-focused group psychotherapy module of an elementary school-based violence prevention/intervention program. In J. D. Osofsky (Ed.), *Children in a violent society* (pp. 223-255). New York: Guilford Press.

National Council of Juvenile and Family Court Judges, Domestic Violence Project (1998). *Battered mothers and their children: Emerging programs.* Reno, Nevada: Author.

Osofsky, J. D. (1999). The impact of violence on children. *The Future of Children, 9,* 33-49.

Peled, E., & Davis, D. (1995). *Groupwork with children of battered women: A practitioner's manual.* Thousand Oaks, CA: Sage.

Pynoos, R. S., & Eth, S. (1986). Witness to violence: The child interview. *Journal of the American Academy of Child & Adolescent Psychiatry, 25,* 306-319.

Roseby, V., Erdberg, P., Bardenstein, K., & Johnston, J. R. (1995, March). *Developmental psychopathology in children in high-conflict divorcing families: Attachment, personality disorder and the Rorschach.* Paper presented at the Biennial Meeting of the Society for Child Development, Kansas City, MO.

Roseby, V., Gentner, B., & Enomoto, E. (1998). *Group treatment manual for preschool children in high-conflict and separating families.* Unpublished manuscript available from Protecting Children from Conflict, P.O. Box 2483, Menlo Park, CA 94026.

Roseby, V., & Johnston, J. R. (1998). Children of Armageddon: Common developmental threats in high-conflict divorcing families. In K. D. Pruett & M. Kline Pruett

(Eds.), *Child and Adolescent Psychiatric Clinics of North America: Child Custody, 7*, (pp. 295-310). Philadelphia: W.B. Saunders.

Roseby, V., & Johnston, J. R. (1997). *High-conflict, violent & separating families: A group treatment manual for school-age children.* New York: Free Press.

Rosenberg, M. S., & Rossman, B. B. (1990). The child witness to marital violence. In R. T. Ammerman & M. Hersen (Eds.), *Treatment of family violence: A sourcebook* (pp. 183-210). New York: John Wiley.

Rutter, M. (1987). Psychological resilience and protective mechanisms. *American Journal of Orthopsychiatry, 57*, 316-331.

Shaffer, M., & Bala, N. (2003). Wife abuse, child custody, and access in Canada. *Journal of Emotional Abuse, 3*(3/4), 253-275.

Shirk, S. R., & Eltz, M. (1998). Multiple victimization and the process and outcome of child psychotherapy. In B. B. Robbie Rossman & M. S. Rosenberg (Eds.), *Multiple victimization of children: Conceptual, developmental, research and treatment issues* (pp. 233-253). New York: The Haworth Press, Inc.

Silvern, L., Karyl, J., & Landis, T. Y. (1995). Individual psychotherapy for the traumatized children of abused women. In E. Peled, P. G. Jaffe & J. L. Edleson (Eds.), *Ending the cycle of violence: Community responses to children of battered women* (pp. 43-76). Thousand Oaks, CA: Sage.

Straus, M., Gelles, R., & Steinmetz, S. (1980). *Behind closed doors: Violence in the American family.* Garden City, NY: Anchor/Doubleday.

Terr, L. (1991). Childhood traumas: An outline and overview. *American Journal of Psychiatry, 148*, 10-20.

Trickett, P. K. (1998). Multiple maltreatment and the development of self and emotion regulation. In B. B. Robbie Rossman & M. S. Rosenberg (Eds.), *Multiple victimization of children: Conceptual, developmental, research and treatment issues* (pp. 171-188). New York: The Haworth Press, Inc.

van der Kolk, B. A., van der Hart, O., & Marmar, C. R. (1996). Dissociation and information processing in posttraumatic stress disorder. In B. A. van der Kolk, A. C. McFarlane & L. Weisaeth (Eds.), *Traumatic stress: The effects of overwhelming experience on mind, body and society* (pp. 303-327). New York: Guilford Press.

Widom, C. S. (1989). Does violence beget violence? A critical examination of the literature. *Psychological Bulletin, 106*, 3-28.

Wolfe, D. A. (1999). *Child abuse.* Vol 10. Second Edition, Developmental Clinical Psychology and Psychiatry. Thousand Oaks, CA: Sage.

Wolfe, D. A., & Jaffe, P. G. (1999). Emerging strategies in the prevention of domestic violence. *The Future of Children, 9*, 133-144.

Wolfe, D. A., Wekerle, C., & Scott, K. (1997). *Alternatives to violence: Empowering youth to develop healthy relationships.* Thousand Oaks, CA: Sage.

Wolfe, D. A., Wekerle, C., Gough, R., Reitzel-Jaffe, D., Grasley, C., Pittman, A., Lefebvre, L., & Stumpf, J. (1996). *The youth relationship manual: A group approach with adolescents for the prevention of woman abuse and the promotion of healthy relationships.* Thousand Oaks, CA: Sage.

Zeanah, C. H., & Zeanah, P. D. (1989). Intergenerational transmission of maltreatment: Insights from attachment theory and research. *Psychiatry, 52*, 177-196.

An Examination of Children
Exposed to Marital Violence
Accessing a Treatment Intervention

Karen M. MacMillan
Lisa L. Harpur

SUMMARY. This study examines the well-being of families accessing treatment due to children's exposure to marital violence. Participants were 47 children, aged 6-12 years, enrolled in a 10-week group treatment intervention and one of their parents who were attending a corresponding parenting group. Measures were administered prior to the commencement of the programs and again in the ninth week of the interventions. Children completed self-report measures of anxiety, depression, posttraumatic stress and associated symptoms, and knowledge of abuse and safety planning. Parents reported on child competence and behavior problems, as well as their own experience of stress. Results indicated elevated rates of clinical scores on several measures compared with normative data. Parental stress was significantly correlated with reported child behavior problems, anxiety, depression, and posttraumatic stress

Address correspondence to: Karen M. MacMillan, 2337-2 Avenue N.W. Calgary, Alberta Canada T2N 0H3 (E-mail: kmmacmil@ucalgary.ca).

The authors would like to thank the anonymous reviewers of the *JEA* Editorial Board for their helpful comments. Special acknowledgments to the staff and clients at the YWCA Family Violence Prevention Centre and Sheriff King Home in Calgary.

[Haworth co-indexing entry note]: "An Examination of Children Exposed to Marital Violence Accessing a Treatment Intervention." MacMillan, Karen M., and Lisa L. Harpur. Co-published simultaneously in *Journal of Emotional Abuse* (The Haworth Maltreatment & Trauma Press, an imprint of The Haworth Press, Inc.) Vol. 3, No. 3/4, 2003, pp. 227-252; and: *The Effects of Intimate Partner Violence on Children* (ed: Robert A. Geffner, Robyn Spurling Igelman, and Jennifer Zellner) The Haworth Maltreatment & Trauma Press, an imprint of The Haworth Press, Inc., 2003, pp. 227-252. Single or multiple copies of this article are available for a fee from The Haworth Document Delivery Service [1-800-HAWORTH, 9:00 a.m. - 5:00 p.m. (EST). E-mail address: docdelivery@haworthpress.com].

10.1300J135v03n03_04

symptoms. Scores at the second assessment indicated significant changes in ratings of child behavior problems, parental stress, and child knowledge. Mediating factors of gender and child physical abuse were examined. *[Article copies available for a fee from The Haworth Document Delivery Service: 1-800-HAWORTH. E-mail address: <docdelivery@haworthpress.com> Website: <http://www.HaworthPress.com> © 2003 by The Haworth Press, Inc. All rights reserved.]*

KEYWORDS. Children, emotional and behavioral concerns, family violence, group treatment, marital violence, parent stress, Posttraumatic Stress Disorder, program evaluation

The impact of children's exposure to marital violence has been subject to repeated investigation over the past two decades, particularly with samples of children residing with their mothers in women's shelters (Mohr, Lutz, Fantuzzo, & Perry, 2000). Barnett, Miller-Perrin, and Perrin (1997) note that there is "extreme variability in outcomes" in this population, including a proportion of children who appear to have no adverse effects from exposure to marital violence (p. 146). However, children who live in maritally violent homes are clearly at risk for numerous problems affecting a variety of domains of functioning including emotional, behavioral, social, cognitive, and physical concerns (Holden, 1998; Kolbo, Blakely, & Engleman, 1996; Pelcovitz & Kaplan, 1994). In fact, previous researchers have conceptualized the deleterious impact of interparental violence on children as a form of emotional or psychological abuse (Cummings, 1998; Hughes & Fantuzzo, 1994; Margolin, 1998). Recent research efforts to gain understanding of the impact of marital violence have expanded and begun to identify posttraumatic stress symptoms in this population of children (Graham-Bermann & Levendosky, 1998; Kilpatrick & Williams, 1998; Lehmann, 1997).

Developmental psychopathology "emphasizes dynamic processes of interaction between multiple intra- and extra-organismic factors" (Cummings, 1998, p. 67). This perspective highlights the process of person-environment interactions over time, such as the unique contextual factors of a child's experience in a maritally violent home and the unique meanings and interpretations that the child ascribes to this experience. Developmental psychopathology points to the need to examine multiple domains of functioning (e.g., emotional, cognitive, behavioral) as well as consider the potential emergence of effects over time. Therefore, in applying this approach to understanding children's exposure to marital violence multiple pathways of influence need to be considered. Hughes and Fantuzzo (1994) conceptualized extant theories of the effects of marital violence on children as reflecting either direct or indirect mechanisms. Direct sources of influence include the modeling of aggression within the home and the stress and trauma associated with living in an unpredictable and violent environment. Indirect mechanisms include parental disciplinary practices and changes in the parent-child relationship.

The importance of investigating the impact of marital violence on children is highlighted when prevalence rates of marital violence are taken into account. The 1999 General Social Survey (GSS) on Victimization in Canada estimated that 7% of people who were married or living in a common-law relationship had experienced some type of violence by a partner during the previous five years (Statistics Canada, 2000). Thirty-seven percent of spousal violence victims in the GSS reported that children had heard or seen violence in the home. That figure translates into "approximately half a million children [that] have heard or witnessed a parent being assaulted during the 5-year period" (Statistics Canada, 2000, p. 5).

Awareness of the prevalence of children's exposure to interspousal violence and the potentially detrimental effects of this experience has led to the development and implementation of interventions for children at women's shelters. A few studies have documented intervention efforts and evaluations of treatment programs with children exposed to marital violence. For example, Jaffe, Wilson, and Wolfe (1988) investigated outcomes for children who had witnessed marital violence and were referred to a 10-week group counselling program. Interviews conducted after the completion of the group indicated that the 88% of mothers in this study believed that their child enjoyed the group and reported that they perceived an improvement in their child's behavioral adjustment. However, despite positive trends in the problem and social competence scales, there were no significant changes on the Child Behavior Checklist between children's pre- and post-intervention scores. Jaffe et al. did detect a significant shift in knowledge variables for the children between the two time periods. After the group intervention, children reported more safety skill strategies as well as more positive perceptions of their mothers and fathers.

Wagar and Rodway (1995) conducted one of the few treatment evaluations with this population of children to utilize a control group. These researchers assessed outcomes for a treatment program (developed by Jaffe, Wilson, & Wolfe, 1986) that involved direct instruction regarding attitudes and responses to anger, knowledge and support around the use of safety skills, and attributions for the responsibility for violence. The children in the treatment group were shown to have significantly improved post-test scores on attitudes and responses to anger, as well as their sense of responsibility for parents and the violence. The variable that the treatment did not appear to have a significant impact on was children's knowledge of safety and support.

More recently, Pepler, Catallo, and Moore (2000) documented an evaluation of a 10-week peer group counselling program for children. Significant differences were found in children's ratings of their anxiety and depression and parental ratings of their childrens' behavioral concerns. Pepler et al. also investigated children's attitudes towards violence and found that children were significantly less likely to condone hitting at the conclusion of the program; however, no significant shifts were found in children's responsibility for violence, their responses to anger, and their reactions to provocation. Within this study a concurrent support group was available for mothers, and it was expected that children of mothers who participated in this program would show more positive adjustment than the children whose mothers did not participate in the support group. However, there was no relation between mothers' participation in counselling and children's improvement. The authors noted that there were some limitations in their study that may have led to this finding.

Children in the present sample accessed a 10-week group treatment intervention while their parents were provided with a coinciding parenting program. The purpose of this study was to describe the well-being and functioning of this sample of children and parents who are living in the community and seeking out treatment. Measures of child affective (depression, anxiety, and posttraumatic stress and associated symptoms), behavioral, and knowledge factors, as well as parental stress are examined in relation to normative data for those measures. Shifts on these parent and child measures are examined over the ten-week treatment period to identify any significant differences between the pre- and post-treatment assessment periods.

It was hypothesized that the child and the parent reports in this sample would reveal elevated rates of clinical scores relative to the normative data for the measurement instruments. Children's levels of depression, anxiety, and posttraumatic stress and associated symptoms were expected to positively correlate with parents' ratings of their children's internalizing behavior concerns. Parents' rating of their own stress was expected to be positively correlated with anxiety, depression, posttraumatic stress symptoms, and behavior problems in children. Also, parental stress was expected to be negatively correlated to children's competence scores. Children with clinical levels of concern on a measure of posttraumatic stress and associated symptoms were expected to be more likely to have elevated scores in measures of their anxiety, depression, and behavior compared to the other children in the sample. Further, it was expected that boys in this sample would have significantly higher scores of behavior problems and significantly lower scores of competence than girls in this sample. In addition, children in this sample who were also identified as being victims of child physical abuse were expected to have lower levels of adjustment compared to the children in the sample without this experience. Finally, significant improvement was expected on parental stress and measures of childrens' depression, anxiety, posttraumatic stress and associated symptoms, behavior, and competence at the post-treatment assessment, while ratings of children's knowledge about abuse were expected to significantly increase at this time.

METHOD

Participants

The present investigation examined 47 children living in the community and accessing treatment through the YWCA Family Violence Prevention Centre and Sheriff King Home in Calgary. This agency provides services, shelter, and counseling to women, men, and children who have witnessed, experienced, and/or perpetrated abusive behavior in intimate relationships. All children were registered in a ten-week group treatment intervention. At least one parent of each child was registered in a corresponding parenting group. Three inclusion criteria were utilized: (a) the child was between the ages of 6 and 12 years at the commencement of the study, (b) this was the child's first time participating in the group program, and (c) parents' written consent and children's verbal consent were given. Consents were obtained for all children registered in the treatment program for the Fall 2000 who met the first two criteria. The children, 24 males and 23 females, had a mean age of 9.02 (*SD* = 1.91) and were from 35 different families.

Within this sample, 15% of the children (*n* = 7) were reported to be mandated by Child and Family Services to the treatment program; the remainder of the families was self-referred, having heard about the programs through community advertising. The child's mother was generally the reporting parent who attended the corresponding parenting group; however, in a few cases the child's father (for 4 children) or a foster parent (for 2 children) fulfilled these roles. Parents in the study ranged in age from 22 to 52 years old, with a mean age of 37. While some parents indicated that they were either married or in a common-law relationship, the parents of the majority of the children (61%) described themselves as either single, divorced, or separated with or without contact with the former partner. Only the parents of five children (10%) reported that they had not completed high school, and the parents of the majority of children (78%) indicated that they were employed. Reported family incomes ranged between $7,200 and $60,000 per year, with a mean of $19,566 (*SD* = $13,937).

Parent reports indicated that of the total sample, 40 children (85%) had been exposed to spousal physical abuse (26 by fathers, 1 by mother, and 13 by both parents). The questionnaires for seven children (15%) in the sample did not provide complete information about the type of abuse witnessed by the child. Additionally, parents reported that 76% of the children in this sample were exposed to marital emotional abuse. Eleven (23%) of the children were reported by their parents to have been physically abused (5 by fathers, 3 by mothers, 2 by both parents, and 1 by another individual). Five (10%) of the children were reported to have experienced sexual abuse (2 by fathers and 3 by other individuals). Finally, 27 children were reported to have been emotionally abused (17 by fathers, 1 by mothers, 8 by both parents, and 1 by another individual).

Interventions

The group programs were developed by staff at the YWCA Family Violence Prevention Centre and Sheriff King Home in Calgary. The children's program is based on the work of Terr (1995), which is focused on addressing posttraumatic stress issues in children by creating a safe and trusting therapeutic environment so that children can express their thoughts and feelings, as well as share their experiences. There is also a psychoeducational aspect to the program, including information about appropriate identification and expression of feelings, safety planning, problem solving, and education in regards to definitions of emotional, sexual, and physical abuse. As well, children are taught relaxation exercises and encouraged to use them as needed. Each of the ten sessions are based on a particular theme and have associated activities; however, facilitators may vary the timing of each topic according to the needs of the group and its individual members.

At least one parent of each child in the group intervention program is required to attend a corresponding parenting group. The parenting program focuses on two main goals. First, there is an emphasis on relationship building between the parent and child. For example, there is an effort to help parents better understand their child's world through the use of empathy. The second goal is to promote positive discipline practices. For example, facilitators attempt to raise the awareness of the long-range consequences of different discipline methods for children. These goals are addressed through the use of experiential activities, videos, and supportive group discussions.

The parent and child programs coincide over a ten-week period, with each session lasting approximately one and one-half hours. The children were organized according to age, with 6-8 children in each group, and a male and a female facilitator were assigned to each group. In this sample sixty-three percent of the children ($n = 30$) and their parents attended ≥ 7 of the 10 sessions. Concerns regarding attrition rates are not unusual in programming for this population of children (Peled & Edleson, 1998; Pepler et al., 2000).

Measures

Parent-Report Measures. Parents completed intake and child history forms asking for qualitative information (e.g., fill in the blanks) at Time 1 only. They completed two other measures at both Time 1 and 2. Parents completed the Child Behavior Checklist (CBCL; Achenbach, 1991), a standardized questionnaire utilized to rate the competence and behavioral concerns of children aged 4 to 18 years. The first twenty questions on the CBCL inquire about a child's competence in their activities, social interactions, and school performance. The second portion of this measure investigates concerns about the child through 118 specific problem questions and 2 open-ended problem questions. This instrument provides subscale behavior problem scores for Internalizing behaviors (i.e., anxiety and depression) and Externalizing behaviors (i.e., aggression). The CBCL is a widely utilized assessment tool and has been used in numerous investigations with this population of children (Hughes, Parkinson, & Vargo, 1989; Levendosky & Graham-Bermann, 1998; Sternberg et al., 1993).

Achenbach (1991) notes that assessments on the CBCL should be at least two months apart to provide sufficient opportunity for behavioral change to develop and be identified. This amount of time between administrations also minimizes the possibility of "practice effects," which is the tendency for scores on rating scales to decline over brief test-retest intervals (Achenbach, 1991). Despite some "practice effects," the test-retest reliability of the CBCL has been demonstrated to be .87 for the competence scales and .89 for the problem scales over a one-week interval. As well, mean scores did not shift beyond chance expectations in studies with intervals of one or two years (Achenbach, 1991). The CBCL Manual also provides strong evidence of construct, content, and criterion-related validity, as well as good internal consistency (Achenbach, 1991). T-scores were calculated for parents' ratings of children's total competence, total behavior problems, Internalizing behaviors, and Externalizing behaviors. The CBCL Manual (Achenbach, 1991) guidelines were utilized to determine clinical cut-off criteria at, or within, the tenth percentile of normative data. Therefore, a T-score of $\geq$ 63 indicated an Internalizing, Externalizing, or total behavior problem score at the clinical level. Similarly, for the total competence score a T-score of $\leq$ 37 was deemed in the clinical range.

The Parenting Stress Index (PSI; Abidin, 1995) assesses parents' experience of stress by their rating of 120 items on a 5-point Likert scale. The instrument provides a Life Stress score rating situational factors affecting the parent, such as the death of a relative or the loss of a job. The PSI also provides a total stress score comprised of a Child Domain score (parent's perceptions of their child's characteristics) and a Parent Domain score (parent characteristics and family context variables). Previous studies have utilized this measure for parents in situations of family violence (Holden & Ritchie, 1991; Levendosky & Graham-Bermann, 1998).

Abidin (1995) identified correlation coefficients for test-retest reliability for the PSI Total Stress score to range between .65 and .96 over intervals of 3 weeks to 1 year. In regards to internal consistency, reliability coefficients for the two domains and the Total Stress score were .90 or greater for the normative sample (Abidin, 1995). The PSI Professional Manual also reviews hundreds of studies that have utilized the PSI, including numerous research efforts examining family violence contexts. Abidin (1995) stated that these studies "provide evidence for the construct and predictive validity of the PSI" (p. 36). According to the PSI Manual (Abidin, 1995), the 85th percentile serves as the cutoff point to delineate clinical scores for the total stress ($\geq$ 258), Parent Domain ($\geq$ 148), Child Domain ($\geq$ 116), and Life Stress ($\geq$ 14) scores.

Child Self-Report Measures. Children completed four separate self-report measures at both assessment times. The Children's Depression Inventory (CDI; Kovacs, 1992) is a 27-item self-report questionnaire assessing symptoms of depression in children aged 7 to 17 years; however, Kovacs (1992) noted that this instrument should be comprehensible to children 6 years old. Each of the items is keyed 0, 1, or 2, providing a total score between 0 and 54. This measure has been utilized in numerous investigations of this population of children (Hughes, 1988; Hughes et al., 1989; Lehmann, 1997; Pepler et al., 2000; Sternberg et al., 1993).

Kovacs (1992) reviewed the expansive literature on the CDI and concludes that it is a reliable and reasonably valid measure of depression for children. "Overall, the weight of the evidence gained from this voluminous literature is that the inventory assesses important constructs which have strong explanatory and predictive utility in the characterization of depressive symptoms in children and adolescents" (Kovacs, 1992, p. 38). The CDI Manual indicates good internal consistency, with reliability coefficients from .71 to .89. In regards to test-retest reliability, the CDI has been demonstrated to have an acceptable level of stability, with a range of .38 to .87 on studies with normal and clinical populations over a period of 1 week to 1 year (Kovacs, 1992). However, Kovacs (1992) also warned that lower CDI scores at a second testing should not be overly interpreted, as several studies have detected a significant drop in CDI scores at a second testing. In correspondence with the CDI Manual (Kovacs, 1992), total CDI T-scores $\geq$ 66 are considered clinically significant in the present study.

The Revised Children's Manifest Anxiety Scale (RCMAS; Reynolds & Richmond, 1985) is a 37-item self-report form that assesses the nature and level of anxiety in children aged 6 to 19 years. Children indicate "yes" or "no" to each of the items; this yields a total anxiety raw score between 0 and 28. The RCMAS has been previously utilized in studies with this population of children (Hughes, 1988; Hughes et al., 1989; Pepler et al., 2000). Reynolds and Richmond (1985) presented numerous studies that have utilized the RCMAS with children in clinical and non-clinical samples. "Reliability and validity of the RCMAS as a measure of chronic anxiety in children seems well established by the existing literature" (Reynolds & Richmond, 1985, p. 41). The RCMAS manual reviews numerous studies and found internal consistency coefficients of .78 to .85 for the total anxiety score. Reynolds and Richmond (1985) illustrated the test-retest stability of the RCMAS with data from two studies of elementary school children. These studies garnered coefficients of .68 over a 9-month interval and .98 over a period of 3 weeks. For purposes of the present study, total RCMAS T-scores $\geq$ 67 are deemed to be at the clinical level as this represents approximately the 95th percentile of normative data presented in the manual (Reynolds & Richmond, 1985).

The Angie/Andy Cartoon Trauma Scales (ACTS; Praver, Pelcovitz, & DiGiuseppe, 1998) are a relatively new instrument designed to measure trauma-related sequelae (posttraumatic stress and associated symptoms) of prolonged, repeated abuse in children aged 6 to 12. This measure consists of 44 statements based on cartoon pictures of a boy or a girl; children are asked how often they feel, think, or act like Angie or Andy. Children may either answer verbally or point to a visual of a 4-point Likert scale in the form of a thermometer. This measure is comprised of 44 items measuring symptoms from seven scales: dysregulation, dissociation, self-perception, system of meaning, avoidance of stimuli, re-experiencing, and somatization. Although research efforts are currently underway, to-date no studies have been published on this version of the ACTS (Multi-Health Services, personal communication, 2001). A study utilizing a previous version of this instrument found a high correlation between the total ACTS score and the degree and frequency of children's exposure to family violence (Praver, DiGiuseppe, Pelcovitz, Mandel, & Gaines, 2000). The ACTS provides a total score between 44 and 176. In correspondence with the interpretive information for the ACTS (provided for research and exploratory purposes) scores $\geq$ 76 are considered to be at the clinical level for the purposes of this investigation.

The Pre-Post Child/Teen Questionnaire/Interview is a condensed version of the knowledge and attitude form utilized by Marshall, Miller, Miller-Hewitt, Sudermann, and Watson (1995) to investigate children's understanding of abuse before and after a group treatment program. The version of this instrument utilized in the present study was adapted by staff at the YWCA Family Violence Prevention Centre and Sheriff King Home in Calgary and consists of two parts. The first section investigates children's knowledge about what actions constitute "abuse" and then explores children's attributions for the responsibility of abuse in the home. The second part of the form identifies children's repertoire of safety planning skills. Therefore, this measure addresses the three main areas of "subtle symptoms" of exposure to marital violence identified by Jaffe, Wolfe, and Wilson (1990, p. 51) that may affect the attitudes and emotional expression of children exposed to marital violence. This version of the Pre-Post Child/Teen Questionnaire/Interview provides a total score of 17, with higher scores denoting greater levels of appropriate knowledge and attitudes. No validity or reliability information has been collected on this measure.

Procedure

Parent and child measures were administered the week prior to the commencement of the group treatment program (Time 1) and in the ninth week of the intervention (Time 2). At each time the children's measures were administered in a one-on-one format with a group facilitator in approximately 40 minutes. Parents completed the intake and child history forms at Time 1 only. The CBCL and PSI were filled out at both times by most parents in a group format with a facilitator; however, some parents were provided with these forms to take with them and return to the agency. Erratic attendance and attrition over the course of the treatment programs affected the amount of data available for analysis. In addition, the lack of returned parent-report forms hampered data collection at both assessment periods.

RESULTS

Description of Sample at Time 1

Figures 1 and 2 show a visual comparison of the sample versus the normative data of the percentage of CBCL and PSI scores that fall in the clinical range. Inspection of these percentages revealed higher rates of clinical scores on the CBCL and the PSI within the present study's sample for both parent-ratings of their children's behavior (Figure 1) and parent-ratings of their own stress (Figure 2) at Time 1. Table 1 shows the means and standard deviations of scores on all instruments completed at Time 1. On the ACTS, forty percent ($n = 19$) of the children in the present sample rated themselves in the clinical range in regards to posttraumatic stress and associated symptoms. Overall, the mean scores were in the clinical range for Internalizing behavior and total behavior problems (CBCL) and posttraumatic stress and associated symptoms (ACTS). Parents in this sample had a mean score in the clinical range for Child Domain stress and Life Stress.

FIGURE 1. Percentage of CBCL Scores at Time 1 Falling in the Clinical Range: Sample (*n* = 39) versus Normative Data

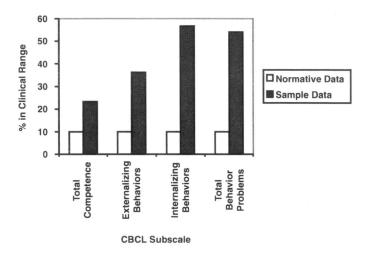

FIGURE 2. Percentage of PSI Scores at Time 1 Falling in the Clinical Range: Sample (*n* = 32) versus Normative Data

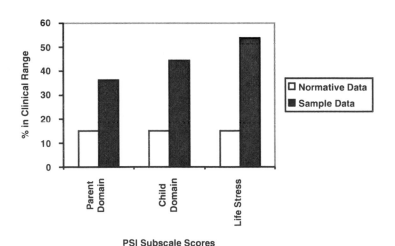

TABLE 1. Mean Scores for Time 1

Score	N	M	SD
Parent Report Measures			
CBCL			
Total Competence T-Score	39	42.5	7.80
Internalizing T-Score	39	66.5*	8.54
Externalizing T-Score	39	60.3	12.12
Total Problem T-Score	39	64.7*	9.17
PSI			
Child Domain Score	42	125.8*	23.87
Parent Domain Score	42	137.0	28.51
Life Stress Score	42	19.4*	11.60
Child Self-Report Measures			
CDI T-score	46	47.3	12.71
RCMAS T-score	46	46.0	12.17
ACTS score	47	76.9*	28.54
Knowledge score	46	10.2	2.54

* The mean score is within the pre-determined clinical range.

A one-way MANOVA revealed that the only significant gender differences evident in this sample were in parent ratings of children's behavior and competence. Boys in this sample were found to have significantly higher behavior problem scores (total and Internalizing) and significantly lower competence scores than girls, in regards to normative data for their gender (see Table 2). The mean scores for boys on all four reported dimensions of the CBCL were in the clinical range. Although the boys' scores were significantly higher than girls' for Internalizing behavior problems, it is important to note that the mean of the girls' Internalizing scores was also in the clinical range. No significant differences were found on the child or parent measures in regards to children who were reported to be physically abused ($n = 11$), and those who were not ($n = 36$).

A bivariate correlation was conducted between parental stress and children's functioning on a variety of measures (see Table 3). Parent stress scores were significantly positively correlated with parent-

TABLE 2. Scores at Time 1 According to Gender

Scores	Boys			Girls			F	df
	N	M	SD	N	M	SD		
Parent Report Measures								
CBCL								
Total Competence T-Score	20	39.7	7.3	19	45.4	7.4	5.92*	1, 37
Externalizing T-Score	20	63.2	10.6	19	57.4	13.2	2.29	1, 37
Internalizing T-Score	20	69.1	8.4	19	63.7	8.0	4.17*	1, 37
Total Problem T-Score	20	68.3	7.9	19	61.0	9.1	7.18*	1, 37
PSI								
Child Domain Score	21	129.9	22.6	21	121.7	25.0	1.24	1, 40
Parent Domain Score	21	139.4	24.1	21	134.6	32.7	.29	1, 40
Life Stress Score	21	20.8	11.2	21	18.0	12.1	.61	1, 40
Child Self-Report Measures								
CDI T-Score	24	47.5	11.8	22	47.1	13.9	.01	1, 44
RCMAS T-Score	24	45.6	11.8	22	46.5	12.8	.06	1, 44
ACTS Score	24	74.9	23.7	22	77.4	33.2	.09	1, 44
Knowledge Score	24	9.9	2.6	22	10.5	2.6	.06	1, 44

* significant difference at $p < .05$

reports of children's functioning on measures of Internalizing behavior and Externalizing behavior, as well as child self-reports of depression, anxiety, and posttraumatic stress and associated symptoms.

Further bivariate correlations revealed that children's ratings of their posttraumatic stress and associated symptoms were highly correlated (≤ 0.01) with their self-reports of their depression and anxiety. However, parent ratings of children's Internalizing behaviors were not significantly correlated with children's self-reports of anxiety, depression, and posttraumatic stress and associated symptoms.

A one-way MANOVA found scores on the ACTS discriminated between the children in terms of their functioning on other measures (see Table 4). Compared to their peers, children with clinical scores on the ACTS had significantly higher scores of depression, anxiety, total problem behaviors, and Externalizing behavior problems. As well, these children were found to have significantly lower levels of parent-rated

TABLE 3. Correlations Between Parent Stress and Child Measures at Time 1

Scores	Pearson Correlation Coefficient
	Total PSI Score
CBCL	
Total Competence T-Score	−.148
Externalizing Problems T-Score	.506**
Internalizing Problems T-Score	.485**
CDI T-Score	.426**
RCMAS T-Score	.474**
ACTS Score	.372*

* significant correlation at the 0.05 level
** significant correlation at the 0.01 level

TABLE 4. Scores at Time 1 According to the Child's Status on the ACTS

Scores	ACTS Non-Clinical Levels			ACTS Clinical Levels			F	df
	N	M	SD	N	M	SD		
Parent Report Measures								
CBCL								
Total Competence T-Score	24	44.5	7.5	15	39.3	7.4	4.54*	1, 37
Externalizing T-Score	24	55.0	10.3	15	68.9	9.8	17.65***	1, 37
Internalizing T-Score	24	65.6	7.3	15	67.9	10.4	0.63	1, 37
Total Problem T-Score	24	61.8	8.6	15	69.3	8.2	7.28**	1, 37
PSI								
Child Domain Score	26	121.5	22.4	16	132.8	25.2	0.39	1, 40
Parent Domain Score	26	134.8	27.5	16	140.5	30.7	2.95	1, 40
Life Stress Score	26	21.9	11.5	16	15.4	10.9	3.18	1, 40
Child Self-Report Measures								
CDI T-Score	28	41.4	6.0	18	56.5	15.0	24.23***	1, 44
RCMAS T-Score	28	40.3	9.1	18	54.9	11.0	22.89***	1, 44
Knowledge Score	28	10.8	2.7	18	9.3	2.1	3.59	1, 44

* significant difference at $p < .05$
** significant difference at $p < .01$
*** significant difference at $p < .001$

competence in relation to children with ACTS scores in the normal range.

Changes Between Time 1 and Time 2

Participant Attrition. Eighteen of the original 47 children were assessed at Time 2. A one-factor ANOVA was conducted to determine if there were differences between the 18 children who remained in the study and those who did not. These two groups of children were compared in terms of the types of abuse they were reported to have endured and in terms of their scores on each of the measures at Time 1. These groups were found to significantly differ on whether the children had been reported to be emotionally abused ($F (1, 44) = 16.86, p < .001$) and in terms of their competence ratings on the CBCL at Time 1 ($F (1, 37) = 12.49, p = .001$).

Analyses on 18 Remaining Participants. A paired t-test, with a Bonferroni adjustment, demonstrated significant differences on five scores between the two assessment periods for the 18 children with complete data sets (parent and child measures) at both times (see Table 5). Children's behavior problems (Externalizing, Internalizing, and total score) were rated by their parents as significantly lowered at Time 2, while children's scores on the knowledge forms were significantly increased. At Time 2, parent ratings of their own stress in the Child Domain were also found to be significantly lowered from the first assessment.

There was also a decrease in the percentages of scores in the clinical range for some measures. Table 6 displays the frequency of clinical scores on parent and child measures for the 18 children at both assessment times, and it becomes clear that many scores dropped out of the clinical range by the second assessment period. These shifts are particularly evident in regards to total and Externalizing behavior problems, as well as parental stress in the Child Domain.

DISCUSSION

This investigation utilized parent and child reports to attain a description of a sample of community children exposed to marital violence accessing treatment services with their parents. This sample was initially found to have elevated rates of clinical scores similar to previous studies of shelter populations on the CBCL (e.g., Holden & Ritchie, 1991;

TABLE 5. Paired T-Test with Scores at Time 1 and 2 (n = 18)

Scores	Time 1 M	SD	Time 2 M	SD	t	df
Parent Report Measures						
CBCL						
Total Competence T-Score	46.7	7.4	46.4	6.9	.22	17
Externalizing T-Score	58.1	9.0	53.3	5.1	3.54*	17
Internalizing T-Score	64.1	8.5	58.2	10.0	4.10**	17
Total Problem T-Score	62.0	8.9	55.7	8.5	5.84**	17
PSI						
Child Domain Score	122.8	20.0	107.8	22.0	4.30**	17
Parent Domain Score	132.4	28.3	128.9	27.9	1.24	17
Life Stress Score	15.2	9.6	14.1	7.9	.51	17
Child Self-Report Measures						
CDI T-Score	46.3	11.8	45.9	10.5	.31	17
RCMAS T-Score	46.8	11.1	44.3	14.9	.96	17
ACTS Score	71.6	24.0	67.2	20.4	1.46	17
Knowledge Score	9.8	2.7	12.9	1.4	−5.32**	17

* significant difference at $p < .05$
** significant difference at $p < .01$

Hughes et al., 1989; O'Keefe, 1994) and the PSI (e.g., Holden & Ritchie, 1991; Levendosky & Graham-Bermann, 1998). As well, similar to previous studies of children exposed to marital violence (Lehmann, 1997; Graham-Bermann & Levendosky, 1998; O'Keefe, 1994), there was a notable prevalence of posttraumatic stress symptomology within this sample. However, in this sample rates of the anxiety and depression scores in the clinical range were not markedly above rates of clinical scores for the normative data provided for the instruments.

Of the 39 children in this sample with complete data for the CDI, RCMAS, CBCL, and ACTS at Time 1, 6 children (15%) did not have *any* scores in the clinical range. According to a developmental psychopathology perspective there is a need to study personal and environmental sources of resilience in the face of adverse experiences (Cummings, 1998; see also Kerig, 2003). Further investigation into those children growing up in maritally violent environments who do *not* develop concerns would be of particular interest. Does this finding mean that their

TABLE 6. Frequency of Clinical Scores at Time 1 and 2 (n = 18)

T-Scores	Time 1		Time 2	
	N in Clinical Range	% in Clinical Range	N in Clinical Range	% in Clinical Range
Parent Report Measures				
CBCL				
Total Competence Score	3	16.7	1	5.6
Externalizing Problems	5	27.8	0	0.0
Internalizing Problems	8	44.4	6	33.3
Total Problem Score	9	50.0	4	22.2
PSI				
Parent Domain	7	38.9	5	27.8
Child Domain	12	66.7	5	27.8
Life Stress	9	50.0	9	50.0
Child Self-Report Measures				
CDI	1	5.6	1	5.6
RCMAS	1	5.6	2	11.1
ACTS	6	33.3	6	33.3

experience of adversity may be reflected in variables not examined in this study? Will these children have concerns at later stages of development? Did these children have less adverse exposure to abuse? Do these children have unique protective factors within themselves or their environment? Studying adaptive outcomes under adverse circumstances may also provide vital information for future treatment efforts.

Consistent with gender trends in previous studies (Margolin, 1998) a greater vulnerability was evident with males compared to females within this sample, as males had significantly elevated scores on the total competence, Internalizing, and total problem scales of the CBCL. In contrast to previous investigations (Hughes et al., 1989; Sternberg et al., 1993), no significant differences were found between children within this sample who were identified as physically abused and those who were not. However, it is possible that the small number of children in the physically abused group (*n* = 11) may have contributed to the lack of significant findings.

A correspondence between parental ratings of their own and their children's well-being is well established in the literature (Holden &

Ritchie, 1991; Levendosky & Graham-Bermann, 1998). In the present study, a strong association was found between parental stress and parent reports of children's functioning as well as parental stress and child self-reports of their own symptoms. This result may be viewed as further credibility to theories that cite parental stress as a factor in children's poorer functioning in situations of domestic violence, or it may reflect the fact that children with problems create increased stress for their parents. Although the pattern of effect is unclear, the influence between the child and parent systems is an important consideration for treatment planning.

The lack of correspondence between parent ratings of their child's Internalizing behaviors and children's ratings of their own internalizing symptoms (anxiety, depression, and posttraumatic stress and associated symptoms) supports the concerns raised by previous investigators (Spaccarelli, Sandler, & Roosa, 1994; Sternberg, Lamb, & Dawud-Noursi, 1998; Sternberg et al., 1993). The inconsistency of these reports highlights the need for multiple sources of information for assessing child well being. In contrast to these other investigations, in the present study parents appear to have identified more internalizing problems in their children than the children reported for themselves. A possible explanation for this finding is that trauma symptoms associated with ongoing, Type II trauma, such as repression, dissociation, and self-anesthesis (Terr, 1991) contribute to children under-reporting their own symptoms. On the other hand, it is also possible that parents generalize their own stress and emotional turmoil and/or become more sensitive to their children's symptoms (Margolin, 1998).

A self-report measure specific to assessing ongoing interpersonal trauma symptoms in young children (the ACTS) indicated high levels of posttraumatic stress and associated symptoms in this sample. The ACTS also discriminated between the children, as significant differences in children's scores (depression, anxiety, competence, and behavior) were found between children with clinical and non-clinical scores on this instrument. Therefore, children with ACTS scores in the clinical range had significantly higher depression, anxiety, and behavior (total and Externalizing) scores and significantly lower competence scores than the other children in the sample. Although it is unclear if any of the children scoring in the clinical range on the ACTS meet the criteria for a DSM-IV-TR (American Psychiatric Association, 2000) diagnosis of PTSD, the present findings are similar to those found by other studies. Lehmann (1997) reported that children exposed to marital violence within his sample who met the PTSD criteria reported significantly higher scores on self-report measures of anger, dissociation, depression, and assault anxiety than the rest of the sample. Graham-Bermann and Levendosky (1998) found that compared with other children of marital violence, children who experienced PTSD symptoms had higher CBCL Internalizing and Externalizing scores. In the present investigation, both child reports of internalizing concerns (anxiety and depression) and parent-reports of Externalizing behaviors were significantly higher in the children within the clinical range on the ACTS. This finding supports the postulation that children traumatized by marital violence display externalizing symptoms, as well as the more expected internalizing symptoms (Graham-Bermann & Levendosky, 1998). The identification of this constellation of symptoms highlights the question of whether this comorbidity represents multiple disorders manifested within a child, or a specific trauma syndrome that has not yet been fully captured by DSM categories (Lehmann, 2000).

Significant shifts in child knowledge and behavior, as well as parent stress, over a ten-week period indicate optimism for outcomes through the parent and child treatment interventions. The decrease in the percentages of scores in the clinical range (particularly children's total and Externalizing behavior problems and parental stress in the Child Domain) are also encouraging. This finding suggests a "clinically significant" result, in addition to statistical significance, as the children were more likely to be functioning within the identified range for the general population (i.e., within the non-clinical range) (Jacobson, Follette, & Revenstorf, 1984). Like other evaluations of group treatment programs, this study demonstrated that children made significant shifts in their knowledge of types of abuse, responsibility for abuse, and safety planning (Jaffe et al., 1988; Marshall et al., 1995; Wagar & Rodway, 1995). This is an encouraging finding as increased knowledge and attitudinal shifts may serve as protective factors for children (Graham-Bermann, 1998; Jaffe et al., 1990).

The lack of control group in this study precludes definitively attributing the child behavioral and parental stress changes solely to the treatment intervention. It is possible that the significant shift in scores reflects factors such as non-specific aspects of treatment. There is also a possibility that some, or most, of the changes evidenced are due to a spontaneous "recovery" over time (Wolfe, Zak, Wilson, & Jaffe, 1986); however, the heterogeneity of the experiences of the families in this study brings this explanation into question, with just ten weeks between assessments. Children in this sample are living in diverse circumstances (e.g., with or without ongoing exposure to marital conflict) and are likely to be at a variety of stages in terms of dealing with their experiences. In addition, four months of living in a violence-free environment does not seem to be enough time to see changes in problem behaviors (Rossman, Hughes, & Rosenberg, 2000).

Parent self-ratings of stress in the Child Domain significantly decreased between Time 1 and Time 2. This finding corresponds with parents' ratings of significantly less behavior problems for their children at Time 2. It is likely that parents' reports of their own decreased stress in the Child Domain and their reports of their child's improved functioning are related. However, it is unclear how parental stress and parental perceptions of child behavior are influencing each other. It is possible that children's reduced problem behaviors (perhaps due to the group intervention) may have led to decreased stress for their parents. Another consideration is that parents are experiencing less stress, perhaps due to the parenting group, and this shift has led to a less severe judgment of their child. Kilpatrick and Williams (1998) noted the possibility that "maternal reports of children's behavioral and emotional problems may more truly be a reflection of the emotional well-being and coping level of mothers than an accurate indication of the children's level of difficulty" (p. 327). A final possibility is that these two pathways to change are both responsible for the significant shifts evidenced between the two assessment periods.

Theoretical models proposed to make sense of the impact that witnessing spousal violence has on children suggest that they are impacted by the direct effects of exposure to marital violence (e.g., trauma, modeling) and/or by indirect factors (e.g., parenting stress, insecure attachments) (Hughes & Fantuzzo, 1994; Margolin, 1998; Rossman et al., 2000). The range of explanations offered for outcomes with this population of children support the postulation that treatment programs targeted at children *and* parents are likely to have the greatest impact. Programs for children may validate their experiences and provide them with helpful skills and information, while interventions focusing on reducing parenting stress and promoting positive parenting behaviors may have a beneficial impact on child adjustment as well. Levendosky and Graham-Bermann (1998) have suggested that "parenting by the non-violent parent may serve as a potential protective/vulnerability factor for children regardless of the mechanisms through which they are affected by the violence" (p. 385). Therefore, intervention efforts for both parents and children are likely to positively influence short-term and long-term outcomes for children exposed to marital violence.

LIMITATIONS

Information about children's abuse histories was not collected in an interview format; thus, these data were not as complete and thorough as possible. For example, due to the use of questionnaires there was no way to verify that parents who did not specifically indicate the presence of marital physical abuse did not have this experience. A more thorough understanding of the duration, frequency, and extent of abuse directed towards themselves or others in the home is needed in order to provide a clearer picture of the factors influencing children's well-being. Information through an interactive process or a quantitative instrument may have better represented the diversity and further clarified the multifonality evident within this group of children. In addition to these definitional issues, there is also a need for external verification of the abusive incidents (Mohr et al., 2000).

The sample under investigation in this study is one of convenience as the families were mostly self-selected to a treatment program. Therefore, the findings are not necessarily representative of the general population of children exposed to marital violence. No comparison or control group was utilized in this study, so normative data for each measure was the only source of comparison. In addition, the use of cross-sectional, correlational data precludes the interpretation of unequivocal causal relationships among the variables investigated. The 47 children in this sample were from 35 different families; therefore, there are concerns about the non-independence of the data as some parents reported results for multiple children. The small sample size available for this study precluded investigating variables that may have further illuminated the present results (e.g., children's age, family socioeconomic status). The sample was further hampered by attrition in the treatment interventions and uncompleted measures.

Finally, the sample was not randomly selected, and the 18 participants investigated over the two points in time were further self-selected by remaining in the program. Therefore, those 18 children and their parents may have been particularly "ready" for treatment and these results may not have been found if all the participants had remained in the program and been assessed at the second time. Analyses showed that the two groups significantly differed on whether the children had been reported to be emotionally abused and in terms of their competence ratings on the CBCL at Time 1. Therefore, the 29 children whose data were not included in the pre- and post-treatment analyses were more likely to have been emotionally abused and had lower competence scores than the other 18 children according to parental reports.

CONCLUSION

The present investigation described the functioning of a group of children and parents accessing treatment intervention programs at two points in time. This study addressed several of the methodological issues affecting previous investigations with children exposed to marital violence (Edleson, 1999). The sample was comprised of families living in the community, not those in crisis residing in shelters, and the role of child physical abuse was specifically examined. Child and parent report measures were utilized, and the majority of instruments were widely recognized and standardized assessment tools. In addition, this study utilized a relatively new instrument specifically designed for use with young children exposed to on-going family violence.

The children and parents in this sample were found to have similar levels of concern found in previous studies with samples of children and mothers residing in shelters for battered women. The rates of clinical scores in this sample highlight the need for resources available to families struggling with family violence who remain in the community. As well, the strong association between children's mental health and parental stress was confirmed in this sample, and this finding emphasizes the need for intervention efforts aimed at both children and parents. The results of this study also support the need for professionals to consider both trauma and behavioral symptoms when preparing interventions and further research. The prevalence of trauma symptoms identified by children in this sample further underscores the detrimental effects associated with exposure to marital violence and supports the categorization of this experience as a form of emotional and/or psychological abuse for children.

This study is unique, as significant shifts were evidenced in children's and parents' functioning on standardized measures over the course of treatment efforts targeting each of these groups. These results suggest optimism for immediate and long-term well-being for some children exposed to marital violence. Efforts to address parental factors in addition to children's emotional, behavioral, and trauma symptoms, as well as their knowledge and attitudes about violence, may also serve to reduce the likelihood of the perpetuation of family violence in subsequent generations.

REFERENCES

Abidin, R. R. (1995). *Parenting stress index (3rd edition): Professional manual.* Odessa, Florida: Psychological Assessment Resources, Inc.

Achenbach, T. M. (1991). *Manual for the child behavior checklist/4-18 and 1991 profile.* Burlington, VT: University of Vermont Department of Psychiatry.

American Psychiatric Association. (2000). *Diagnostic and statistical manual of mental disorders* (4th ed-TR.). Washington, DC: Author.

Barnett, O. W., Miller-Perrin, C. L., & Perrin, R. D. (1997). Children exposed to marital violence. In O. W. Barnett, C. L. Miller-Perrin, & R. D. Perrin (Eds.), *Family violence across the lifespan: An introduction* (pp. 135-157). Thousand Oaks, CA: Sage Publications.

Cummings, E. M. (1998). Children exposed to marital conflict and violence: Conceptual and theoretical directions. In G. W. Holden, R. Geffner, & E. N. Jouriles (Eds.), *Children exposed to marital violence: Theory, research and applied issues* (pp. 55-93). Washington: American Psychological Association.

Edleson, J. L. (1999). Children's witnessing of adult domestic violence. *Journal of Interpersonal Violence, 14*(8), 839-870.

Graham-Bermann, S. A. (1998). The impact of woman abuse on children's social development: Research and theoretical perspectives. In G. W. Holden, R. Geffner, & E. N. Jouriles (Eds.), *Children exposed to marital violence: Theory, research and applied issues* (pp. 21-54). Washington: American Psychological Association.

Graham-Bermann, S. A., & Levendosky, A. (1998). Traumatic stress symptoms in children of battered women. *Journal of Interpersonal Violence, 13*(1), 111-128.

Holden, G. W. (1998). Introduction: The development of research into another consequence of family violence. In G. W. Holden, R. Geffner, & E. N. Jouriles (Eds.), *Children exposed to marital violence: Theory, research and applied issues* (pp. 1-18). Washington: American Psychological Association.

Holden, G. W., & Ritchie, K. L. (1991). Linking extreme marital discord, child rearing, and child behavior problems: Evidence from battered women. *Child Development, 62,* 311-327.

Hughes, H. M. (1988). Psychological and behavioral correlates of family violence in child witnesses and victims. *American Journal of Orthopsychiatry, 58*(1), 77-90.

Hughes, H. M., & Fantuzzo, J. W. (1994). Family violence-child. In M. Hersen, R. T. Ammerman, & L. A. Sisson (Eds.), *Handbook of aggressive and destructive behavior in psychiatric patients* (pp. 491-507). New York, NY: Plenum Press.

Hughes, H. M., Parkinson, D., & Vargo, M. (1989). Witnessing spouse abuse and experiencing physical abuse: A "double whammy"? *Journal of Family Violence, 4*(2), 197-209.

Jacobson, N. S., Follette, W. C., & Revenstorf, D. (1984). Psychotherapy outcome research: Methods for reporting variability and evaluating clinical significance. *Behavior Therapy, 15,* 336-352.

Jaffe, P., Wilson, S., & Wolfe, D. A. (1986). Promoting changes in attitudes and understanding of conflict resolution among child witnesses of family violence. *Canadian Journal of Behavioural Science, 18*(4), 356-366.

Jaffe, P. G., Wilson, S. K., & Wolfe, D. (1988). Specific assessment and intervention strategies for children exposed to wife battering: Preliminary empirical investigations. *Canadian Journal of Community Mental Health, 7*(2), 157-163.

Jaffe, P. G., Wolfe, D. A., & Wilson, S. K. (Eds.). (1990). *Children of battered women* (Vol. 21). Newbury Park, CA: SAGE Publications.

Kerig, P. K. (2003). In search of protective processes for children exposed to inter-parental violence. *Journal of Emotional Abuse, 3*(3/4), 149-181.

Kilpatrick, K. L., & Williams, L. M. (1998). Potential mediators of post-traumatic stress disorder in child witnesses to domestic violence. *Child Abuse and Neglect, 22*(4), 319-320.

Kolbo, J. R., Blakely, E. H., & Engleman, D. (1996). Children who witness domestic violence: A review of empirical literature. *Journal of Interpersonal Violence, 11*(2), 281-293.

Kovacs, M. (1992). *Children's depression inventory CDI manual.* North Tonawanda, New York: Multi-Health Systems, Inc.

Lehmann, P. (1997). The development of posttraumatic stress disorder (PTSD) in a sample of child witnesses to mother assault. *Journal of Family Violence, 12*(3), 241-257.

Lehmann, P. (2000). Posttraumatic Stress Disorder (PTSD) and child witness to mother-assault: A summary and review. *Child and Youth Services Review, 22*(3-4), 275-306.

Levendosky, A. A., & Graham-Bermann, S. A. (1998). The moderating effects of parenting stress on children's adjustment in woman-abusing families. *Journal of Interpersonal Violence, 13*(2), 383-397.

Margolin, G. (1998). Effects of domestic violence on children. In P. K. Trickett & C. J. Shellenbach (Eds.), *Violence against children in the family and the community* (pp. 57-101). Washington, DC: American Psychological Association.

Marshall, L., Miller, N., Miller-Hewitt, S., Sudermann, M., & Watson, L. (1995). *Evaluation of groups for children who have witnessed violence.* (Available from the Community Group Treatment Program at the London & Middlesex Children's Aid Society, P.O. Box 6010, Depot 1 London, Ontario Canada N5W 5R6).

Mohr, W. K., Lutz, M. J. N., Fantuzzo, J. W., & Perry, M. A. (2000). Children exposed to family violence: A review of empirical research from a developmental-ecological respective. *Trauma, Violence, and Abuse, 1*(3), 264-283.

Multi-Health Systems (March, 2001). Personal communication.

O'Keefe, M. (1994). Adjustment of children from maritally violent homes. *Families in Society, 75,* 403-415.

Pelcovitz, D., & Kaplan, S. J. (1994). Child witnesses of violence between parents: Psychosocial correlates and implications for treatment. *Child and Adolescent Psychiatric Clinics of North America, 3*(4), 745-758.

Peled, E., & Edleson, J. L. (1998). Predicting children's domestic violence service participation and completion. *Research on Social Work Practice, 8*(6), 698-712.

Pepler, D. J., Catallo, R., & Moore, T. E. (2000). Consider the children: Research informing interventions for children exposed to domestic violence. In R. A. Geffner, P. G. Jaffe, & M. Sudermann (Eds.), *Children exposed to domestic violence: Current issues in research, intervention, prevention, and policy development* (pp. 37-57). Binghamton, NY: The Haworth Maltreatment & Trauma Press.

Praver, F., Pelcovitz, D., & DiGiuseppe, R. (1998). *Angie/Andy cartoon trauma scales.* Toronto, Ontario: Multi-Health Systems.

Praver, F., DiGiuseppe, R., Pelcovitz, D., Mandel, F. S., & Gaines, R. (2000). A preliminary study of a cartoon measure for children's reactions to chronic trauma. *Child Maltreatment, 5*(3), 273-285.

Reynolds, C. R., & Richmond, B. O. (1985). *Revised children's manifest anxiety scale manual*. Los Angeles, CA: Western Psychological Services.

Rossman, B. B. R., Hughes, H. M., & Rosenberg, M. S. (2000). *Children and interparental violence: The impact of exposure*. Philadelphia, PA: Taylor & Francis.

Spaccarelli, S., Sandler, I. N., & Roosa, M. (1994). History of spouse violence against mother: Correlated risks and unique effects in child mental health. *Journal of Family Violence, 9*(1), 79-98.

Statistics Canada. (2000). *Family violence in Canada: A statistical profile*. Canadian Centre for Justice Statistics. Available on line at: http://statcan.ca.

Sternberg, K. J., Lamb, M. E., & Dawud-Noursi, S. (1998). Using multiple informants to understand domestic violence and its effects. In G. W. Holden, R. Geffner, & E. N. Jouriles (Eds.), *Children exposed to marital violence: Theory, research and applied issues* (pp. 121-156). Washington, DC: American Psychological Association.

Sternberg, K. J., Lamb, M. E., Greenbaum, C., Cicchetti, D., Dawud, S., Cortes, R. M., Krispin, O., & Lorey, F. (1993). Effects of domestic violence on children's behavior problems and depression. *Developmental Psychology, 29*(1), 44-52.

Terr, L. C. (1991). Childhood traumas: An outline and overview. *American Journal of Psychiatry, 148*(1), 10-20.

Terr, L. C. (1995). Childhood posttraumatic stress disorder. In G. O. Gabbard (Ed.), *Treatments of Psychiatric Disorders* (Vol. 1, pp. 287-299). Washington, DC: American Psychiatric Press, Inc.

Wagar, J. M., & Rodway, M. R. (1995). An evaluation of a group treatment approach for children who have witnessed wife abuse. *Journal of Family Violence, 10*(3), 295-306.

Wolfe, D. A., Zak, L., Wilson, S., & Jaffe, P. (1986). Child-witnesses to family violence between parents: Critical issues in behavioral and social adjustment. *Journal of Abnormal Child Psychology, 14*(1), 95-104.

LEGAL ISSUES
AND POLICY IMPLICATIONS

Wife Abuse, Child Custody
and Access in Canada

Martha Shaffer
Nicholas Bala

SUMMARY. In Canada, custody and access decisions continue to be made on the basis of the highly discretionary "best interests of the child" test, with only one province having legislation that requires judges to take account of spousal abuse in making decisions about children. This article reports on a study of Canadian family law cases from 1997-2000 that had spousal abuse issues ($N = 45$). Judges tended not to grant custody to a man who has abused his partner if the woman's claims of abuse were accepted as valid, but routinely granted abusive men access to their children on an unsupervised basis. This is problematic as many of the factors

---

Address correspondence to: Professor Martha Shaffer, Faculty of Law, University of Toronto, Toronto, Ontario M5S 2C6 (E-mail: m.shaffer@utoronto.ca).

[Haworth co-indexing entry note]: "Wife Abuse, Child Custody and Access in Canada." Shaffer, Martha, and Nicholas Bala. Co-published simultaneously in *Journal of Emotional Abuse* (The Haworth Maltreatment & Trauma Press, an imprint of The Haworth Press, Inc.) Vol. 3, No. 3/4, 2003, pp. 253-275; and: *The Effects of Intimate Partner Violence on Children* (ed: Robert A. Geffner, Robyn Spurling Igelman, and Jennifer Zellner) The Haworth Maltreatment & Trauma Press, an imprint of The Haworth Press, Inc., 2003, pp. 253-275. Single or multiple copies of this article are available for a fee from The Haworth Document Delivery Service [1-800-HAWORTH, 9:00 a.m. - 5:00 p.m. (EST). E-mail address: docdelivery@haworthpress.com].

10.1300J135v03n03_05

which create a risk in awarding custody to a batterer may endanger the mother or child if there is unsupervised access. Canada is in the midst of a contentious process of reforming child custody and access laws. Legislation should make specific reference to spousal abuse as a factor in making child related decisions, including consideration of the effect of any custody or access order on the safety of children and victims of spousal abuse. *[Article copies available for a fee from The Haworth Document Delivery Service: 1-800-HAWORTH. E-mail address: <docdelivery@haworthpress.com> Website: <http://www.HaworthPress.com> © 2003 by The Haworth Press, Inc. All rights reserved.]*

KEYWORDS. Wife abuse, family law, child custody and access, visitation, law reform

BACKGROUND:
RESPONDING TO WIFE ABUSE IN THE 1980s

In 1988, Judge Freeman, then of the Nova Scotia County Court, and since promoted to the Nova Scotia Court of Appeal, rendered a decision in which he displayed a disturbing lack of understanding about the dynamics of wife abuse and its effects on children. In *Peterson v. Peterson* (1988), the mother applied to vary an interim court order which her husband had obtained two months earlier on an *ex parte* basis (without notice to her), giving the husband custody of the couple's two young children. Judge Freeman noted that "[f]rom outward appearance . . . the family appeared to be a stable and happy one with superior material benefits and a favored way of life" (p. 109). In reality, there was ample evidence that Mr. Peterson was a violent and controlling man who had abused Mrs. Peterson both before and during their marriage. The judge observed that she "tolerated" his conduct through eight years of marriage without complaint, and commented that, "it could have come as no surprise to her that he had such a predisposition" (p. 109) since there was evidence of violence even before they had married.

Mr. Peterson's violence culminated in a particularly brutal incident which brought an end to the marriage. Following what the court described as a "quarrel" in which Mr. Peterson "applied physical force to his wife" (p. 110), Mrs. Peterson left the home and arranged to meet a male friend (Mr. Smith), with whom there was no evidence of her having prior sexual involvement, in order to "get away from the home environment" (p. 111). At about 11:00 p.m. that night, Mr. Peterson kicked in the door of the motel room where Mrs. Peterson had met her friend. Upon finding her in bed with Mr. Smith, Mr. Peterson attacked both of them with a metal bar. Mrs. Peterson was left with several injuries, including a laceration in her head which required eight stitches.

The incident did not end there, however. Displaying what the judge referred to as a "lack of parental wisdom" (p. 113), Mr. Peterson had taken the couple's 7-year-old son, Jeffrey, and their 3-year-old daughter, on his search for Mrs. Peterson. After beating Mrs. Peterson, who was then lying naked and bleeding on the motel room floor, Mr. Peterson had Jeffrey brought to the motel room door, took him by the hand and told him to look at his mother.

In addition to evidence of Mr. Peterson's violence towards Mrs. Peterson, the judge also had evidence before him of other incidents in which Mr. Peterson had assaulted his son, Jeffrey. One assault on Jeffrey occurred when he was four years old and Mr. Peterson became enraged by the young boy's crankiness and crying. Mr. Peterson stormed up the stairs and hit Jeffrey three times. This incident was described by Mrs. Peterson's sister, a school teacher, who was in Jeffrey's room comforting him at the time that his father stormed in. The aunt testified that Mr. Peterson raised his hand over his head and swung it down on the small boy. When she intervened to try to protect the child, Mr. Peterson drove her head through a wall, causing the aunt to suffer a black eye and facial swelling. The father testified that this was the only time he "spanked" the boy, though the judge did not accept his characterization of this incident, or that this was his only assault on the boy. Another incident occurred one day before Jeffrey left for school. Mr. Peterson became angry with Jeffrey and kicked him in the chest. His anger persisted after the child left for school; the father was so agitated that he shoved his hand through a door.

In court, Mrs. Peterson argued that she should have interim custody of the children because Mr. Peterson's violence was relevant to his ability to parent, and because the children were afraid of him. The judge, however, did not accept this argument and concluded that it was in the best interests of the children to continue to reside with their father. In awarding him interim custody, Judge Freeman reasoned that the father had, with the help of his mother, taken good care of the children in the two months since Mrs. Peterson had fled the matrimonial home. He also held that Mrs. Peterson's proposal for caring for the children was inferior to Mr. Peterson's, as she was living in her parents' modest home and was involved with Mr. Smith, whom the court considered a "destabilizing influence" (p. 115). While the judge expressed concerns over Mr. Peterson's decision to bring his son to the motel room door, he felt held that Mr. Peterson's past conduct involving the children had "been laid to rest," and that Mrs. Peterson was primarily responsible for breaking up the marriage and for bringing the "ideal lifestyle" (p. 117) of the children to an end. Despite evidence that since the separation, Mr. Peterson had restricted Mrs. Peterson's access to the children, the court held that "there is a greater likelihood of the children retaining an affectionate relationship toward both parents if they continue to reside with the father" (p. 117).

The willingness of the judge in *Peterson* to grant custody to a man whom the evidence clearly showed had abused his wife and children during their eight year marriage displayed a distressing lack of understanding of the relationship between wife abuse and parenting. Unfortunately, the *Peterson* decision is typical of judicial or societal responses to wife abuse in Canada in the late 1980s when wife abuse was believed to be irrelevant to custody or access decisions. A man could, it was thought, abuse his wife, yet be a wonderful father (Canadian Panel, 1993).

THIS STUDY: CANADIAN FAMILY LAW CASES 1997-2000

Since the *Peterson* case was decided, a significant body of research has documented the damaging effects to children of exposure to wife abuse. This research reveals children exposed to wife abuse to be at greater risk of suffering various types of psychological and physical harm than children who are not exposed to domestic violence. Children who are exposed to spousal abuse are at greater risk of suffering behavioral, academic and emotional problems, as well as problems with social functioning (Dauvergne & Johnson, 2001; see also Kalil, Tolman, Rosen & Gruber, 2003; Onyskiw, 2003). In terms of physical harm, researchers have established that many men who abuse their wives also abuse their children (Edleson, 1999), as occurred in *Peterson*. Children are also at risk of physical harm when they try to intervene to protect their mother from violence or when they are in the "cross-fire" of objects or blows intended for the mother.

There has also been a growing awareness of wife abuse among Canadian judges and lawyers in the past decade (Bala, 2000). In this study, we sought to assess how far Canadian family law courts have come in understanding the relevance of wife abuse to child custody and access (visitation) determinations in the 14 years since the *Peterson* case was decided. In particular, we sought to examine the following questions. First, whether the attitudes underlying *Peterson* (i.e., that a man could batter his spouse yet be a good father) were still alive and well, or whether the judiciary had demonstrated an awareness of the psychological research on the impact of exposure to wife abuse on children. Second, we sought to examine in what circumstances, and on what terms, abusive men were being granted access to their children. Specifically, we wanted to examine the circumstances in which courts would deny or suspend an abuser's access to the children, and when courts would opt for supervised access. More generally, we were also interested in assessing judicial attitudes towards claims of wife abuse brought in the context of custody and access proceedings. We sought to discern whether judges were generally skeptical of these claims, and tended to perceive them to be unfounded, exaggerated or brought for strategic purposes.

METHOD

To answer the above questions, we performed a computer search of child related family law cases reported on Quicklaw, a leading Canadian computer data base, over a 3 1/2 year period from January 1997 to May 2000. The search generated only 45 cases, a small number given the number of custody or access cases Canada-wide in which wife abuse was likely to have been an issue. Quicklaw claims to include all legal decisions in which written reasons are produced; the cases with written reasons tend to be ones that are more complex or contentious, or that raise novel legal issues. Cases that are relatively routine may only result in oral reasons from the judge that are "unreported" on computer or print data bases, though the outcomes of these unreported cases could often be determined from a laborious search of court files.

Although we cannot be certain of how representative these reported cases are of all cases in which abusive men made custody or access claims, our principal conclusions about judicial decisions are consistent with those reached in a recent unpublished study by a New Brunswick research team (Neilson, 2001) looking at patterns in a much larger sample of reported and unreported judicial decisions in that province. That research also reveals that in many cases a woman's allegations of abuse are not even put before a judge. Some lawyers will, for example, discourage women from introducing evidence about wife abuse, considering it "irrelevant" if there is no evidence of the children also being abused.

RESULTS AND DISCUSSION

The Cases

Of the 45 cases located, 42 were cases in which women were the party primarily raising abuse allegations. In many of these 42 cases, men also asserted that they had been abused by their female partners, an issue we will discuss in greater detail below.

Three cases differed from the pattern of the primary allegations of abuse being against the male partner. One was a case in which the father claimed custody on the basis that the mother had entered into a new relationship in which both she and the children were being abused by her new partner (*Collins v. Collins,* 1998). The court found this claim to be unfounded. The other two cases were ones in which the men were alleging that their former wives were violent and should not receive custody. In one of these three cases (*F. (D.) v. F. (W),* 1998), the mother had twice been convicted of assault, once for assaulting her mother and once for assaulting the husband's new girlfriend. She also suffered from substance abuse problems. In the other case (*Ouimet v. Ouimet,* 1997), the judge concluded that while the wife had yelled at the husband and occasionally pushed him, the husband had psychologically abused his wife through the use of demeaning language and by calling her a "fat cow" and a "pig."

The remaining 42 cases, in which women were primarily making allegations of abuse against their male partners, revealed a wide spectrum of abusive conduct. The abuse ranged from extreme levels of chronic physical (and sexual) violence, to cases of some physical violence accompanied by other forms of controlling and abusive behavior, to cases in which the abuse was confined to emotional and verbal abuse without a physical component.

The cases reflect many of the characteristics of abusive relationships discussed in the psychological literature. For example, many of the cases involved men who were serial abusers, abusing their female partners in successive relationships, and many of the cases showed men engaging in a host of controlling behaviors including isolating women from family and friends and emotionally denigrating the women.

Many of the men in the 42 cases in which they were alleged to have been abusive minimized or denied their violent behavior, for example, by proposing improbable explanations for the woman's injuries (including one man who asserted his wife's injuries were caused when she repeatedly fell down while wearing high heels), or claiming that if they had harmed their wives, they had done so in self-defense. Generally, where these kinds of claims were raised, the courts were quick to reject them *so long as* the physical violence against the woman was extreme or well documented. In these cases, courts frequently noted that the husband's strength or physical size relative to his spouse made his self-defense claims incredible. There was, however, a tendency in some of the cases where the violence was less extreme to view the violence as mutual. Finally, the cases revealed situations in which the abuse continued after separation, including cases of stalking and physical assaults, emotional manipulation, and serious attempts to denigrate and undermine women's parenting abilities.

Overall, the cases demonstrate a greater sensitivity towards issues of wife abuse and a greater awareness of the link between spousal abuse and harm to children than there was when *Peterson* was decided in 1988. At least at a rhetorical level, the cases are replete with statements that exposure to wife abuse is harmful to children, judicial statements that were infrequently made as recently as a decade ago. Our research reveals that judges rarely grant custody to a man who has abused his partner when the woman's claims of abuse have been accepted (see Table 1). While this is a positive development, there continue to be problematic judicial statements about wife abuse, and questionable approaches to some of the cases that raise spousal abuse issues. In addition, judges routinely grant abusive men access to their children on an unsupervised basis. Granting an abusive man unsupervised access may be problematic, as the same factors which make it risky to award custody to an abusive man may endanger the mother and child if there is no supervision of access, or at least of the exchange of the care of the child.

Problematic Judicial Attitudes About Wife Abuse

In 11 of the 42 cases in which women raised allegations of spousal abuse, the court found the allegations to be exaggerated or unfounded. In some of these cases, the court gave no reasons for concluding that the women had fabricated or embellished their claims, making the validity of these judicial conclusions impossible to assess. It is possible that the courts were correct and the claims had been fabricated or exaggerated. It is also possible, however, that judges failed to recognize abuse be-

TABLE 1. Abuse Allegations and Custody/Access Outcome

1997-2000 Canadian Custody– Access Cases with Spousal Abuse Alleged	Mother Granted Custody	Father Granted Custody	Joint Custody Granted
11 Court finds Mother's allegations of abuse by husband to be exaggerated or unfounded	3	3	5
30 Mother's allegations of abuse accepted by court	28	0	2
1 Court makes no finding on abuse	0	1	0
3 Father alleges mother abusive partner & mother not alleging abuse by father	1	1	1
N = 45 cases	32	5	8

cause it was not well documented or because the abuse took a predominantly emotional, rather than physical, form.

In the absence of medical records, police reports or witnesses to the abuse, judges may have difficulty finding that abuse occurred, and in fact, judges mention this as a problem in some of the cases. In part this may be a function of the law's requirement that the person making an allegation of abuse prove it true on the balance of probabilities (the equivalent of the American standard of proof on a preponderance of evidence). Often the only adult witnesses to spousal abuse are the spouses. While children often see or hear spousal abuse (Statistics Canada, 2001), there are a variety of evidentiary and ethical concerns about calling them as witnesses. Many women do not disclose their abuse, report it to doctors, or call the police (Statistics Canada, 2001); therefore, it may be difficult to prove abuse in many cases. Absent evidence corroborating the woman's allegations, judges may be reluctant to find that abuse has been proven to the court's satisfaction. Judges may decide the allegations are "unfounded" simply because the woman cannot muster sufficient evidence that it has occurred.

Judges may also conclude that allegations are unfounded where woman raise allegations of emotional or verbal abuse rather than physical violence. Many judges conceive of abuse as involving significant physical violence. If the abuse is primarily emotional or verbal, courts may have difficulty conceptualizing the conduct as abusive, viewing it instead as mutual conflict or discord.

In some cases, the judge's conclusion that the abuse was "exaggerated" appeared suspect in light of the description of the relationship provided by the court. In *T. (S.L.) v. T. (M.L.)* (1997), for example, the wife alleged that the husband had hit and pushed her, dragged her down a flight of stairs, hit her with a belt, thrown objects at her, and threatened to kill her and throw her body in the river that ran behind the house. Her description of the abuse was supported by each of her three children. After separation, the husband was charged criminally with five counts relating to wife abuse, and he subsequently pled guilty to "unlawfully committing an assault upon the [wife] 'on several and diverse occasions.'" The wife and the children also alleged that the husband frequently hit the children, sometimes with a studded belt, and that he kept a belt at his side at the kitchen table or in his lap. The husband admitted to pushing and shoving the wife, but claimed that this violence was "mutual." He also admitted to hitting the children with a strap on a few occasions. The judge accepted that the husband had abused the wife during the marriage, including strapping her with a belt in the presence of one of the children, and that he had threatened to kill her. Nonetheless, the judge concluded that the wife had "greatly exaggerated" her fear of her husband. Given the level of violence that the court found to have existed in the relationship, and the judge's ultimate decision that the father should only have supervised access, the conclusion that the woman's fears were "exaggerated" seems both questionable and gratuitous.

Finally, some of the comments which judges make continue to provide cause for concern about judicial sensitivity to woman abuse issues. In one 1999 Alberta case, for example, the judge noted that the on three separate occasions the wife left the husband and went to a women's shelter, one time remaining there for two months (*W. (J.W.) v. W. (N.)*, 1999). The court did not discuss the reasons for the woman's decision to take refuge in a shelter, stating instead that "these were troubled times" for the spouses and that the "parties made allegations one against the other." The failure to address the wife's reasons for fleeing to a shelter is problematic, given that violence is the primary reason women do so, and the woman was making allegations of abuse against her estranged husband. More problematic was the court's decision to apply s.16(9) of the *Divorce Act*, which directs judges not to consider parental conduct unless it is "relevant to the person's ability to act as a parent." If in fact the wife had gone to a shelter because of abuse, the comment that s.16(9) "governs" is reflective of the same lack of understanding of the relevance of wife abuse to parenting as the *Peterson* court expressed a decade earlier.

Wife Abuse and Custody

In contrast to the 1988 decision in *Peterson*, the more recent cases we examined showed that courts generally did not grant either sole or joint custody to an abusive husband, *provided* that the court determined that he physically abused her. Usually the fact that there had been spousal abuse was not the only reason for denying the father's custody claim, but it was one of several factors supporting a decision to grant custody to the mother. These factors frequently included the fact that the mother had been the child's primary caregiver and that the father had engaged in other destructive conduct relevant to his parenting abilities, such as putting his own interests ahead of the children, or abusing alcohol or drugs. Nonetheless, courts frequently stated that wife abuse was relevant to a man's parenting ability as it made him a poor role model for the children and possibly posed a risk of physical harm to the children were they to be placed in his custody.

There were, however, three exceptions to the general trend of denying custody to batterers. In two cases, the court awarded joint custody to men found to have abused their wives. In one of these cases (*M. (G.E.) v. M. (C.)*, 1999), the court's decision may be explained by the fact that it was responding to the mother's own request for joint custody, with her also having primary care of the child, and rejecting the claim of an abusive husband for sole custody. In making the joint custody order, the judge observed that "this is really an abuse case" (para 40) and that "Mr. G.E.M. has a severe anger problem and absent any admission of this problem, and absent any evidence of treatment of this problem, I am fearful that the health safety and indeed the best interests of the children, could be placed at risk by Mr. G.E.M. gaining sole custody" (para 41). While the judge may have felt constrained to order joint custody because the parties had previously agreed to joint custody, and the mother had requested it, abused women may often feel pressured to agree to joint custody, even when this arrangement may be unworkable, and contrary to the interests of their children. We discuss this problem in more detail later.

In *Mbaruk v. Mbaruk* the court awarded joint custody with primary care and control to the father, notwithstanding the fact that the father was a "rigid and domineering" (para 33) person who had physically abused the mother during the marriage, refused to take responsibility for the abuse by claiming that the mother's injuries were self-inflicted or sustained by falling while wearing shoes with high heels, and that he continued to denigrate and demean the mother after separation, including in the courtroom during the trial. The judge expressed concern that the father would attempt to undermine the mother's relationship to the children by limiting access, but opined that a joint custody order would give her the leverage she needed to protect their on-going relationship. In awarding the father primary residence, the court was influenced by the fact that the children had been living with the father for 16 months preceding the decision, because the mother had difficulty coping with the demands of her job and of raising the two children. This decision is disturbing given that it puts inordinate weight on the "status quo," a situation that was established when the mother was experiencing the sort of adjustment problems many women face when extricating themselves from an abusive relationship. More generally, women who have been abused by their husbands often have difficulty effectively protecting their interests and those of their children within the context of a joint custody arrangement, a situation Mrs. Mbaruk seemed certain to face.

In one case, *A. (B.) v. T. (A.)* (1997), the judge awarded custody to a man alleged to have been abusive without concluding that the woman's abuse allegations were false or significantly exaggerated. In that case, the mother suffered from serious mental health problems and appeared to have "suffered a break from reality" (para 161) while on the witness stand. The mother's mental health issues made her testimony difficult for the court to accept and made awarding her custody impossible. Despite awarding the father custody, the judge had sufficient concerns about the father's conduct that he personally reported the case to the local child protection agency, which apprehended the child as soon as the custody order took effect.

These cases aside, the general picture in terms of custody in the cases we surveyed was that abusive men were not succeeding in getting either sole or joint custody, provided that the court accepted the allegations of abuse. Joint custody orders were made in five cases where the court concluded that the allegations were unsubstantiated or at least not proven to the court's satisfaction. This is a concern, in that even if a judge concludes that the allegations of spousal abuse are exaggerated, they are indicative of a high conflict separation, and an absence of the co-operative relationship that is needed for a good joint custody situation. In three cases, where the woman's abuse allegations were considered by the judge to be unfounded, the father was awarded sole custody. However, the fact that the mother made allegations that were considered false was not the only reason for denying her custody. In three other cases in which the judge regarded the mother's allegations of spousal abuse to be substantially exaggerated, she was nevertheless awarded custody.

Wife Abuse and Access

While Canadian courts are generally recognizing the significance of wife abuse when dealing with custody issues, the situation is quite different when dealing with access. Most of the men found to have abused their wives were granted access rights to their children, usually on an unsupervised basis. When there are significant abuse concerns, unsupervised access may expose a child to the risk of further emotional or physical harm. Further, the father may use access to question the child about the mother, and attempt to continue to exert control over her life. Access was denied in only seven cases of the 31 cases in which the court did not reject the mother's allegations of spousal abuse. These seven cases were ones in which the mother had been subjected to extreme levels of physical violence, where the children had also been exposed to the risk of serious physical harm, or where there was clear evidence that the children had been traumatized by exposure to the violence.

The case of A. (P.) v. A. (F.) (1997) is a good example of the degree of abuse necessary before the abuser's access will be suspended. The wife alleged that the husband had subjected her to physical, sexual, and emotional abuse for 12 years. Although the abuse is not described in the judgment, the court noted that the wife had given detailed descriptions of beatings that had occurred throughout the marriage. The wife's account of abuse was supported by the couple's four children. The wife and children also alleged the husband had physically abused the couple's two sons and sexually abused their two daughters. The husband beat the boys with a cane and an electrical cord. Once when one of the boys attempted to stop the father from beating the mother, the father force the child's head into the toilet and flushed. The sexual abuse of the girls, aged 6 and 9, consisted of fondling them in the bath, inserting his fingers into their vaginas, and fondling them through their clothing. The father denied the allegations, calling the wife "crazy" and maintaining that the children were fabricating.

Even on these facts, the father had initially been granted supervised access. After a few visits the children refused to participate, because they were afraid of their father, fearful for their mother's safety and because they felt guilty for not being able to protect her. The court denied the father access until he could show that he had taken counseling to help him understand the impact of his abusive behavior on his wife and children.

Two other examples serve to illustrate the kinds of cases in which access is denied. Access was denied in *D. (C.L.) v. D. (B.E.)* (1999) where the three children were found to be exhibiting signs of "post-traumatic distress" and would sometimes enter into a "dissociative, trance-like state at the mention of the father's name." Similarly, access was denied in *B. (M.J.) v. B. (W.P.)* (1999) where the husband had repeatedly assaulted his wife in the presence of their young children, and the children were ultimately so frightened of their father that they would hide when they saw a car the same color as their father's.

As these cases demonstrate, courts will deny access in cases of chronic, serious violence and where the children have experienced extreme trauma. Generally, however, men who have abused their female partners are granted unsupervised access to their children. Supervised access was ordered in six cases, generally with the objective of allowing the father to re-establish a relationship with the children where the relationship had lapsed or where the children were fearful of their father. For example, in *Cadeau v. Martell* (1998), supervised access was ordered for a father who had not seen his two year old daughter for over a year and in *H. (P.G.) v. H. (K.D.)* (1999), supervised access was ordered where a 10-year-old girl felt insecure about visiting her father as a result of his drinking and abusive behaviour.

In some cases unsupervised access may be appropriate despite a finding of spousal abuse, for example, where it is clear that there is little likelihood of a recurrence of abuse and the children do not fear their father. However, in some of the cases in which unsupervised access orders were made, the orders seemed problematic because they appeared to subject the children to the same risks of harm that exist when an abusive man is granted custody. In *L. (C.R.) v. L. (R.F.)* (1998), for example, the court awarded unsupervised access on alternate weekends to a man who had not only abused his wife and her child from a previous relationship, but had also abused women in three other intimate relationships. The violence against the wife included punching her in the abdomen when she was eight months pregnant with the couple's first child and punching her in the head while she was holding the child. The violence ultimately escalated until it was occurring once a week or once every other week. The allegations of child abuse involved the father punching the child in the arms and legs, and during one access visit "disciplining" the child by putting him outside in the snow in his bare feet. The father admitted to using physical force to discipline the child, but said he had not done so maliciously. He also admitted that there had been physical altercations in his relationships with each of the four women, but refused to take responsibility for the violence. Instead, he asserted that all four women suffered from emotional difficulties and attributed the violence to their emotional problems.

The mother initially agreed to the father having access two evenings a week and every other weekend, but then sought to restrict access to non-overnight, supervised access. In part, her decision to seek supervision was motivated by the results of two assessment reports. The first, prepared as a result of a court order, recommended that the father have supervised access with only one overnight visit at Christmas because the father had been violent and refused to accept responsibility for his violence. It was the assessor's opinion that until the father completed a counseling program on alternatives to violence, he would not be well suited to meeting the children's developmental needs. In addition, because the father made a complaint that the mother's new partner was physically abusing the children and sexually abusing the daughter, a child protection worker investigated the family. The worker found the father's concerns to be unsubstantiated, but became concerned about the *father's* parenting ability. He determined that the father was a violent person who took out his frustrations through violence and who had frequently assaulted the mother in front of the children. Due to the protection worker's concern that the father would abuse the children, he recommended only short visits and none overnight.

Despite this evidence, the court denied the mother's request to limit the father's access. The court reasoned that the mother had agreed to unsupervised access and, although she complained that the father continued to attempt to control her, she could not conclusively demonstrate that access had been harmful to the children. The court also noted that access had gone well for over a year and concluded that denying the children continued access would be "adverse" to their interests.

While the fact that the arrangement existed without reported incident for a lengthy period might make a change to supervised access seem unnecessary, in this case, the court's refusal to order supervised access is troubling. Women who are victims of abuse frequently feel pressured into agreeing to unsupervised access, even if this arrangement gives rise to concerns about the safety of themselves or their children (Neilson, 2001). There were aspects of this case which suggest that unsupervised access may not have been appropriate. The two assessment reports revealed a continuing concern for the children's welfare if they were exposed to the father without supervision. The father was a serial abuser who had not only refused to seek treatment, but refused to acknowledge his problem. Given the father's history of spousal abuse, there is every reason for concern that the children would again be exposed to violence in the father's new intimate relationship or that the children themselves might be the target of his abuse. Supervised access until the father successfully completed some treatment should have been a minimum step towards trying to reduce the risk.

Similar concerns arise in the case of *C. (A.C.) v. G. (I.C.)* (1999), in which the court awarded unsupervised weekend access to a father despite concluding that there was "overwhelming evidence" (para 106) that the father had been physically and emotionally abusive to the mother and had exercised a "reign of tyranny" (para 107) over her. The physical abuse involved slapping and kicking the mother, pushing her down into a chair, and on one occasion, striking her in the head with such force that she suffered a permanent hearing loss. The father's emotional abuse included calling the mother names such as "whore, slut, retard, lesbian, incompetent, liar" (para 6), telling her she was an incompetent mother, accusing her of molesting the child, and constantly accusing her of infidelity. The physical and verbal abuse often occurred in the presence of the child, who developed a habit of hitting and slapping herself. The father also isolated the mother from her family and friends, and threatened the mother by saying that he would hurt or kill her if she ever left him and took the child. Shortly after the separation, when the mother called to arrange to pick up the child, the father threatened if she took the child: "I will hunt you down and kill you" (para 82). The judge described the father's testimony in court as a "continuation of his abuse" of the mother (para 129).

The evidence also revealed a pattern of troubling behavior on the part of the father as well as some deeply disturbing attitudes about women. He testified that he held to "a 19th century moral code," that all women found him attractive, that his mother-in-law was sexually interested in him, and that he had tried to "train" the mother. He had been abusive to at least one other female partner, and had three convictions for assault and aggravated assault which were unrelated to either intimate relationship. One of these convictions was for assaulting a woman who was a stranger. The father admitted to using violence in his intimate relationships, but claimed that the women had been the aggressors, asserting that "[e]very woman I get involved with wants to beat me up" (para 91).

The father's explanation for the assault convictions was that he had been wrongly convicted. Finally, when asked about his plan for caring for the child if he succeeded in his claim for custody, he responded by saying simply that his daughter was his "best friend."

Despite concluding that the father had a "weakened capacity to act as an appropriate role model and custodial parent" (para 121) due to his abuse of the mother, the judge awarded him unsupervised access every second weekend. This order seems to have been based in part by the fact that the mother did not request supervised access. While there is no indication why she did not do so, one possibility is that she had received legal advice that she would likely not be successful as the father had been exercising unsupervised access since the separation. Shortly after separation the mother had been hospitalized twice, having experienced what was diagnosed as a psychotic episode precipitated by the break up of an abusive relationship and the use of marijuana and alcohol. As a result of her 6-week hospitalization, the mother consented to the child residing with the father 5 days a week and with her own mother (the child's maternal grandmother) for the other two days. This arrangement had been in place for six months by the time the mother's custody claim was heard.

In light of the father's abusive behavior, and his unwillingness to accept responsibility for it or to change it, the access order is troubling. There are good reasons for suspecting that the child would be exposed to abuse during access visits, or that the child would become the target of the father's emotional abuse and manipulation. There are clear risks of harm arising from unsupervised access by a man with a history of woman abuse who describes his three year old daughter as his "best friend." This seems to be a situation in which supervised access would be warranted.

In cases in which there is a history of spousal abuse, unsupervised access should only be awarded if there is no likelihood of a recurrence of physical or emotional abuse of the mother or child, and the child is not afraid of the father. The court should also ensure that there is no risk to the custodial mother from the exchange of the child; in some cases of exchange, supervision may be needed. There can be difficulties in arranging suitable supervision of access or the exchange of the child, though recently a number of programs have been established in some parts of Canada to supervise visitation or the exchange of children.

APPLICATIONS

The Practice of Family Law

In order to fully understand how spousal abuse is dealt with by the Canadian justice system, it is necessary to look beyond the reported cases to get a sense of the actual practice of family law, considering both unreported judicial decisions and how cases are settled. It is difficult to get an accurate picture of how cases that are unreported are resolved. However, it is very important to attempt to get some understanding of these cases, as the cases that go to trial (i.e., reported) are just a tiny fraction of all the cases in which parents have separated and there are spousal abuse issues. The cases involving survivors of abuse who go to trial are not typical; they tend to be those where victims have the most effective or supportive counsel, or where the women have the emotional strength to withstand the pressures to settle.

Although all Canadian provinces have legal aid schemes, and most give some priority to domestic abuse cases in determining whether to provide representation, the level of funding per case is inadequate for the complex demands of these cases (Doucette, 2001). While there are some highly competent lawyers who deal with domestic violence cases, and a few clinics that specialize in these cases, many of the lawyers who represent women in these cases lack the training and resources to deal adequately with them.

Some lawyers may advise at least some of their women clients who claim to have been victims of spousal abuse not to raise abuse issues in their court documents (Neilson, 2001). Some lawyers do this because they consider spousal abuse irrelevant to custody and access issues if there is no direct abuse of the children. In other cases, there is a concern that if the issue of spousal abuse is raised but not proven, that this will reflect poorly on the mother's claim for custody, suggesting that she is an "unfriendly parent" who will thwart the father's access to the children for selfish reasons.

Despite the fact that the Canadian legislation makes clear that the actual test for determining whether there is to be access is the "best interests" of the child, in practice many judges, lawyers, and mediators continue to operate on the presumption that all spouses, including those who are abusive, have a right to have access to their children (Neilson, 2000). Abusive men demand the "right" to regular access, threatening violence, or at least protracted litigation, if they do not get what they want. In the absence of clear evidence of child abuse, many lawyers (in negotiations), judges (in pre-hearing settlement conferences) and mediators pressure victims of spousal abuse into agreeing to on-going access to a child (Neilson, 2001). Indeed, as a result of financial and psychological pressures to settle cases, spouse abuse victims may feel pressure to settle even if they have on-going concerns about inadequate care, possible child abuse, or high risk behavior by the non-custodial parent during access visit. Despite fears for the safety of their children during visits many women will "consent" to regular unsupervised access.

Judges and lawyers feel the pressure of heavy caseloads and are aware that a contested trial can be a financially and emotionally draining experience; they continue to refer parental disputes to mediation, especially those involving access disputes, despite the presence of allegations of spousal abuse (Neilson, 2001). While the guidelines for Canadian mediators require that cases involving domestic violence should be screened out (Landau, 1995), in practice some mediators do deal with cases where there are spousal abuse issues. Busy staff mediators may pressure abused women into agreeing to accept generous access terms, without dealing adequately with the fears and safety concerns of the women and their children.

It is also apparent that many custodial mothers feel pressured by mediators or their lawyers to settle cases on the basis of some form of "joint custody," despite on-going issues of spousal abuse. While in cases without violence issues, joint custody can be appropriate, abusive men often use joint custody as a means of maintaining control over their former partners. Further, women who have been abused often lack the psychological resources to effectively represent the interests of their children or themselves in a continuing joint custody arrangement.

Responding More Effectively to Spousal Abuse in Family Law Cases

All justice system professionals who work with divorcing couples, including lawyers, judges, police, assessors and mediators, need the knowledge and training to deal effectively with situations where spousal abuse is at issue, and in particular should be aware of the risks faced by victims of abuse and their children. These professionals must appreciate that spousal abuse covers a broad range of conduct. While physical abuse represents the most obvious danger, emotional abuse can also be extremely destructive.

Given the wide range of abusive spousal conduct and the high portion of separations and divorces that involve at least one incident of spousal violence, the justice system and the professionals who work in it need to develop differentiated responses that take account of the specific situation of abuse, and its effect on the particular parents and children involved. While there are clearly some judges who are less sensitive to the issue, leading Canadian precedents now recognize the importance of spousal abuse as a factor in custody and access disputes. Domestic violence issues are now a topic that is regularly covered in judicial education programs in Canada, though generally attendance at these programs is optional. Many judges now appreciate the need for differentiated responses, depending on the nature of the abuse, the effects of that abuse on the children and the prognosis for the future, as well as on the risk of immediate harm. It is, however, also clear that too often judges, lawyers, mediators, assessors, police and other professionals fail to adequately recognize and deal with spousal abuse issues, and that too often children and victims are endangered as a result.

In comparison to the late 1980s there are more resources for shelters, supervised visitation centers, and a range of programs to support victims and their children. There is, however, also a clear need for more resources, and for more effective mandatory interdisciplinary professional training. Too often victims of abuse are pressured by circumstances, a lack of resources, and a lack of effective advocacy into accepting resolutions that leave them and their children vulnerable to further abuse (see DeVoe & Smith, 2003).

In terms of legislative reform, Canada is in the midst of a contentious process of reform of the child related provisions of its *Divorce Act*, the federal legislation that deals with child related issues when parents divorce. Provincial statutes that deal with child related issues in contexts in which parents are not getting a divorce, usually because they have not married, are also under review.

There is real concern about how issues of domestic violence were dealt with by the 1998 Special Parliamentary Committee, both in the hearings and its Report, *For the Sake of the Children* (Canada, 1998). Although the Committee heard from a range of professionals and academics, and both victims of spousal abuse and those who work with them, the Committee seemed much more sympathetic to fathers who appeared before it to raise the issue of false allegations of spousal abuse than it was to victims of family violence (Bala, 1999). The most inadequate aspects of the *Report* are its treatment of spousal violence issues, which reflect the "pro-father" tone of the hearings, and the sympathies of some of the key Committee members. The *Report* deals more extensively with the issue of false allegations by mothers and abuse perpetrated by women than with the much more prevalent and serious problem of male abuse of women and children. There are some recommendations that address spousal abuse concerns, but they are very problematic.

One recommendation was that the best interests test should include "*proven* family violence" as a factor in making determinations about children. This clearly reflects the Committee's pro-father slant as the qualifier "proven" is not used to modify any other listed best interests factors. The Committee may have expected a criminal conviction before spousal abuse would be taken into account. The Committee's approach was undoubtedly influenced by its Co-Chair, Member of Parliament Roger Gallaway, who in a recent speech remarked (Gallaway, 2001):

> women are statistically about as violent as men. But violence is for the criminal courts: it has no place in our divorce or family courts in terms of culpability . . . [the] philosophy of violence being overwhelmingly a men's trait is . . . in itself discriminatory in that it leads to contempt for . . . men. (p. 2)

These ill-informed comments are, unfortunately, reflected in the Committee *Report.*

In its May 1999 *Response* to the Committee *Report*, the Department of Justice made an effort to distance itself from the approach of the Committee to domestic violence and the issue of false allegations of abuse, writing (Canada, 1999):

> The Government of Canada strongly believes that it is important to send a message that all aspects of the family law system must take into account incidents of family violence involving the child or a member of the child's family. Ensuring the safety of all parties involved must be the guiding principle. (p. 21)

Subsequent to the release of its *Response* to the Committee *Report*, the federal Department of Justice undertook a process of public consultation (Canada, 2001) on the reform of custody and access laws. This consultation process also became extremely contentious, with women's groups refusing to attend meetings hosted by the Department of Justice if men's groups were also invited, and expressing deep concern about the Department's lack of commitment to gender equality (Ontario Women's Network, 2001). At the time of writing, the Minister of Justice still had not announced what legislative reforms, if any, are to be proposed by the government.

CONCLUSION

In our view, for cases where there has been spousal violence, Canadian legislation should be modelled after that of England, Australia, New Zealand and many American states. Violence should not just be another "best interests" factor that judges may take into account. Rather, courts should be satisfied that any parenting arrangements do not pose a significant risk to the safety of a child or parent, emphasizing the importance of this factor for justice system professionals and parents (Bala, 1998).

All Canadian jurisdictions should enact statutes that would specifically acknowledge the significance of domestic violence for child-related proceedings, as has occurred in Newfoundland and most American states. The enactment of such legislation would clarify the law. Perhaps more important, such legislation would facilitate the education of lawyers, judges and other professionals, as well as the public.

Changing statutes is only a relatively small part of a process of reform that is needed to improve the protection afforded to victims of domestic violence and their children. Enforcement issues are critical. In particular, ensuring that the remedies afforded to victims of domestic violence, such as restraining orders, are effective (Alberta Law Reform Institute, 1995). The protection of victims must be a priority. There is also a need for appropriate support services for victims of domestic violence, including counseling for victims and the children of these families, as well as programs for abusive spouses, and facilities to supervise access. Model programs like the spousal assault criminal courts in Ontario, intended to improve the efficiency and effectiveness of the court system, should be monitored and, if successful, replicated.

REFERENCES

Alberta Law Reform Institute (1995). *Domestic abuse: Toward an effective legal response.* Available online at: http://www.law.ualberta.ca/alri/pdfs/reports_disc/rfd015.pdf.

Bala, N. (2000). A differentiated legal approach to the effects of spousal abuse on children: A Canadian context. *Journal of Aggression, Maltreatment & Trauma, 3*(1), 301-328.

Bala, N. (1999). A report from Canada's gender war zone: Reforming the child related provisions of the Divorce Act. *Canadian Journal of Family Law*, 16, 163-227.

Bala, N. (1998). *Spousal violence in custody and access disputes: Recommendations for reform*. Ottawa: Status of Women Canada.

Canada, Department of Justice. (2001). *Consultation: Custody, access and child support in Canada–Putting children's interests first*. Available online at: http://canada.justice.gc.ca/en/cons/ConsultationDocument.pdf.

Canada, Department of Justice. (1999). *Government of Canada's response to the report of the special joint committee on child custody and access*. Available online at: http://canada.justice.gc.ca/en/dept/pub/cca/sjcarp02.html.

Canada, Special Joint Committee on Custody and Access. (1998). *For the sake of the children: Final report*. Available online at: http://www.parl.gc.ca/InfoComDoc/36/1/SJCA/Studies/Reports/sjcarp02-e.htm.

Canadian Panel on Violence Against Women. (1993). *Changing the landscape: Ending violence, achieving equality*, Ottawa: Canada Communications Group.

Dauvergne, M., & Johnson, H. (2001). "Children witnessing family violence." *Juristat* (Statistics Canada), *21*(6).

DeVoe, E., & Smith, E. (2003). Don't take my kids: Barriers to service delivery for battered mothers and their young children. *Journal of Emotional Abuse, 3*(3/4), 277-294.

Doucette, M. (2001). *Family legal aid: A comparative study*. (Charlottetown, P.E.I.: Women's Network PEI).

Edleson J. L. (1999). Children's witnessing of adult domestic violence. *Journal of Interpersonal Violence, 14*(8), 839-870.

Gallaway, R. (2001). Speaking notes for talk to GRAND Society, as distributed by his Office, Parliament of Canada (Ottawa, 28 April 2001).

Kalil, A., Tolman, R., Rosen, D., & Gruber, G. (2003). Domestic violence and children's behavior in low-income families. *Journal of Emotional Abuse, 3*(1/2), 75-101.

Landau, B. (1995). The Toronto forum on woman abuse: The process and the outcome. *Family & Conciliation Courts Review, 33*, 63-78.

Neilson, L. (2000). Partner abuse, children and statutory change: Cautionary comments on women's access to justice. *Windsor Yearbook of Access to Justice, 18*, 115-152.

Neilson, L. (2001). *Spousal abuse, children and the legal system*. From University of New Brunswick Web site: http://www.unb.ca/arts/CFVR/spousal_abuse.pdf.

Ontario Women's Network on Custody and Access (2001). *Brief to the Federal, Provincial, Territorial to the Federal, Provincial, Territorial Family Law Committee on Custody, Access and Child Support*. (Toronto). Available online: http://www.owjn.org/custody/brief-e.htm.

Onyskiw, J. E. (2003). Domestic violence and children's adjustment: A review of research. *Journal of Emotional Abuse, 3*(1/2), 11-45.

Statistics Canada. (2001). *Family violence in Canada: A statistical profile 2001*. Available online at: http://www.statcan.ca:80/english/freepub/85-224-XIE/0100085-224-XIE.pdf.

CASES

A.(B) v. T.(A)., [1997] N.S.J. No. 323 (Fam. Ct.) (QL), varied by *Nova Scotia (Minister of Community and Social Services v A.(B),* [1997] N.S.J. 453 (Fam Ct.) (QL).

A.(P.) v. A.(F.), [1997] B.C.J. No. 1566 (S.C.)(QL).

B.(M.J.) v. B.(W.P.), (1999) 139 Man.R. (2d) 288, [1999] M.J. No. 314 (Q.B., Fam. Div.) (QL).

C.(A.C.) v. G.(I.C.), [1999] B.C.J. No. 963 (Prov. Ct.)(QL).

Cadeau v. Martell, [1998] N.S.J. No. 159 (Fam. Ct.) (QL).

Collins v. Collins, [1998] A.J. No.160 (Q.B.) (QL).

D.(C.L.) v. D.(B.E.), [1999] N.B.J. No. 436 (Q.B.)(QL).

F.(D.) v. F.(W), [1998] O.J. No. 3198 (Gen. Div.) (QL).

H.(P.G.) v. H.(K.D.), [1999] B.C.J. No. 173 (S.C.) (QL).

L.(C.R.) v. L.(R.F.), [1998] S.J. No. 20(Q.B.) (QL).

M.(G.E.) v. M.(C.), [1999] M.J. No. 273 (Q.B.), aff'd [2000] M.J. No. 142 (C.A.)(QL) .

Mbaruk v. Mbaruk (1997), 27 R.F.L. (4th) 146, [1997] B.C.J. No. 125 (S.C.)(QL).

Ouimet v. Ouimet, [1997] B.C.J. No. 2127 (S.C.) (QL).

Peterson v. Peterson (1988), 85 N.S.R. (2d) 107.

T.(S.L.) v. T.(M.L.) (1997), 119 Man. R. (2d) 200, [1997] M.J. No. 285 (Q.B.) (QL).

W.(J.W.) v. W.(N.), [1999] A.J. No. 946 (Q.B.) (QL).

Don't Take My Kids:
Barriers to Service Delivery
for Battered Mothers and Their Young Children

Ellen R. DeVoe
Erica L. Smith

SUMMARY. Using focus group methodology, we explored experiences of and barriers to help-seeking among battered mothers of children under six years of age. Forty-three women who had experienced recent domestic violence from diverse socio-economic backgrounds participated in a series of focus groups. The findings suggest that women perceived punitive consequences upon reporting domestic violence, declined to seek services out of fear of child removal, and encountered few, if any, appropriate services for their young children exposed to domestic violence. The inherent tensions in practice philosophies among battered women's advocates and child protective services are discussed with specific attention to the conceptualization of exposure to domestic violence as a form of child abuse

Address correspondence to: Ellen R. DeVoe, PhD, Columbia University School of Social Work, 622 West 113th Street, New York, NY 10025 (E-mail: ed156@columbia.edu).

The authors would like to thank Dr. Kathryn Conroy, the editors, and three anonymous reviewers for their helpful comments on earlier drafts of the manuscript.

This research is funded by a B/START award (R03MH61762-01) from the National Institute of Mental Health to the first author.

[Haworth co-indexing entry note]: "Don't Take My Kids: Barriers to Service Delivery for Battered Mothers and Their Young Children." DeVoe, Ellen R., and Erica L. Smith. Co-published simultaneously in *Journal of Emotional Abuse* (The Haworth Maltreatment & Trauma Press, an imprint of The Haworth Press, Inc.) Vol. 3, No. 3/4, 2003, pp. 277-294; and: *The Effects of Intimate Partner Violence on Children* (ed: Robert A. Geffner, Robyn Spurling Igelman, and Jennifer Zellner) The Haworth Maltreatment & Trauma Press, an imprint of The Haworth Press, Inc., 2003, pp. 277-294. Single or multiple copies of this article are available for a fee from The Haworth Document Delivery Service [1-800-HAWORTH, 9:00 a.m. - 5:00 p.m. (EST). E-mail address: docdelivery@haworthpress.com].

10.1300J135v03n03_06

(i.e., neglect, failure to protect, emotional abuse). Implications for service delivery and policy are suggested. *[Article copies available for a fee from The Haworth Document Delivery Service: 1-800-HAWORTH. E-mail address: <docdelivery@haworthpress.com> Website: <http://www.HaworthPress.com> © 2003 by The Haworth Press, Inc. All rights reserved.]*

KEYWORDS. Domestic violence, neglect, failure to protect, emotional abuse, battered mothers

Between 3.3 and 10 million children are estimated to witness domestic violence during childhood (Carlson, 1984; Fantuzzo, Boruch, Abdullahi, Atkins, & Marcus, 1997; Straus, 1992). Even though not all children are adversely affected, exposure to domestic violence can result in damaging consequences for young children (Jaffe & Geffner, 1998). For example, in some studies, over half of children exposed to domestic violence display traumatic stress symptoms, and many are at risk of perpetuating violence themselves (Bell, 1995; DeVoe & Graham-Bermann, 1997; Lehman, 1997; Rossman & Ho, 2000). However, because victims, perpetrators, and child witnesses of domestic violence potentially interface with multiple systems (e.g., child welfare, criminal justice, and women's advocacy programs, and shelter systems), it is difficult to approach the problem with simple or single system solutions. Abused mothers seeking assistance often face numerous barriers as they attempt to escape the violence. For example, victims may encounter a lack of or inadequate services, insensitive workers, and/or punitive agency consequences, such as the threat of child placement, as they navigate helping systems. As a result, many women are deterred from reporting the violence or leaving batterers (Beeman, Hagemeister, & Edelson, 2001; Levin, 1999; Magen, Conroy, Hess, Panciera, & Simon, 2001; Shepard & Raschick, 1999).

One major relationship that may be compromised in the context and aftermath of domestic violence is the mother-child unit (Mills et al., 2000). Preserving this supportive relationship can provide a critical buffer for young children against the potential risks associated with exposure to domestic violence (Magen et al., 2001; Mills et al., 2000; Whitney & Davis, 1999; see also Kerig, 2003). Unfortunately, remedies currently offered to victims seeking help lack sufficient focus on and support for addressing battered women's needs as mothers. Whitney and Davis (1999) note, "[t]he safety and well-being of children in domestic violence cases is usually linked to the safety and well-being of the mother" (p. 160). In addition, services for very young children (under six years of age) who are exposed to domestic violence are extremely scarce.

In addition to the negative effects of being exposed to intimate partner violence, children living in violent homes are also at greater risk of being victims of abuse themselves. This overlap of child abuse with domestic violence is well documented. For example, research indicates that in families where there has been severe domestic violence, there is an elevated risk of severe child maltreatment (Beeman, Hagemeister, & Edleson, 2001; Magen et al., 2001; Mills et al., 2000; Shepard & Raschick, 1999). Likewise, a pattern of abuse to the woman is also present in 70% of child abuse fatality cases (Mills et al., 2000). Although studies present empirical data correlating domestic violence and child abuse, many current service systems continue to treat the problems as unrelated. By contrast, other system responses rely on a definition of child maltreatment that includes exposure to domestic violence. These conflicting perspectives result, in part, from unresolved tensions between advocates for battered women and the child protection system (Fleck-Henderson, 2000; Mills et al., 2000; Shepard & Raschick, 1999) and from the failure of service providers, policymakers and researchers to reach consensus regarding whether and when exposure to domestic violence should be considered a form of child maltreatment.

CURRENT RESPONSES TO DOMESTIC VIOLENCE

Two major gateways to service for victims of domestic violence are battered women's advocacy programs and child protective services (CPS). Although there is consensus that coordinated service response and delivery are necessary, these systems are not yet in place in most parts of the country. Further, there is a significant gap between the mission of women's advocates and that of CPS in efforts to protect the best interests of children. This gap often results in ineffective interventions in cases of domestic violence whereby children are removed from the home. Thus, children already at risk as a result of exposure to violence may be further traumatized by separation from the non-offending parent (often the mother). In many cases, child welfare responses have been punitive toward women by failing to hold perpetrators of domestic violence responsible for their abusive actions. On the other hand, advocacy responses have been protective of resources targeting women with only recent recognition of women's roles as mothers and the needs of their children. There is an emerging consensus in the literature that these individual responses to domestic violence are inadequate to meet the needs of both mother and child (Clark, Burt, Schulte, & Maguire, 1996; Sullivan & Allen, 2001), and are sometimes at cross-purposes (Schechter & Edelson, 1995). Thus, while advocates for victims place an emphasis on empowering women through independence to escape violence, CPS agencies focus on the safety and well-being of the child, which may be operationalized by removal of children from the violent environment. Both perspectives are valid, but strategies for each view often place the needs of mothers and children in conflict (Fleck-Henderson, 2000; Lennett & Colten, 1999; Magen et al., 2001). Finally, neither system has developed supportive responses to the full range of women's choices about their involvement in abusive intimate partnerships nor have they developed solutions that address the needs of mothers and children simultaneously.

The institutional belief that domestic violence is beyond the scope of CPS's mandate remains a significant hurdle for system change (Fleck-Henderson, 2000; Magen et al., 2001; Mills et al., 2000; Shepard & Raschick, 1999; Whitney & Davis, 1999). In instituting its mandate, CPS historically has issued sole responsibility for protection of children to mothers. The responsibility of the batterer for perpetrating the abuse often is not brought to light in securing safety for children. Thus, children can be removed from the mother due to neglect, failure to protect, or emotional abuse, when in fact it is the batterer who is compromising the safety of the children. In cases of domestic violence, it seems that mothers must bear the burden of protecting their children even though they are unable to protect themselves.

One major factor in mothers' reluctance to seek help for their own abuse arises from their fear of losing their children (Mills et al., 2000). These fears are not unfounded (Bernstein, 2002; Glaberson, 2002). As child abuse is more likely to occur in families experiencing domestic violence and vice versa, there *should be* a higher rate of child welfare intervention and possible child removal in these families (Beeman, Hagemeister, & Edelson, 2001). At issue, however, is the controversial CPS policy or practice in many districts that identifies children's exposure to domestic violence as a specific form of child maltreatment (i.e., neglect, failure to protect or emotional abuse) for which child removal is deemed an appropriate response.

Paradoxically, CPS workers often miss, ignore, or overlook domestic violence in their assessment of possible child maltreatment (Magen et al., 2001; Mills et al., 2000; Whitney & Davis, 1999). Whitney's (1999) study of integrated practice, in which women's advocates and child welfare agents worked together in a CPS setting, indicated that 71% of serious CPS cases of abuse and neglect of children referred to the study involved domestic violence, while only 50% of those cases had been previously identified as domestic violence cases. Much of the literature attributes this oversight to lack of training in domestic violence, failure to screen, overloaded agencies, and overworked agents (Magen et al., 2001; Mills et al., 1999; Shepard & Raschick, 1999).

Fleck-Henderson (2000) notes that the integration of advocacy for battered women and the child welfare mandate of protecting children's best interests is not an easy task and is not feasible in the current delivery system. Some studies find that overcoming the distrust between women's advocates and CPS workers is the first step to a successful program (Beeman, Hagemeister, & Edleson, 2001; Fleck-Henderson, 2000; Levin, 1999; Mills et al., 2000). Only recently have a few innovative studies described successful collaboration between battered women's advocates and child protection workers (Lennett & Colten, 1999; Mills et al., 2000). In one study, four schools of social work were funded to develop community-integrated interventions for domestic violence and child abuse (Magen et al., 2001). At one site, researchers at Columbia University focused on heightening awareness of domestic violence and its related consequences among CPS workers. These researchers created a training curriculum and manual for city CPS workers, as well as a website for information about domestic violence and its victims. Using a pre-post test design to assess the effectiveness of a two-day training, the researchers determined change in worker attitudes toward greater awareness of domestic violence and measured positive participant satisfaction. These and similar efforts focused on training CPS workers about domestic violence and accomplished a successful collaboration between women's advocates and CPS workers (Magen et al., 2001; Mills et al., 2000). Only with such collaboration can the mutual goal of victim and child safety be reached.

CURRENT STUDY

The complexity of the issues facing battered women who are also mothers of young children led us to explore women's experiences of help-seeking in the current study. Specifically, we employed focus group methodology to examine whether women perceived a need for services for themselves and/or their young children, whether they had sought services, what barriers to help-seeking they had encountered, and the quality of responses women experienced from the service delivery system. Exploration of other aspects of battered women's experiences of parenting in the context of domestic violence, including their perceptions of the impact of domestic violence upon their children and the challenges they faced in parenting specific to the circumstances of domestic violence are reported elsewhere (DeVoe & Smith, in press).

METHOD

Participants

The sample consisted of 43 mothers who reported having experienced domestic violence within the last 18 months. Women ranged in age from early twenties to mid-thirties. Target children ranged in age from 22 months to six years, although many women had more than one child. Mothers identified their race/ethnic background as follows: 53% African-American (*n* = 23), 23% Latina (*n* = 10), 12% multiracial (*n* = 5), 5% Asian (*n* = 2), and 2% White (*n* = 1). The average income reported by mothers was $373 per month, with a range from no income or benefits to $2,468 monthly. Half the sample had not completed high school or obtained a GED.

The average length of the relationship with an abusive partner was six years, with a wide range from two months to 17 years. Many women continued to have contact with the batterer, on average three times per month. Some women had ended all contact with their former partners, and others estimated that they had contact with batterers as many as nine times per month.

Procedure

During the summer of 2000, women were recruited for participation in the study from three sites within a large social and legal services agency that serves victims of domestic violence and their families throughout New York City. Several methods of recruitment were used, including presentations by female project staff to community meetings of women receiving services related to domestic violence, direct referrals from agency staff, and postings describing the study. Potential participants were informed that the purpose of the project was to learn as much as possible about the needs of young children who have been exposed to domestic violence so that services could be designed to meet these specific needs. Women also were informed of the eligibility criteria, namely the experience of partner violence and having a child under six years old. Initially, we had sought women with recent partner violence (i.e., within one year); however, this criterion was extended because many women were recruited from a long-term shelter and had been away from their abusive partners for more than one year.

Women were invited to participate in a focus group with other women from the same recruitment site; however, groups were not segmented by race/ethnicity. A total of 43 women participated in one of five focus groups. The size of the focus groups ranged from nine to 16 participants. One group, comprised of four women, was conducted in Spanish. The focus groups were conducted at three different sites in Manhattan and the Bronx, New York. Groups were offered during the day and evening to accommodate participants' schedules. Each group was audiotaped with the knowledge and consent of participants and later transcribed verbatim. On-site child-care was provided for all children regardless of age, and a meal or snack was supplied for both children and mothers. The focus groups were conducted by the principal investigator and trained female research assistants enrolled in a graduate program in social work who had experience working with domestic violence issues. Two female facilitators and one observer were present for each group except for the Spanish-language group, which did not have an observer. For each session, one facilitator assumed the lead role in posing focus group questions while the second facilitator was responsible for probing, clarifying and summarizing participants' responses. The third observer attended to the dynamics of group process, monitored equipment, and assisted children who periodically entered to check in with their mothers.

Prior to beginning the focus groups, informed consent was obtained from each participant. Each participant received $20 and a Metrocard for each herself and her children. Next, facilitators explained that participation in the study and views expressed by the women in the focus groups would not impact services they received with the agency. The focus group was introduced with the following statement: "The goal of today's discussion is to learn more about how you think children may be affected by domestic violence, and how counselors and programs could be more helpful to mothers of young children." The focus group questions were centered around four areas of women's perceptions and concerns related to their preschool children and parenting in the context of domestic violence: (1) witnessing domestic violence and impact on young children; (2) communication with young children about domestic violence; (3) parenting and sources of parenting stress; and (4) support and intervention. The protocol included specific probes to encourage elaboration on these topics but they were not necessary because the women in each group were detailed in their descriptions of how children are exposed to and affected by domestic violence, the difficulties they faced in communicating with young children about violence, the challenges of parenting in the context of domestic violence and broken relationships, and the limitations of current service systems to address the needs of their families.

Because the results of the focus group discussion could not be brought back to the participants of each focus group once the analysis was complete, a member checking procedure was conducted within each focus group session as follows: near the end of the group, the facilitators summarized the themes from the focus group discussion and invited clarification, elaboration and additions to the list. Facilitators asked, "Did we capture the issues you've raised? What did we leave out or miss?" Women also were asked to rate which themes were the most important to them. At the completion of the groups, women completed a 20-minute survey as previously described. Debriefing was accomplished on an individual basis. As women completed the survey, project staff approached them individually to address any issues raised during the focus group and to discuss referral needs.

Data Analysis

The focus groups were audiotaped and transcribed verbatim. Focus group data were analyzed based on a modification of the coding system described by Krueger (1994, 1998) as follows. The authors served as the analysts for focus group data. First, we identified a preliminary set of analytic coding categories by reading the transcripts from each of the five focus groups. Next, we developed a list of themes and concepts from across groups that were used as an organizational framework for subsequent coding. Specifically, we identified three conceptual spheres or code families, which followed from our series of questions. The first two code families, level of child's exposure to domestic violence and parenting in the context of domestic violence are discussed at length elsewhere (see DeVoe & Smith, in press). The third code family broadly included the mothers' experiences with the service delivery system. Within the "services" code family, several sub-themes emerged and are discussed below: (1) The difficulty of finding services for young children, (2) The experience of punitive consequences for seeking assistance, and (3) Lack of trust in the social services/mental health systems to provide appropriate and non-punitive assistance and support.

Once code families were established, analysts reviewed the transcripts independently to identify themes and patterns (e.g., codes) within these categories regarding experiences of help-seeking, perceptions of barriers to service, and service needs. All disagreements about the coding categories were discussed until agreement was reached.

FINDINGS

All women who participated in the focus groups reported psychological abuse by an intimate partner within the last year. With regard to physical violence, thirty-nine women (90%) indicated that they had experienced mild physical abuse, such as a slap or push, and 24 women (55%) reported severe violence, including the use or threat of use of a weapon. Similarly, 24 women (55%) had experienced sexual violence at the hands of their partners.

Within the conceptual sphere of help-seeking, participants identified two central themes with respect to their experiences with the service delivery system: (1) punitive consequences for seeking help; and (2) system mistrust. The segment of the focus groups in which help-seeking and service delivery were explored began with a question to mothers about where they can turn for help and support. Since all women in the sample had accessed services through the study site, participants reported a wide variety of experiences with multiple delivery systems and a range of service providers (e.g., police, child protection workers, counselors, social workers, shelter staff).

Many women described positive encounters with individual counselors, support group facilitators, shelter staff, and hotline operators. However, the dominant tone of the discussions across groups was one of negativity when help-seeking efforts and experiences with providers were recounted. First, of those women who did seek services for their young children, very few reported that they had been able to locate providers with appropriate developmental and domestic violence expertise. In fact, it was disturbing to hear that some women had been told by providers that their very young children were "too young to be affected." Furthermore, many women reported that they had not sought services in a timely manner for their children because they feared the removal of their children from their custody and placement into foster care. Others recalled that when they tried to obtain assistance for their children, they felt punished or blamed, or were met with insensitive responses from service providers.

Punitive Consequences for Seeking Help: Child Removal

Many women recognized the need for help and sought assistance for themselves in the context of domestic violence. In most cases, women described reaching out for help during an acute battering incident and requesting assistance in having the batterer removed from the home. Unfortunately, a number of women described that upon making a report about the violence, their children were removed from their custody. Women captured the inherent contradiction in the act of seeking help, such that they and their children were punished as a consequence of their attempts to deal with or escape the violence:

> When I did call the police I got my child taken away. And it took me 17 years to call the police. I–I had my son three years ago. He's three years old, right? I'm just coming home and I'm saying to myself, "I'm not gonna take no more." You know what I'm saying? I get home and a couple of months later we have this blow-out. And the first time I call the police in 17 years, I have my son taken away from me.

> I called the cops to have him removed from the house, right? Okay, and then we had to go to court and everything but they made me plead guilty to neglect. You know what I'm saying? So I don't think that's helping anybody. And then they took my child from me. You know what I'm saying? And that affected him real bad 'cause when I went to pick him up he was like in another world . . . I don't understand today, why would they take him from me, when I called the cops on him (the batterer) to be removed from the house?

> We had an argument and I called the cops 'cause I thought he was gonna hit me. And the cops came, right? And my baby was sleeping . . . We ended up in court and I had to plead to neglect. Why is that? I just don't understand how that's–I feel that I pleaded to

something I didn't do. They told me that I had to plead to neglect . . .
So I felt that I never should have called the cops. That's how I feel.
'Cause I'm left with guilt.

In these cases, women described punitive consequences for their help-seeking efforts and observed negative effects on their children as a result of the separation. Many of the women whose children were removed expressed anger and frustration at the system, and feelings of helplessness and guilt related to losing custody of their children as a consequence of attempting to escape from or stop the violence.

System Mistrust: Fear of Child Removal

The fear of being charged with neglect or failure to protect and the threat of losing custody of their children caused many victims of domestic violence to delay or avoid altogether seeking help or protective services for themselves or their children. Women reported that they needed services to help them cope with the stress of domestic violence, parenting, and the impact of domestic violence upon their children, and that they often were aware of resources that might have been helpful (DeVoe & Smith, in press). However, a deep mistrust based on perceptions that their children would be removed from their custody if they revealed the domestic violence or a need for help with parenting stress caused many women to view programs with skepticism.

> *You need help alright. ACS (The New York City Administration for Children's Services) gonna help you take them kids outta there. You know you could be the best caregiver but just need a few minutes for yourself or you in the situation that you really can't control at that time and the system take your kids away from you.*

> *They scared the system gonna find out what's going on. They even got this crap that I see in the bus* [public service advertisements]. *If you need a break from your child, drop your kid off. You know damn well you're not coming back to get him. There'll be somebody waiting for you, standing right there at that door. You think you going to go get your little baby outta there. It's a set up.*

Some women who had been successful in locating help for themselves worked with providers who shared their skepticism about seeking assistance with or respite from parenting. As one woman related:

There was this one time that I wanted to take my daughter for help. There is this place in the city and I was so stressed out because I was in the shelter . . . And I just needed a break, by myself. And I spoke to my counselor about it . . . and she was concerned that they might conclude that I'm not capable to take care of her during that time. And she was skeptical that they would take her away from me for a period of time until I recover.

Other women described altering their reports about domestic violence out of fear of punitive consequences, such as the removal of their children. For example, one mother of two had called the police to intervene in an altercation but changed her story during her interview with police. She explained:

Like one of the officers was saying, 'Well, if you press charges then . . . blah blah blah.' But I was hip to the fact that if I press charges, that's going to reflect negatively on me. So I basically started to cover myself. I basically started to lie. I started to say, 'Oh no, it wasn't as bad as they made it out . . . We were just arguing. No, the kids weren't able to see anything.' And then you start getting into self-protection mode because you don' want to lose yourself or your kids. That's the joy of your life. And it's not that your kids are being abused, you're the person being abused.

In another case, a mother stated that she had been afraid to leave the batterer because of her fear that her child would be removed upon her becoming homeless (in order to enter the shelter system). She risked this consequence and left when the batterer directly abused her child:

I dealt with the battering for 3 years . . . And I was scared that if I left from this house–because it's a stable home, it was my apartment but it was a stable home–to go into a shelter they gonna say, "Well, we taking him from you because you don't have your apartment." I was like what the fuck I'm gonna do? And when he hit my child, the first time he hit him, I wrapped him (the child) in a sheet and I left.

Participants recognized that as mothers, they were generally held responsible for the well-being of their children and identified the impossible task of protecting their children from exposure to their partners' violence while simultaneously dealing with their own victimization.

Many expressed anger that abusive men were not being held accountable for placing their children in harm's way:

> *. . . Because we as mothers are responsible. Fathers are not responsible. We are held fully responsible for anything that happens to our children. And that's another bad thing about domestic violence. We're trying to get out of having bad feelings, and the depression, and all the emotions that we have in domestic violence, but we still receive it once the man leaves. Because now we have to handle everything on our own.*

> *As mothers, like I said, we are held responsible for anything and everything as far as our children are concerned: their health, their well-being, their lifestyle, everything. If we turn to an agency or someone who is supposed to provide us with services and help as far as for us or our children, the worst thing that they can possibly do is neglect to give us the services we're asking for and do like they've done to a few of us in this room—remove our child. You understand?*

DISCUSSION

> *The system is so screwed up. It's like damned if you do, damned if you don't. (Group: for real!) And a lot of women are scared that "I gonna ask for help and they gonna help me a little bit too much and take my children away!"*

The mothers in this sample had encountered a wide range of services in their efforts to address domestic violence. As noted, many women reported positive experiences with individual providers or agencies along the way. These constructive experiences, however, were overshadowed by what women perceived as punitive consequences for obtaining help and a deep mistrust of "the system." Specifically, many described the experience of having their children removed from their custody on the basis of exposure to domestic violence alone. Similarly, these women talked of the humiliation of pleading neglect because of their inability to shield their children from the violence of their partners. Even more disturbing was that the fear of child removal intensified women's reluctance to seek help for themselves and their children. In essence, system responses exacerbated women's distrust of and appeared to promote an underutilization of available services, particularly those services related to assistance with parenting and child well-being. Even if actual system responses begin to change to become more supportive of preserving the mother-child unit, battered women's perceptions of negative consequences for reporting domestic violence may remain a significant barrier to seeking help for themselves or their children.

Women who did obtain assistance typically entered the service delivery system via agencies for battered women where their children's needs and their own needs as mothers did not always receive appropriate attention. That is, since many women were in crisis at the point of entry into the service system, immediate safety was the first priority. However, for many women, assistance with decision-making about whether to return to the relationship, grieving the lost relationship, addressing complex feelings about leaving the fathers of their children, and dealing with the concrete realities of economic self-sufficiency and housing in New York City was sorely needed. Furthermore, support for addressing the impact of both domestic violence and the demise of their relationships with partners on their children is critical and was often missing. Finally, mothers who specifically sought mental health or counseling intervention for their children to deal with the effects of exposure to domestic violence were frustrated by the lack of providers with appropriate expertise to offer developmentally and clinically sound treatment for their youngest children.

Setting Dynamics and Limitations

Several issues related to focus group methodology and this study in particular warrant mention. First, we sampled from a pool of battered women who were actively engaged in either shelter-based or non-residential services. The sample was quite diverse along a number of dimensions, including demographic variables (e.g., race/ethnicity, religion), domestic violence experiences, and relationship status. However, because groups were not segmented by race/ethnicity, culturally-specific information may have been lost in favor of descriptions of experiences common to many group members. In addition, the stories described here cannot be generalized beyond the study population, although it is noteworthy that women with diverse life experiences shared much common ground in this study.

On the whole, group discussions were spirited. In order to minimize any perception of blaming mothers, the first several questions were carefully phrased to focus on children in general, rather than asking directly about participants' children. However, group members immediately described their perceptions about their own children. Three aspects of the group process were especially challenging but not unanticipated. First, because of a highly successful recruiting effort by agency partners, several groups were quite large (the largest group included 16 women). With smaller groups, women would have had a greater opportunity to discuss and elaborate on the topics. In addition, focus group questions were designed to investigate several critical issues related to parenting and the needs of young children in the context of domestic violence. Thus, although facilitators used a variety of techniques designed to encourage and ensure participation from all group members, greater depth of discussion about barriers to service, including the view of domestic violence as a form of child abuse, was not possible.

Second, women were at all levels of resolution of their relationships with their abusive partners, including some women who had chosen to stay with the partner, others who were temporarily or recently separated, and still others who had ended the relationship. Not surprisingly, many women were interested in sharing their stories with other women in similar circumstances and sometimes had to be redirected to the topic. Third, in order to minimize any discomfort among the children of focus group participants, children were shown where their mothers were meeting, and were brought to the meeting rooms if they were unusually upset by separation from their mothers. Thus, young children periodically visited the focus group to check in with their mothers. Although these interruptions were sometimes disruptive, they were necessary to ensure that children were not unduly distressed during the focus group.

Implications for Service Delivery and Policy

Clearly, not all battered mothers are adequate parents. Indeed, some children are in need of protective services intervention that includes child removal from a maltreating mother who also is abused. Certainly, any child who is a *direct target* of physical, sexual or emotional abuse by either parent requires protective services intervention. Furthermore, given the impact of domestic violence on women, it would not be surprising to find that some battered mothers are temporarily unable to parent because of their own traumatization. However, several studies of parenting among battered women suggest that many mothers are able to attend to their children's needs appropriately despite their own victimization in the context of domestic violence (Holden, Stein, Ritchie, Harris & Jouriles, 1998; Levendosky & Graham-Bermann, 2000). Future inquiry into the parenting capacities of battered women will provide important information regarding how best to support battered mothers as parents while they address their own difficulties. While additional research on the parenting of battered women will be useful, it is also critical to understand parenting patterns and abilities among battering men and to examine the influence of violent men on their children.

Until there is consensus among service providers, policymakers, and researchers regarding whether and when exposure to domestic violence crosses the line to become a form of child abuse or neglect, it is likely that a wide range of child protective services interventions in cases of domestic violence will continue. While the authors recognize the potentially profound negative impact of exposure to domestic violence on children's functioning and well-being, we do not agree that violence exposure in the absence of direct child victimization should be viewed and treated as a form of child abuse or neglect, including emotional abuse. However, if our service delivery and legal systems are to allow formal or informal policies or practices that maintain that exposure to domestic violence is a form of child maltreatment per se (e.g., emotional abuse, neglect or failure to protect), then it is the perpetrators of such violence who should be so charged, not mothers who are also victims. Furthermore, consequences should be aimed at perpetrators rather than at children and women. While many battered mothers could benefit from supportive and preventive services related to parenting and understanding the impact of domestic violence on their children as components of child maltreatment prevention (DeVoe & Smith, forthcoming), separation of young children from their non-maltreating mothers as a standard practice is misguided.

Efforts to protect the best interests of young children must also address the needs of their mothers *in the context of domestic violence*. There is agreement that a redefinition and restructuring of mandates and services will provide remedies to the problems that mothers and children confront in the face of domestic violence. The development of services that truly address the preservation of the mother-child unit exposed to domestic violence is critical. Finding ways to enhance the potentially protective element of the mother-child bond may boost the resilience of young children exposed to violence. Supporting this critical relationship by building the strengths of the mother-child unit is a more humane and potentially effective remedy than removing infants, toddlers and preschoolers from their primary caregivers at such a critical period in their development.

REFERENCES

Beeman, S., Hagemeister, A., & Edelson, J. (2001). Case assessment and service receipt in families experiencing both child maltreatment and woman battering. *Journal of Interpersonal Violence, 16*(5), 437-458.

Bell, C. C. (1995). Exposure to violence distresses children and may lead to their becoming violence. *Psychiatric News, 15,* 6-8.

Bernstein, N. (March 8, 2002). Harsh light is shed on way city treats abused mothers. *New York Times,* Section B, p. 1.

Carlson, B. E. (1984). Children's observations of interparental violence. In A. R. Roberts (Ed.), *Battered women and their families* (pp. 147-167). New York: Springer.

Clark, S. J., Burt, M. R., Schulte, M. M., & Maguire, K. (1996). *Coordinated community responses to domestic violence in six communities: Beyond the justice system.* Washington, DC: Urban Institute.

DeVoe, E. R., & Graham-Bermann, S. A. (June, 1997). *Predictors of posttraumatic stress symptoms in battered women and their children.* Poster presented at the Second International Conference on Children Exposed to Family Violence. London, Ontario, Canada.

DeVoe, E. R., & Smith, E. L. (in press). The impact of domestic violence on urban preschool children: Battered mothers' perspectives. *Journal of Interpersonal Violence.*

Fantuzzo, J. W., Boruch, R., Abdullahi, B., Atkins, M., & Marcus, S. (1997). Effects of interpersonal violence on the psychological adjustment and competencies of young children. *Journal of the American Academy of Child and Adolescent Psychiatry, 36,* 116-122.

Fleck-Henderson, A. (2000). Domestic violence in the child protection system: Seeing double. *Children and Youth Services Review, 22*(5), 333-354.

Glaberson, W. (March 5, 2002). Judge rebukes city officials for removing children from homes of battered women. *New York Times,* Section B, p. 3.

Holden, G. W., Stein, J. D., Ritchie, K. L., Harris, S. D., & Jouriles, E. N. (1998). Parenting behaviors and beliefs of battered women. In G. W. Holden, R. Geffner & E. N. Jouriles (Eds.), *Children exposed to marital violence: Theory, research and applied issues* (pp. 289-336). Washington, DC: APA Press.

Jaffe, P. G., & Geffner, R. (1998). Child custody disputes and domestic violence: Critical issues for mental health, social service, and legal professionals. In G. W. Holden, R. Geffner, & E. N. Jouriles (Eds.), *Children exposed to marital violence: Theory, research, and applied issues* (pp. 371-408). Washington, DC: APA Press.

Kerig, P. K. (2003). In search of protective processes for children exposed to interparental violence. *Journal of Emotional Abuse, 3*(3/4), 149-181.

Krueger, R. A. (1994). *Focus groups: A practical guide for applied research* (2nd ed.). Thousand Oaks, CA: Sage.

Krueger, R. A. (1998). *Analyzing and reporting focus group results. Focus Group Kit* 6. Thousand Oaks, CA: Sage.

Lehman, P. (1997). The development of posttraumatic stress disorder (PTSD) in a sample of child witnesses to mother assault. *Journal of Family Violence, 12,* 241-257.

Lennett, J., & Colten, M. (1999). A winning alliance: Collaboration of advocates and researchers on the Massachusetts mothers survey. *Violence against Women, 5*(10), 1118-1139.

Levin, R. (1999). Participatory evaluation: Researchers and service providers as collaborators versus adversaries. *Violence against Women, 5*(10),1213-1227.

Levendosky, A. A., & Graham-Bermann, S. A. (2000). Trauma and parenting in battered women: An addition to an ecological model of parenting. *Journal of Aggression, Maltreatment, & Trauma, 3*(1), 25-36.

Magen, R., Conroy, K., Hess, P., Panciera, A., & Simon, B. L. (2001). Identifying domestic violence in child abuse and neglect investigations. *Journal of Interpersonal Violence, 16*(6), 580-601.

Mills, L., Friend, C., Conroy, K., Fleck-Henderson, A., Krug, S., Magen, R., Thomas, R., & Trudeau, J. (2000). Child protection and domestic violence: Training, practice, and policy issues. *Children and Youth Services Review, 22*(5), 315-332.

Rossman, B. B. R., & Ho, J. (2000). Posttraumatic stress response and children exposed to parental violence. *Journal of Aggression, Maltreatment & Trauma, 3*(1), 85-106.

Schechter, S., & Edleson, J. L. (1995). In the best interest of women and children: A call for collaboration between child welfare and domestic violence constituencies. *Protecting Children, 11*, 6-11.

Shepard, M., & Raschick, M. (1999). How child welfare workers assess and intervene around issues of domestic violence. *Child Maltreatment, 4*(2), 148-156.

Straus, M. A. (1992). Children as witnesses to marital violence: A risk factor for lifelong problems in a nationally representative sample of American men and women. *Report of the Twenty-Third Ross Roundtable*. Columbus, OH: Ross Laboratories.

Sullivan, C. E., & Allen, N. E. (2001). Evaluating coordinated community response for abused women and their children. In S. A. Graham-Bermann & J. L. Edleson (Eds.), *Domestic violence in the lives of children* (pp. 269-282). Washington, DC: American Psychological Association.

Whitney, P., & Davis, L. (1999). Child abuse and domestic violence in Massachusetts: Can practice be integrated in a public child welfare setting? *Child Maltreatment, 4*(2),158-166.

Index

SPECIAL 25%-OFF DISCOUNT!

Order a copy of this book with this form or online at:
http://www.haworthpress.com/store/product.asp?sku=4943
Use Sale Code BOF25 in the online bookshop to receive 25% off!

The Effects of Intimate Partner Violence on Children

___ in softbound at $29.96 (regularly $39.95) (ISBN: 0-7890-2161-7)
___ in hardbound at $44.96 (regularly $59.95) (ISBN: 0-7890-2160-9)

COST OF BOOKS _____	❏ **BILL ME LATER:** ($5 service charge will be added)
Outside USA/ Canada/ Mexico: Add 20% _____	(Bill-me option is good on US/Canada/ Mexico orders only; not good to jobbers, wholesalers, or subscription agencies.)
POSTAGE & HANDLING _____	
(US: $4.00 for first book & $1.50 for each additional book)	❏ **Signature** _____
Outside US: $5.00 for first book & $2.00 for each additional book)	❏ **Payment Enclosed: $** _____
SUBTOTAL _____	❏ **PLEASE CHARGE TO MY CREDIT CARD:**
in Canada: add 7% GST _____	❏ Visa ❏ MasterCard ❏ AmEx ❏ Discover ❏ Diner's Club ❏ Eurocard ❏ JCB
STATE TAX _____	**Account #**_____
(NY, OH, & MIN residents please add appropriate local sales tax	
FINAL TOTAL _____	**Exp Date** _____
(if paying in Canadian funds, convert using the current exchange rate, UNESCO coupons welcome)	**Signature**_____
	(Prices in US dollars and subject to change without notice.)

<table>
<tr><td colspan="3">PLEASE PRINT ALL INFORMATION OR ATTACH YOUR BUSINESS CARD</td></tr>
<tr><td colspan="3">Name</td></tr>
<tr><td colspan="3">Address</td></tr>
<tr><td>City</td><td>State/Province</td><td>Zip/Postal Code</td></tr>
<tr><td colspan="3">Country</td></tr>
<tr><td>Tel</td><td>Fax</td><td></td></tr>
<tr><td colspan="3">E-Mail</td></tr>
</table>

May we use your e-mail address for confirmations and other types of information? ❏Yes❏ No
We appreciate receiving your e-mail address. Haworth would like to e-mail special discount offers to you, as a preferred customer. **We will never share, rent, or exchange your e-mail address.** We regard such actions as an invasion of your privacy.

Order From Your Local Bookstore or Directly From
The Haworth Press, Inc.
10 Alice Street, Binghamton, New York 13904-1580 • USA
Call Our toll-free number (1-800-429-6784) / Outside US/Canada: (607) 722-5857
Fax: 1-800-895-0582 / Outside US/Canada: (607) 771-0012
E-Mail your order to us: Orders@haworthpress.com

Please Photocopy this form for your personal use.
www.HaworthPress.com

BOF03